Viral Times

This book explores the relationship between COVID-19 and AIDS. It considers both how the earlier HIV pandemic informed our engagement with COVID-19, as well as the ways in which COVID-19 has changed how we remember and experience AIDS.

Individual sections focus on sexual and intimate relationships, inequalities and injustice, the progressive biomedicalisation of the response (in the absence of a vaccine or effective treatment or cure), and professional, practitioner and community perspectives on the pandemics. The authors come from a wide variety of backgrounds – including public health, nursing, law and legal studies, political studies, and the humanities and social sciences. The book contains contributions by established writers such as Dennis Altman, Shalini Bharat, Tim Dean, Deborah Lupton, Shubhada Maitra, Pauline Oosterhoff and Michael Tan, as well as chapters by Chris Ashford and Gareth Longstaff, Bernard Kelly, Dean Murphy and Kiran Pienaar, and Theodore (ted) Kerr.

This thought-provoking and timely volume includes case studies from Australia, Austria, Brazil, Canada, Germany, India, Indonesia, the Philippines, the UK, the USA and Vietnam. It has been written for students and scholars from a wide range of disciplinary backgrounds, including sociology, healthcare, public health, social work, anthropology, and gender and sexuality studies. The book will also be of interest to the general reader who wants a better understanding of the social and cultural dimensions of modern-day pandemics and the personal and community responses to which they give rise.

Jaime García-Iglesias is a Chancellor's Fellow in the Usher Institute at the University of Edinburgh, UK.

Maurice Nagington is a lecturer, researcher and registered nurse at the University of Manchester, UK.

Peter Aggleton holds senior professorial positions at The Australian National University, UNSW Sydney, and UCL. He is an adjunct professor in the Australian Research Centre for Sex, Health and Society at La Trobe University in Melbourne.

Sexuality, Culture and Health series

Edited by Peter Aggleton[1], Richard Parker[2], Sonia Corrêa[3], Gary Dowsett[4], and Shirley Lindenbaum[5]

[1]UNSW Sydney, Sydney, Australia
[2]Columbia University, New York, USA
[3]ABIA, Rio de Janeiro, Brazil
[4]La Trobe University, Melbourne, Australia
[5]City University of New York, USA

This series of books offers cutting-edge analysis, current theoretical perspectives, and up-to-the-minute ideas concerning the interface between sexuality, public health, human rights, culture and social development. It adopts a global and interdisciplinary perspective in which the needs of poorer countries are given equal status to those of richer nations. Books are written with a broad range of readers in mind and will be invaluable to students, academics and those working in policy and practice. The series also aims to serve as a spur to practical action in an increasingly globalised world.

Culture, Health and Sexuality: An Introduction
Edited by Peter Aggleton, Richard Parker

Gay Science: Intimate experiments with the problem of HIV
Kane Race

Young People and Sexual Citizenship
Edited by Peter Aggleton, Rob Cover, Deana Leahy, Daniel Marshall and Mary Lou Rasmussen

Sexualities, Transnationalism, and Globalization: New Perspectives
Edited By Yanqiu Rachel Zhou, Christina Sinding and Donald Goellnicht

Sex, Sexuality and Sexual Health in Southern Africa
Edited by Deevia Bhana, Mary Crewe and Peter Aggleton

Sex and Gender in the Pacific: Contemporary Perspectives on Sexuality, Gender and Health
Edited by Angela Kelly-Hanku, Peter Aggleton and Anne Malcolm

Viral Times: Reflections on the COVID-19 and HIV Pandemics
Edited by Jaime García-Iglesias, Maurice Nagington, and Peter Aggleton

For more information about this series, please visit: https://www.routledge.com/Sexuality-Culture-and-Health/book-series/SCH

Viral Times

Reflections on the COVID-19 and HIV Pandemics

Edited by Jaime García-Iglesias, Maurice Nagington and Peter Aggleton

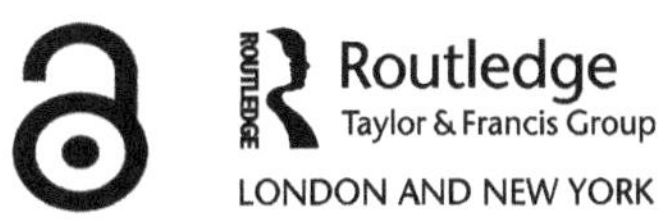

Designed cover image: © Getty, lowball-jack

First published 2024
by Routledge
4 Park Square, Milton Park, Abingdon, Oxon OX14 4RN

and by Routledge
605 Third Avenue, New York, NY 10158

Routledge is an imprint of the Taylor & Francis Group, an informa business

Funded by the Economic and Social Research Council [ES/X003604/1].

British Library Cataloguing-in-Publication Data
A catalogue record for this book is available from the British Library

ISBN: 978-1-032-34556-7 (hbk)
ISBN: 978-1-032-76498-6 (pbk)
ISBN: 978-1-003-32278-8 (ebk)

DOI: 10.4324/9781003322788

Typeset in Times New Roman
by MPS Limited, Dehradun

Contents

Figures

Table

Contributors

Peter Aggleton has a background in the social sciences as applied to well-being, education and health. He holds senior professorial positions at The Australian National University, UNSW Sydney, and UCL. He is an adjunct professor in the Australian Research Centre for Sex, Health and Society at La Trobe University in Melbourne. In addition to his academic work as a researcher, teacher, editor and writer, Peter has served as a senior adviser to several UN system organisations.

Dennis Altman is a Vice Chancellor's Fellow at La Trobe University in Melbourne, Australia and President of the AIDS Society of Asia and the Pacific. His most recent books include *Unrequited Love: Diary of an Accidental Activist* (2019) and *Death in the Sauna* (2023).

Chris Ashford is Professor of Law and Society at Northumbria University in the UK. Chris is a queer theorist and has published widely on the area of law and sex/sexuality. His research has focused on challenging normative assumptions about sexuality, particularly in relation to public sex, barebacking, pornography, and relationship structures.

Shalini Bharat is the former Director/Vice Chancellor of the Tata Institute of Social Sciences, Mumbai, India. Her research focuses on equity and access issues with specific reference to the reproductive and sexual health of women and young people; the social determinants of HIV and TB, including stigma; migration and health; and demographic transition in minority communities.

Marie A. Brault is an assistant professor at the UTHealth Houston School of Public Health (Texas, USA). Her research largely focuses on sexual, reproductive and mental health programming for adolescents and young adults. She has also conducted mixed methods and social determinants of health research across the lifecourse.

Tim Dean is James M. Benson Professor in English at the University of Illinois, Urbana-Champaign, USA. He has published eight books, including *Unlimited Intimacy: Reflections on the Subculture of Barebacking* (2009) and, with Oliver Davis, *Hatred of Sex* (2022). Currently, he is completing *In the Wake of Pandemics*.

Jaime García-Iglesias has degrees in literature and cultural studies and sociology. His work focuses on the sociology of sexual health as it intersects with technology and sexual and gender minorities. He currently holds a Chancellor's Fellowship in the Usher Institute at the University of Edinburgh in the UK. His most recent book is *The Eroticising of HIV: Viral Fantasies* (2022).

Amalia Puri Handayani is a researcher in the University Centre of Excellence – ARC Health Policy and Social Innovation at the Atma Jaya Catholic University of Indonesia (UCoE – ARC HPSI AJCUI), Jakarta, Indonesia.

Benjamin Hegarty is senior research associate in Global Health Equity and Justice in the Kirby Institute for Infection and Immunity in Society at UNSW Sydney, Australia.

Tu Anh Hoang is a founder and director of the Center for Creative Initiatives in Health and Population (CCIHP) in Vietnam working in emerging contexts such as the COVID-19 pandemic and climate change. She currently chairs the Vietnam Gender-based Violence Prevention and Response Network (GBVNet) and is a core member of the Gender Equality Asia Regional Network. She has worked extensively with marginalised and vulnerable communities to tackle inequity and injustice using an intersectionality framework and an affirming approach.

Bernard Kelly is the HIV Team Lead at St George's University Hospital in London. He has nearly 40 years' experience in the HIV sector as an activist, counsellor, educator and service provider. During COVID-19, Bernard facilitated support groups for healthcare teams facing the brunt of the pandemic.

Theodore (ted) Kerr is a Canadian-born, Brooklyn-based writer and organiser. He is co-author of *We Are Having This Conversation Now: The Times of AIDS Cultural Production* (2022) with Alexandra Juhasz. He is a founding member of the collective What Would an HIV Doula Do?

Carmen H. Logie holds a Canada Research Chair in Global Health Equity and Social Justice with Marginalized Populations and is a professor in the Factor-Inwentash Faculty of Social Work, University of Toronto, Canada. She is an adjunct professor at the United Nations University Institute for Water, Environment and Health and a scientist at the Centre for Gender & Sexual Health Equity at UBC.

Gareth Longstaff is a senior lecturer in media and cultural studies at Newcastle University. Gareth is a queer theorist and has published widely in the fields of gender, masculinities, sexualities, porn, and celebrity culture. His research focuses on the interconnections between public and private spheres of desire, sexual self-representation, pornography, and queer archival spaces.

Deborah Lupton is a SHARP Professor and leader of the Vitalities Lab and the Australian Research Council Centre of Excellence in Automated Decision-Making and Society in the Centre for Social Research in Health and the Social Policy Research Centre at UNSW Sydney, Australia.

Frannie MacKenzie is Research Coordinator in the Factor-Inwentash Faculty of Social Work at the University of Toronto, Canada. Her work supports community-based research with a focus on the intersections of sexual reproductive health and planetary health among refugee and displaced youth and key populations.

Shubhada Maitra is a professor in the Centre for Health and Mental Health in the School of Social Work at the Tata Institute of Social Sciences, Mumbai, India. She is the director of two field action projects – *Muskaan,* the Child and Adolescent Guidance Centre, and *Tarasha,* a community-based recovery and reintegration project for women living with mental health issues. Her work focuses on mental health, sexual and gender-based violence, reproductive and sexual health, and counselling among other issues.

Anna-Greta Mittelberger is a sociologist and sex educator. In her postgraduate work in the field of gender studies, she qualitatively explored how individuals with vulvas experience their vulva, particularly in a sexual context, from an intersectional constructivist feminist perspective. She lives in Vienna and is passionate about de-tabooing research on sexuality in science.

Max Morris is a senior lecturer in criminology at Oxford Brookes University, UK. Their research draws on queer theory to explore the role of law and society in constructing identities. They have published widely on topics including HIV, homophobia, LGBTQ+ inclusion, and sex work in the digital age.

Dean Murphy is a senior research fellow in the Australian Research Centre in Sex, Health and Society at La Trobe University in Melbourne. His work focuses on meanings of HIV diagnosis and biomedical technologies. He is the author of *Gay Men Pursuing Parenthood Through Surrogacy: Reconfiguring Kinship* (2015).

Maurice Nagington is a lecturer, researcher and registered nurse at the University of Manchester in the UK whose interdisciplinary work leverages critical social science perspectives to address health issues such as death, palliative care, cancer and chemsex.

Sandeep Nanwani is the Chief Medical Officer at the Kebaya Foundation in Yogyakarta, Indonesia.

Pauline Oosterhoff is a senior research fellow in the Institute of Development Studies and a visual artist and film maker. She lived and worked in Vietnam for eight years between 2003 and 2011. Her recent work – *Nails* – involved the creation of an interactive art installation that explores the fraught dynamics of the beauty industry, race and migration. With Tu Anh Hoang, she has published on transgender men and women, LGBT organising, gender-based violence, and the role of civil society in managing the HIV and COVID-19 pandemics.

Richard Parker is Professor Emeritus of Sociomedical Sciences and Anthropology and a member of the Committee on Global Thought at Columbia University in New York, as well as Director of the Brazilian Interdisciplinary AIDS Association (ABIA), Co-Chair of Sexuality Policy Watch (SPW), and Editor-in-Chief of *Global Public Health*. He has published very widely including *Sexuality, Health and Human Rights* (authored with Sonia Corrêa and Rosalind Petchesky, 2008), and the *Routledge Handbook on the Politics of Global Health* (co-edited with Jonathan Garcia, 2019).

Kiran Pienaar is a senior lecturer in sociology in the School of Social Sciences and Humanities at Deakin University, Australia. She is the author of *Politics in the Making of HIV/AIDS in South Africa* (2016) and co-edited a recent edited collection entitled *Narcofeminisms: Revisioning Drug Use* (2023) with Fay Dennis and Marsha Rosengarten.

Ignatius Praptoraharjo is the Director of the University Centre of Excellence – ARC Health Policy and Social Innovation at the Atma Jaya Catholic University of Indonesia (UCoE – ARC HPSI AJCUI), Jakarta, Indonesia.

Barbara Rothmüller is a sociologist and senior scientist in the Faculty of Psychology at Sigmund Freud Private University Vienna, Austria. Her research focuses on gender and sexuality studies, social inequalities and the work of Pierre Bourdieu.

Michael Lim Tan is a medical anthropologist and veterinarian. He was Chancellor of the University of the Philippines Diliman from 2014 to 2020 and is currently an emeritus professor at that same and a National Academician. He writes a weekly op-ed column in the *Philippine Daily Inquirer*, the country's largest English-language daily newspaper.

Acknowledgements and permissions

This work was supported by the Economic and Social Research Council [ES/X003604/1].

We thank Sarah Hoile for her editorial assistance and support.

We thank the authors and publishers who gave permission to reprint material included in this volume:

Dung Beetle Books, for permission to reprint the image 'evening virtue signalling' from *We do Lockdown* published by Dung Beetle Books ©Miriam Elia 2020.

Anthony Ellis, Luke Telford, Anthony Lloyd and Daniel Briggs, for permission to reprint the image 'Conceptualising the relationship between the "sacred" and "sacrificed"', in Ellis, A., et al., 2021. For the greater good: Sacrificial violence and the coronavirus pandemic. *Journal of Contemporary Crime, Harm, and Ethics*, 1 (1), 1–22. doi:10.19164/jcche.v1i1.1155.

Taylor & Francis, for permission to reprint, in a revised form, Chasing targets in a pandemic: The impact of COVID-19 on HIV outreach workers for MSM (men who have sex with men) in Jakarta, Indonesia, by Benjamin Hegarty, Amalia Handayani, Sandeep Nanwani & Ignatius Praptoraharjo (2021) *Global Public Health*, 16 11), 1681–1695, doi: 10.1080/17441692.2021.1980599

1 Viral times

HIV, COVID-19 and beyond

Jaime García-Iglesias, Maurice Nagington, and Peter Aggleton

For many people, COVID-19 brought to the fore something that had not been widely recognised beforehand, namely, our close and enduring relationship with viruses. Despite limited recognition of the fact, the reality is that we have always lived in viral times. As the activist motto in the communities most affected by HIV goes, 'AIDS is still a crisis.' The viruses that surround us penetrate us and live within each of us shape our existence in ways that themselves become viral. Writing about HIV, Jeffrey Weeks argued that gay men's lives during the early days of the AIDS crisis were marked by an easy slippage from 'the idea that homosexuals caused "the plague" [...] to the idea that homosexuality itself was a plague' (Weeks 1986, p. 115).

The extent to which COVID-19 has revealed how viruses shape and challenge our existence is such that the Spanish philosopher Paul B. Preciado wrote about how, after becoming sick with COVID-19 in Paris, the virus compels us to consider 'under what conditions and in which ways is life worth living?' (Preciado 2020). The seismic transformations brought about by COVID-19 force us to recall the earlier AIDS crisis about which Sarah Schulman wrote, '[It] was a phenomenon so broad and vast as to permanently transform the experience of being a person in the world' (Schulman 2012, p. 42). Both authors underscore how viruses have the potential to transform our thinking about life. Surviving and thriving together demand policies, systems and social relationships that recognise and honour our interdependence and facilitate empowerment, care, inclusion and collective struggle against the forces that seek to degrade human dignity.

There are of course differences between HIV – the virus that causes AIDS if left untreated – and SARS-CoV-2 – the virus that causes COVID-19. Some of these differences are biological (reflecting variation in modes of transmission, symptoms, incubation periods, etc.) and some are social (in terms of stigma, the collective and individual response, perceptions of who is most affected, etc.). Despite these differences, since the earliest days of COVID-19, we as editors felt there were profound political, affective, social and cultural connections between HIV and COVID-19. On 10 March 2020, Jaime and Maurice – both of whom had been working on HIV and health for several years – met in a coffee shop in Manchester's' Northern Quarter (at the only

DOI: 10.4324/9781003322788-1

table available in a café packed to the brim by patrons, months before it would close, and weeks before protective facial masks were mentioned). In that meeting, we agreed that there was a lot to be said, discussed, fought for and written about HIV and COVID-19. However, we left still unsure about where to start (should it be a paper, a blog post, a book, what about and with whom?) and with the certainty that many other scholars had the same feeling.

On the back of that meeting, and with the support of Peter Aggleton, we embarked on developing a special issue of the journal *Culture, Health and Sexuality*. Our goal was to provide a space to think through the relationships between HIV and COVID-19. The timing of the journal issue, published in 2021, meant that our thinking and writing was not just about COVID-19, it took place amidst it. As waves of infection came and went, the authors prepared their contributions under varying states of lockdown, at a time when effective prevention was a distant hope. With time, however, vaccines transformed the situation and by October 2021 we felt that COVID-19 had changed so much since the early days that much more could be written. Moreover, we wanted to provide space for a longer-term critical engagement that would move beyond the present to address a future living with or beyond COVID-19.

We were inspired in our efforts by Douglas Crimp's (1987) book *AIDS: Cultural Analysis/Cultural Activism* that spoke both to the moment at which it was written and to the world that was to come. Thus, we came up with the initial title of this book, *Viral Times: HIV, COVID-19 and Beyond.* Importantly, several of the contributors to this book were forced to reflect on what exactly that 'beyond' might mean in the summer of 2022, when the advent of the mpox pandemic once more prompted critical reflection on how we have lived, and will always live, in viral times.

With the passing of time, however, it has become clearer to us what 'going beyond' might mean, not just in terms of writing more about the relationships between HIV and COVID-19 but also in enquiring into how and why those relationships have become apparent – for whom, and with what effects. As Jaime and Maurice (García-Iglesias and Nagington 2020) argued in the first piece they wrote on the matter, whether the lessons learned from HIV came to be applied or ignored during COVID-19 reveals just whose lives are worth remembering and whose deaths are seen as irrelevant, whose sacrifices and knowledges are to be recognised, and whose are to be forgotten.

However, in this book, we want to go beyond thinking about memories of HIV and COVID-19. Memory is far from neutral: our collective memory is a profoundly inter-subjective and contextual phenomenon that does not simply mirror the past. Remembering (and forgetting) does not simply engage with one singular set of events but generates co-temporal narratives about both the past and the present. The relationship between HIV and COVID-19 is far from simple and unidirectional. Instead, and throughout the chapters that follow, authors explore how COVID-19 compels us to revisit (and, perhaps, remake) our memories and knowledges about HIV, demanding that we develop new understandings and affective attachments to them.

At the same time, some might say that doing theory amidst the frustration, fear and devastation of COVID-19 might be an uncommon response. There were moments when we wondered whether our efforts were rightly directed in editing another book. Some of us (and some of the authors included here) moved countries, faced major health crises or lost their jobs or loved ones during the COVID-19 pandemic. As we write, we are also (still) trying to survive a devastating pandemic which some have claimed is over. In times like these, it may feel that theory is at a loss, that it cannot grasp the magnitude of the task, or sufficiently incorporate feelings of urgency. And yet, as Paula Treichler earlier argued in relation to HIV, it is in times of crisis that theory can reach its full potential (Treichler 1999).

This book aims to capitalise upon this by bringing into conversation as many different voices as we could manage: some of the authors are scholars who are early in their careers while others have been leading voices within the field of social health for decades. Some write from countries in the Global North, where vaccines and treatments are widely available, others from parts of the world where healthcare or testing cannot be taken for granted. Some authors write from positions that have provided them with special insights and appreciations: as people living with HIV, as policy advisors, or as gay men, for example. Others adopt more discipline-based or professional perspectives. Some engage with viral times in relation to inspiration drawn from the humanities, others examine policy and legislation, yet others are informed by the writers' perspectives as givers of support and care to those living with and dying from HIV and COVID-19.

Overall, this book aims to provide a judicious blend of theory, empirical research and personal and community experience that looks at HIV and COVID-19, and beyond. It is divided into three sections that speak to different areas of work, focusing on intimate relationships; biomedicalisation; and professional, practitioner, and public perspectives, respectively.

Intimate relationships

The first section of the book, on intimacy, contains five chapters which, although methodologically different, all speak to the profound impact that both HIV and COVID-19 have had on people's practices of intimacy. Together, they evidence how these changes are not minor impacts of pandemics but are deeply important for people as well as revelatory of the socio-political contexts in which pandemics arise. More importantly, the authors in this section not only demonstrate how the intimate impacts of COVID-19 had clear antecedents in HIV (despite differences between them), but also how similar seismic shifts in intimate and sexual life are likely to happen again in the future.

In their chapter on the navigation of intimacy during COVID-19, Barbara Rothmüller and Anna-Greta Mittelberger focus on the effects of social distancing in Austria and Germany. They argue that different groups of people adapted their intimate practices to the pandemic in specific and meaningful ways. For some, this involved a turn to monogamy ('Coronamonogamy'), and for others it implied a heightening of relational closeness within couples. Dating and meeting new partners also changed, with people often rethinking their relationship to social expectations, an increased stigmatisation of queer and non-binary people, and with cis-gender heterosexual men looking for dates beyond their usual social circles. In making sense of these changes, Rothmüller and Mittelberger argue that memories of past pandemics played an important role in these adaptations and stress how 'pandemic times shed light on the profoundly social dimensions of human sexuality.'

In the next chapter, Chris Ashford and Gareth Longstaff examine how the 'queer mundane' – or the ordinary ways in which queer people express desire – challenges assumptions about sex during viral times. The authors explore this idea in the context of HIV and COVID-19. At first, both pandemics caused confusion about risk. Laws and sociocultural limits were placed on gay intimacy, often based on narrow assumptions informed by heterosexual models of sex and intimacy. With the passage of time, laws about HIV that focused on condom use alone did not keep up with science, just as COVID-19 rules banned aspects of queer life in a way that precluded more pragmatic approaches to intimacy. In both cases, resistance to legal regulation and these new norms emerged. Drawing on the example of the '75 Loads Guy,' a young Black US man who engaged in anonymous sex with a large number of men, principally as the receptive sexual partner, and whose social media posts about his sexual activity 'went viral,' the authors show how real queer desire disrupts the rules imposed during both pandemics, opening up new and more radical possibilities.

Deborah Lupton's chapter on narratives of pandemic life looks at literary portrayals of experience during outbreaks of infectious disease in writing produced before HIV, during the HIV pandemic and during COVID-19. Lupton argues for the need to properly 'theorise the social' through these and other means given the cultural and biological dimensions of disease outbreaks. She identifies similar themes in the works she explores including fear, visual horror, stigmatisation, and government inaction and inefficiency. In particular, work produced during COVID-19 is characterised by despair and the need to 'come to terms with sudden change' in everyday life. Ultimately, a recurrent theme across the different narratives on concerns the question of 'how to live with others in intimate relationships and the domestic space' in deeply viral times.

Dennis Altman's contribution explores the similarities and differences between HIV and COVID-19 across a range of contexts, from the personal to the global. The chapter begins on a personal note as the author recounts the collapse of a transcontinental romance during COVID-19. This reminds him of how, during HIV, there had been a similar 'loss of faith in a predictable future.' While acknowledging the differences between both pandemics, Altman describes how COVID-19 and HIV share similarities politically (such as in the dominance of a neo-liberal response) and in relation to their threat to human security. He offers a fascinating account which moves from 'a personal account of living through an epidemic' to an understanding of its 'broader socio-political impacts.'

The final chapter in this section is Tim Dean's discussion of how the 'counternarratives of viral intimacy' that emerged in relation to HIV may provide a departure point from which to think about our co-existence with COVID-19. It starts by asking whether the airborne nature of COVID-19 requires us to radically rethink the human relationship with viruses via notions of the 'virosphere.' It then moves to explore how barebacking as a sexual practice may provide a useful paradigm for thinking about the ways in which COVID-19 has transformed relationality, as it exists within the larger 'biopolitics of respiration.'

Biomedicalisation

The second section of this book addresses patterns of progressive biomedicalisation and the neglect of the social that is evident in responses both to HIV and COVID-19. Authors in the section explore how social and political discourses framing our understanding of pandemics are fluid and evolve over time. Together, chapters focus on the progressive shift that has been especially apparent in the case of HIV from the social to the biomedical and the individual. A rather different pattern of response can be seen in the case of COVID-19 where a focus on the social, economic and political determinants of infection has been downplayed from the start.

Max Morris' chapter offers an autoethnography of living with HIV during COVID-19 which explores questions of blame, vulnerability and antiviral medication. A key theme in the chapter is one of horror and dystopia, with Morris weaving insights from dystopic fiction into their own effort to make sense of COVID-19. Informed by their diary writing, Morris reflects on how marginalisation and stigmatisation were mobilised as part of the response to both pandemics, to justify whose lives were valuable.

In their chapter, Kiran Pienaar and Dean Murphy offer a 'diffractive reading' of experience from HIV to make sense of later responses to COVID-19 (and mpox). They suggest that grounded 'historical engagements' with HIV can assist in developing more socially informed responses to contemporary outbreaks of new infections. Using 'diffractive reading' to move beyond binary readings and focus instead on how different phenomena may be 'mutually constituted,' they apply this to the concepts of risk and crisis during HIV, COVID-19 and mpox. These terms, they argue, necessarily construct 'stratified health publics' through which privilege is entrenched and which construct the need for 'urgent, decisive responses' that open the way for 'panic icons.'

Comparing responses to HIV and COVID-19 socially and politically is the goal of Richard Parker and Peter Aggleton's chapter. They describe the history of HIV in terms of a series of waves and outline the social and political character of each, identifying in both cases a progressive individualisation and biomedicalisation of the response. The social insights gained from HIV had little impact on government or international responses to COVID-19. As a result, hundreds of thousands of people died unnecessarily in ways patterned by deep-seated inequalities and suggestive of the need for a better understanding of the social organisation of death (not life) in a globalised world.

Finally, Michael Lim Tan describes how HIV programmes in the Philippines in the 1990s enacted progressive policies that sought to destigmatise at-risk groups and encourage civil society participation. This is contrasted with the highly restrictive laws on movement and association enacted in the same country during the COVID-19 pandemic. Coupled with opaque and corrupt state practices in the purchasing of personal protective equipment and the absence of social protection for healthcare workers, Tan suggests that the COVID-19 response was authoritarian and divisive, undermining the engagement with civil society that had characterised earlier HIV responses. Yet amidst this, 'stubborn disobedience' against the authoritarian regime fostered self-help projects as 'a way to survive' and even 'thrive' amidst adversity and precarity.

Professional, practitioner, and public perspectives

The final six chapters remind us that remembering is a complex affair, one fraught with the power of who remembers what and when, and also who determines which lessons are learned or applied at a system-wide level. Both individually and collectively, authors explore the importance of learning from and building on the activism, community engagement and social justice claims developed in previous pandemics. They highlight how advocacy, anti-stigma campaigning and the actions of affected populations and civil society are important ways to mobilise learning. They demonstrate how authoritarian top-down approaches to pandemic management too frequently obscure the lessons learned from previous pandemics. They also suggest the need for ongoing spaces where activists can highlight and reveal social injustices. Remembering in such circumstances requires openness, creativity and partnership with the most-affected communities, and a sharing of power between professionals, practitioners and publics.

In a deeply personal reflection that weaves theory with emotion, Bernard Kelly explores rituals and mourning in the HIV and COVID-19 pandemics, critiquing the weekly public 'Clapping for Carers' that took place in the UK during the first COVID-19 lockdown. Kelly suggests this spectacle of communal applause served to cover up profound injustices while transforming the living into an audience for their own performance. He contrasts this with the more 'authentic' forms of mourning evident during the HIV pandemic, such as scattering the ashes of those who died from AIDS on the lawn outside The White House in the USA, which gave rise to anger and solidarity alongside legitimate demands for social justice.

Remembering and memorialisation form the core arguments of Theodore (ted) Kerr's chapter which centres on a 2018 pop-up overdose prevention site by activists close to Toronto's AIDS memorial. Kerr notes how HIV memorials are more than physical sites at which to mourn and remember, but act as resources to draw from in responding to other crises, such as the opioid overdose epidemic in Canada. Kerr sees value in COVID-19 and HIV memorials that go beyond passive commemoration to foster empowerment and change in relation to injustices such as food insecurity, police violence against Black people, and the war on drugs. In this way, memorials can become active processes, sites of public collaboration and places of resistance and contestation, contributing to more liveable lives while memorialising the dead.

Thinking about processes of social change, Carmen H. Logie and Frannie MacKenzie's chapter explores the concept of 'critical hope' in community and arts-based responses to HIV and COVID-19. Drawing on the work of Freire, Giroux and hooks, the authors see critical hope as the pursuit of equality and justice while resisting the passivity of pessimism. They suggest critical hope fuelled HIV activism, and like the Denver Principles' assertion of the right to 'to die – and to LIVE – in dignity,' critical hope must be positioned in struggles against inequality. Similarly, during COVID-19, social movements have leveraged ethics of hope and care to meet needs; spark solidarity across differences; refuse the binary of giver and receiver of care; and ignite calls for systemic change. Linking HIV and COVID-19 care networks and practices, they argue critical hope can once again 'catalyse engagement in social justice, care and mutual aid' in pandemic times.

In their chapter, Benjamin Hegarty et al. examine HIV outreach work with men who have sex with men in Indonesia during 2020–2021. Drawing on an ethnographic study, the authors show how peer outreach creatively combined virtual and in-person care amidst COVID-19 restrictions. While still expected to meet donor targets focused on biomedical outcomes within a context of limited resources, peer outreach workers' labour on relationship building within the community often went unrecognised, as did the precarity they faced when conducting outreach during COVID-19. By foregrounding participants' insights and ethics of care, their chapter signals the limitations of biomedical models of response that refused to acknowledge peer outreach workers' own vulnerability, as well as the insights gained into how HIV testing and treatment might successfully function during COVID-19.

Pauline Oosterhoff and Tu Anh Hoang contrast Vietnam's responses to the HIV and COVID-19 pandemics. Drawing on their own involvement in Vietnam's response to HIV, they highlight how the country's success with the HIV pandemic derived not so much from the authoritarian approaches adopted, but its engagement with at-risk and stigmatised populations. This, coupled with arrival of anti-retroviral therapy from 2004, meant that inclusion rather than isolation could become the guiding logic behind the management of the HIV epidemic. In contrast, the top-down response to COVID-19 in Vietnam, whilst initially successful in limiting infection, sought limited involvement with civil society. When initial success gave way to rapid growth in the COVID-19 epidemic, a weakened civil society led to a weakened pandemic response, and a loss of trust in the ability of the state to protect its citizens.

Finally, Shubhada Maitra, Shalini Bharat and Marie A. Brault, drawing on the work of Goffman and Foucault, examine stigma in relation to the HIV and COVID-19 pandemics in India. Stigmatised groups, perceived as 'spreaders,' were initially blamed for infection in both cases, but identities, identifications and the public response differed. In the case of HIV, stigma was attached primarily to gender and sexuality, while with respect to COVID-19 it fuelled xenophobia and bias against religious minorities, migrants and even health workers. While HIV increased support for affected groups through engagement and civil society action, COVID-19 triggered top-down restrictions. However, in state contexts where the more inclusive lessons from HIV came to be applied, success could be seen in reducing stigma. Maitra et al. see value in applying the lessons from HIV to strengthen pandemic preparedness and to proactively reduce the stigma to which future health crises will give rise.

Beyond viral times

Taken together, the contributions within this volume provide a rich, interdisciplinary examination of the complex relationships between HIV and COVID-19 across intimate, biomedical, professional, activist and public contexts. The chapters critically explore how these two pandemics, while differing in important ways, also share profound connections. In detailing these linkages from diverse scholarly, activist, community and practitioner perspectives, the authors collectively achieve the goal of creating a space for critical reflection on viral times – not only one that looks back at the lessons of HIV for COVID-19, but which also looks ahead to envision more just and equitable responses in future pandemics. Importantly, the authors represented here do not see COVID-19 as the end-point of discussions but rather it as a departure point: a springboard to inquire about how viruses partake in our intimate lives, how they influence social and political discourses, and how viral activism functions in our world. The voices included offer nuanced perspectives, yet find common ground in their commitment to understanding the social organisation of viral life, the value of community resilience and activism, and the importance of sustained conversations about social justice in viral times. We hope you enjoy reading it as much as we have enjoyed working on it.

References

Crimp, D., ed., 1987. *AIDS: Cultural analysis/cultural activism.* Cambridge: MIT Press.

García-Iglesias, J. and Maurice Nagington, M., 2020. From AIDS to Coronavirus: Who has the right to care? *The European Sociologist*, 45 (1). https://europeansociology.org/european-sociologist/issue/45/discussion/4f67896e-1a82-4996-8e5e-ff2d17574bf8

Preciado, P.B., 2020. The losers conspiracy. *Artforum* [online], 26 March. www.artforum.com/slant/the-losers-conspiracy-82586

Schulman, S., 2012. *The gentrification of the mind.* Berkeley: University of California Press. 10.1525/9780520952331

Treichler, P.A., 1999. *How to have theory in an epidemic.* Durham: Duke University Press.

Weeks, J., 1986. *Sexuality.* London and New York: Routledge.

Part I

Intimate relationships

2 Navigating dating and sexual intimacy in viral times

How people adapt their sexual relationships to pandemic risk

Barbara Rothmüller and Anna-Greta Mittelberger

Sexual intimacy can be an intense experience that shapes people's identities and their belonging to communities. Since second-wave feminism, cultural theory has critically analysed the normalisation of coupled forms of sexual intimacy and has called for an investigation of 'how public institutions use issues of intimate life to normalize particular forms of knowledge and practice and to create compliant subjects' (Berlant 1999, p. 288). More recently, the COVID-19 pandemic and pandemic mitigation efforts have sought to restructure the social context of intimacy in society. Contact restrictions have impacted sexual relationships and transformed the legitimacy of social closeness and distance within social communities, with negative (as well as partly positive) effects on mental and sexual health. Initially, when SARS-CoV-2 (the causative virus) spread rapidly, little was known about the consequences of efforts to promote social distancing, nor could anyone predict how long populations worldwide would have to cope with a global pandemic.

Nevertheless, scholars from different academic disciplines anticipated some of the unintended effects of pandemic mitigation that were yet to come. Researchers working on the social aspects of HIV, on racial discrimination as well as on gender and sexuality warned that pandemic mitigation through avoidance and distancing might increase the stigmatisation of social minorities (Logie and Turan 2020; Dionne and Turkmen 2020; Inman et al. 2021). Moralising, policing and disciplining allegedly infectious groups has been a common response to cope with diseases such as HIV and other sexually transmitted infections (Nelkin and Gilman 1988; Dionne and Turkmen 2020; Roberto et al. 2020) and has often resulted in the blaming of already discriminated against minorities (Joshi and Swarnakar 2021). Some early HIV prevention policies promoted mononormativity (sticking to one faithful partner) and sometimes also heteronormativity, portraying heterosexual marriage as normal, good and filled 'with inherent protective properties' (Esacove 2010, p. 85). Similarly, in the case of the COVID-19 pandemic in Austria and Germany, early disease prevention strategies sought to privilege

DOI: 10.4324/9781003322788-3

particular relationship arrangements, especially those typical of monogamous heterosexual couples living in the same household.

Under the impact of COVID-19, changes in the social context had an impact on sexual practices. The majority of studies of sexual intimacy during the pandemic showed a decrease in sexual satisfaction, sexual desire, number of sexual contacts and frequency of sexual activities (Estlein et al. 2022; Toldam et al. 2022). These declines were attributable to lack of household privacy for couples with or without children during shutdowns, and health-related anxieties and stress, particularly in healthcare workers and women with multiple care obligations, among other factors (Panzeri et al. 2020). Furthermore, the pandemic negatively impacted close relationships with friends and communities. LGBTIQA+ individuals were among those most likely to experience loneliness, particularly if they were not in a partnered relationship during a lockdown (Herrmann et al. 2022). Yet, we know little about how different social groups adapted their sexual practices and intimate relationships during the pandemic and the meanings they attributed to these transformations. Did social distancing during the pandemic have a lasting impact on sexual behaviour, or has there been a reversion to older practices? What new sexual and intimate practices has COVID-19 given rise to? In this chapter, we aim to explore the unanticipated effects of social distancing on sexual relationships and dating. Informed by empirical data, this chapter maps change in two different contexts: 1) within the intensified intimate spaces of couple relationships; and 2) in the gendered structure of dating within the context of social distancing. We end by discussing what our findings might mean for the transformation of intimate spaces in pandemic times.

Method

The chapter draws on empirical data from four interrelated studies conducted in Austria and Germany.[1] Three survey studies and one qualitative interview study took place between the beginning of the COVID-19 pandemic and June 2022 (see Figure 2.1). Two of the survey studies (studies 1 and 2) collected anonymous data from a total of 10,070 cases on reported changes in intimate and sexual relationships under the impact of COVID-19 from respondents contacted via daily channels, primarily radio and newspapers. In study 3, participants in study 2, who were living in Vienna and had agreed to be contacted for a follow-up study, were recruited for interview. Data were elicited by means of a problem-centred interview, a commonly used approach in Germany and Austria characterised by an open narrative interview stimulus followed by more structured questions on the issue being examined (Witzel 1989). Fifteen interviewees (see Table 2.1) were initially selected based on gender and age with the aim of maximising contrast, and then by (self-defined) minority status (disability, ethnicity, sexual orientation or other), using a theoretical sampling approach. During the interviews, conducted via a videoconference tool, we asked how their sexual and intimate relationships

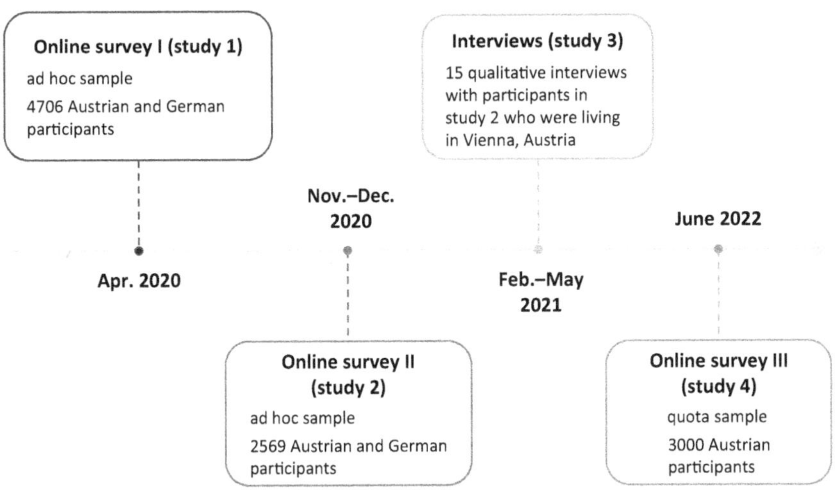

Figure 2.1 Timeline of data collection.

Table 2.1 Qualitative sample (study 3)

Pseudonym	*Gender identity*	*Age*	*Intimate relationship*
Philipp	Man	23	Committed relationship, moved in with male partner during the pandemic
Maria	Woman	34	Committed relationship, lives with male partner
Emelie	Woman	24	Committed relationship, lives with male partner
Alex	Gender fluid	35	Polyamorous marriage, lives with husband
Eva	Woman	52	Committed relationship with a man, lives alone
Hannah	Woman	32	At the beginning of the pandemic, polyamorous arrangement with female partner with children in the same household, then new committed exclusive relationship with a woman, lives alone
Isabella	Woman	38	At the beginning of the pandemic, casual sexual relationships, then new committed exclusive relationship with a man, lives in shared apartment
Ella	Woman	21	Single, lives alone next to her parents' flat
David	Man	59	At the beginning of the pandemic, in a committed relationship with a woman, after a break-up single looking for a new partner, lives alone
Linda	Woman	43	Committed relationship, lives with male partner and child(ren)

(*Continued*)

Table 2.1 (Continued)

Pseudonym	*Gender identity*	*Age*	*Intimate relationship*
Helena	Woman	49	At the beginning of the pandemic, polyamorous arrangement with two male partners, then exclusive relationship with a man during the pandemic, lives alone
Kaya	Woman	31	New committed relationship during the pandemic with a man, lives alone
Julia	Woman	39	In committed relationship, lives with male partner and child(ren)
Ben	Man	28	At the beginning of the pandemic, in a committed relationship with a woman, after break-up single looking for a new partner, lives in shared apartment
Daniel	Man	56	Lives alone, found a new female partner during the pandemic

had changed since the beginning of the pandemic, followed by more focused questions about dating, partnerships and friends. In study 4, data collection of 3,000 cases took place as part of a larger survey on sexual pleasure conducted by one of the authors of this paper in Austria. National data were collected via an online panel convened by a market research institute. Quota sampling included age, gender, education and national federal district. In each case, data were collected with informed consent and all studies were approved by the Research Ethics Committee of Sigmund Freud University.

The transformation of sexual and romantic relationships in a time of crisis

Analysis of our empirical data reveals the extent to which the pandemic has led to changes in desires, practices and routines. While for some people contact with their partner intensified, respondents with multiple partners restricted their sex life, particularly at the beginning of the pandemic.

Coronamonogamy: Unconventional intimate arrangements and the moralisation of sex

Respondents in studies 1 and 2 perceived an increased personal sense of responsibility for the health and safety of others, which led to social pressure particularly when the search for new sexual partners during the pandemic was presented as a violation of social norms. Social distancing in particular triggered the moralisation of casual sex in Austria and Germany (Rothmüller 2021a). Consequently, for some respondents, the revival of a previously ended relationship became one of the few options left to them during nationwide shutdowns. Others looked for a temporary 'Corona partner' and framed their relationship as having a 'commonality of purpose.' Interestingly, our empirical data provided evidence that some of these temporary arrangements transformed themselves into more serious commitments over time as described below.

An intensified focus on commitment was also found in the case of less conventional relationships. In study 1, several respondents who had reported being in previously consensual non-monogamous relationships observed a newly established Coronamonogamy:

> My intimacy and physical needs were spread over a number of people before the pandemic. This included casual sexual contacts, sexual friendships, rope partners, play partners, but also asexual cuddling-closeness partners. Due to the pandemic, this relationship complexity reduced to one person.
>
> (Non-binary respondent, aged 36, queer, casual sexual partners, study 1)

Of respondents who previously had multiple sexual partners, 45% had limited their contact to just one partner only at the time of study 2.

Our interviews in study 3 provided insight into why pandemic times were perceived to require monogamy. In Hannah's case, uncertain and unstable times created the desire for greater stability and support, putting an end to her previous polyamorous relationships. After she had terminated her arrangement with two women, she took a break from dating and sought a monogamous relationship with a new partner. Evaluating her decision to do so, she said:

> I then decided for myself that I, that I would no longer look for a polyamorous relationship but that I would search for a monogamous relationship again so that I have more back-up in life, so to speak. And I wonder how COVID probably had an influence on that subconsciously, that I, that I was looking for more support in a relationship again and … then I found a partner again very quickly via online dating … just in time before the next lockdown, so to speak [laughs] [interviewer giggles]. It was then really nice that I was not alone, that I am not alone, and this has now become a very intense relationship, and we still see each other almost every day.
>
> (Hannah)

In Hannah's view, this rapid development of commitment stemmed from the fact that political measures favoured monogamous partnerships over other forms of intimacy. Her search for relationship stability was typical of the experiences of other respondents who had previously been living alone but who decided to spend the lockdown together with just one partner.

A contrasting theme for some interviewees was the desire to have more than one sexual relationship, but with the adoption of new health and safety measures. One couple made the decision to open their marriage during the pandemic and looked for a partner 'using the [new] possibilities we had' (Alex). These included the use of COVID-19 antigen and PCR testing which enabled them, once it became easily accessible, to safely meet with another woman to enjoy sexual relationships and cuddling. Two other interviewees decided to date partners again once testing and vaccination became widely available. In Vienna, where the qualitative study was conducted, COVID-19 PCR testing was free of charge and exceptionally well organised. Thus, based on risk awareness and new forms of risk management, the re-growth of polyamorous and complex dating networks became possible without jeopardising an individual's health. While a shift towards monogamy was particularly intense at the start of the COVID-19 pandemic (Rothmüller 2021a), many polyamorous participants reverted to multiple dating when risks became more manageable.

The new intensity of intimate couples' spaces

The intensification of intimacy within new relationships is exemplified by several interviewees in study 3, some of whom, like Isabella, decided to move in with a partner together just a few months after getting to know each other.

> Normally, when you enter a new relationship, you might just do more outside actually, so to speak, but that just sort of dropped, and so we just, I think, both [of us] had the feeling now, simply because we're constantly on top of each other at home, that we have … can already estimate quite well … . that we would be able to cope with living together.
>
> (Isabella)

Despite seeing her behaviour as challenging romantic scripts, Isabella appreciated the probation period the shutdowns offered her. Another couple that had lived together during the lockdowns decided to do so permanently because the lockdown time was 'very nice, I thought, and a lot of fun' (Philipp). In these and other cases, the large amount of time spent together sparked the desire to live together once the lockdown was over. Another interviewee argued that sharing a difficult time of crisis with a partner at the beginning of a relationship generated a feeling of trust: 'You also get to know the other person really well in real depth. If I had been together with someone for two years, I probably wouldn't know them as well as I do now over this one year, because we have already gone through a lot together' (Kaya).

For long-term couples, pandemic shutdowns also provided opportunities for relational closeness and intimacy, sometimes resulting in an increase in sexual activity and pleasure. In 2022, we found in study 4 that 22% of the Austrian population experienced sex as more pleasurable during the first two years of the pandemic than before. Interestingly, these and other positive outcomes were not so rare as one might expect (Rothmüller 2021b). In study 2, fully 8% of the participants indicated that they fell in love in between the first two lockdowns, 4% found new sex partners or a new affair, and another 4% transformed a casual contact into a committed relationship. However, in order to realise the positive unintended effects during lockdown, certain preconditions had to be in place, including having a place to retreat to, having more spare time due to the loss of social obligations, and experiencing financial stability through paid short-term employment or furlough during the shutdowns in Austria and Germany (Rothmüller 2021b).

In the absence of these factors, relationship conflicts were more likely to occur. In total, 9% of the participants in study 2 separated or were in the process of ending a committed and/or a casual relationship during the pandemic. Restricted living conditions while working from home and social distancing could also negatively impact sexual intimacy, as was noted by our interviewees. A decrease in sexual desire was for example experienced by couples who had children living with them in the same household. Due to distance learning, the children were often at home and parents did not find the time to have uninterrupted sex as 'it's different to be intimate with your partner when a fourteen-year-old child is sleeping in the next room than when you have the place all to yourself,' explained Julia.

So far, this chapter has shown that changes to sexual relationships under the impact of COVID-19 were complex. Not everyone was affected by pandemic policies in the same way. It is noteworthy that many couples experienced neither a positive nor a negative new intensity in their relationship. Fully 71% of the participants in study 2 indicated that their relationship status remained unchanged within the first year of the pandemic, and every second Austrian interviewed did not perceive any change in sexual pleasure two years into the pandemic in study 4. Thus, not experiencing a significant change in sexual relationships was common, raising the question whether people remember the impact of the pandemic on intimacy in quite the same way.

We turn now to consider how sexual intimacy changed for a group of people that were particularly badly affected, namely, singles who were looking for a new partner within the context of the nationwide shutdowns.

Finding new partners during pandemic distancing

COVID-19 mitigation policies not only transformed sexual and romantic relationships, but also forced people to adjust their dating behaviour due to social distancing regulations. A significant number of people stopped looking for partners during the first two lockdowns. For example, 32% of study 1 respondents and 20% of study 2 respondents who used online dating apps stopped dating. Women and LGBTIQA+ respondents were twice as likely to stop as heterosexual male respondents. Moreover, 9 out of 10 respondents who were looking for a partner had adapted their dating routines to pandemic regulations by the end of 2020. This often involved going for a walk together instead of meeting indoors at a public venue. Changes in dating strategies were still ongoing in 2022. In study 4, 36% of Austrians who were actively searching for a new partner (or partners) indicated that the pandemic had changed their dating behaviour. Among the most frequently experienced changes were intensified communication before a first date, the search for emotional closeness, and dating people only if they shared the same attitude towards pandemic mitigation and/or if they were vaccinated.

Pandemic self-reliance and the dangers of female outdoor dating

Ella, a 21-year-old cisgender female student living alone, saw the biggest impact of the pandemic on her life in the fact that 'during this time, I managed to mentally detach myself from the idea that I had to participate in everything all the time, and that I had to be part of everything … and that has actually helped me.' Describing herself as a 'people pleaser' with a strong fear of missing out, she recalls in the interview that the pandemic provided her with relief from the stressful expectations of being social and excessive partying. During the first year of the pandemic, Ella stopped dating, wondering whether COVID-19 had made her 'incapable of feeling desire for someone.' Reflecting on her negative pre-pandemic dating experiences, including sexual assault, during the quest to 'have as many sexual partners as possible,' she found out that 'I would actually like to have intimacy again.' During a time when contact restrictions in Austria were eased, she met three selected dates and went for a walk. None of these dates resulted in any intimate or sexual activity.

> I'm actually not the kind of person who [usually] goes for a walk … , that's just not the ideal setting for me, especially not for Tinder, because I would not have downloaded Tinder, if it wasn't for the pandemic I would say: Okay let's meet at a bar [Interviewer: yes] let's meet for dinner, whatever. And because of the fact that this is not possible now, and because of that, you will know anyway, as a woman you always have to be a bit careful. I won't invite someone to my house for the first date and I certainly won't go to someone else's, and that's also what a lot of men on Tinder don't understand … . That … somehow … makes it even more complicated because as a woman you completely lose every possibility of meeting someone without danger … That's just something you have to consider, and yes that makes it difficult.
>
> (Ella)

Here, Ella elaborates on some of the emotional barriers to sexual intimacy, among them the pandemic mode of dating outdoors, which made her feel unsafe and eventually refrain from hooking up with strangers. In her case, the dating excitement in finding new sex partners decreased to be replaced by a new focus on self-reliance, close friendship and family ties. Reflecting on women's sexuality in society, she decided to give more time to herself. She pleasured herself more often through masturbation, invested in her (sexual) self by going to psychotherapy and enjoyed her time alone at home during the lockdowns.

While the literature on hook-ups suggests that partying and experimenting before settling down is part of emerging adulthood (Garcia et al. 2015, p. 207), for Ella the pandemic provided a window of opportunity to rethink social expectations and preferences. Similarly, more introverted and asexual people found the release from social expectations and the opportunity to avoid difficult social situations during lockdown, provided them with a sense of relief. They were able to enjoy more time alone, focus on self-care, and rest (Rothmüller 2021b).

The theme of danger for women was present in other interviews, too. Helena's entire dating routine was based on spatial and social opportunity structures. Being a 49-year-old woman with two adult children living alone, she enjoyed multiple romantic relationships following her divorce. However, she stopped dating during the first lockdown because she used to take male hook-ups to a hotel room first, instead of meeting them at home, for security reasons. When the hotels had to close, she took a break from dating completely. However, as soon as hotels reopened in the summer 2020, she resumed online dating again, eventually meeting the person who would become her future regular partner in the next lockdown.

For whom is the public space a safe space? Queer dating experiences

While many people spent more time outdoors so as to meet potential partners and friends in a safe way, our findings show that doing so carried risks not only for women. Queer and non-binary study participants described fear, or experiences, of harassment when they displayed intimacy in public space. In study 2, the proportion of people who said that they could display affection in public without any anxiety ranged from just 28% among lesbian and gay respondents to 37% among queer participants, while 73% of heterosexual respondents completely agreed that they could go for a walk holding hands with their partner free of anxiety during lockdown.

Pandemic-specific risks of meeting sexual partners outdoors could be witnessed in the case of Philipp, a gay man who found himself criminalised for seeing his partner in a park at a time when only romantic relationship partners or people living in the same household were allowed to meet in person.

> During the first lockdown an incident with the police happened to us. They did not believe that we were a couple and we were reported [to the authorities], although we said that we were a couple five times! And uhm, then we got a fine of 500 Euros per person.
>
> (Philipp)

After this incident, Philipp developed a feeling of insecurity in public places and recalled that 'every time a police car passed by, I immediately felt intimidated.' Even though the couple had a very small apartment, they did not leave their flat for two weeks. Philipp filed a complaint about homophobic behaviour with the provincial police directorate. The responsible authority eventually responded to the complaint saying it had not been obvious enough to the police officers that they were a couple. Two weeks later, the couple were reported again despite showing the police a picture of them kissing as a 'proof' of their close and loving relationship.

> We didn't go far, sat down on a park bench, my partner smoked a cigarette, and then the police drove by and stopped, and there were several people sitting on the benches anyway, and then I said: 'I bet they're coming to us' [Interviewer: mhm] and, because it was just us two young men next to each other and everyone else was rather older heterosexual couples, of retirement age. And I was right, they only came to us, checked our ID and then we said: 'Yes, we're together' … I then immediately started to cry, because [Interviewer: yes] I was again so upset … The argument [of one policeman] was then just like: 'Well, everyone who is with friends on the road can tell that' and I said to myself: Well, not everybody would tell that he is gay. [Both laugh] And, yes, that was a bit tedious.
>
> (Philipp)

In study 2, we found additional evidence of discrimination towards queer people. For example, a woman aged 20 reported that 'at the beginning of the lockdown, my ex-partner and I primarily met outdoors but were confronted with homophobic comments and looks that made us feel uncomfortable.' Together, these experiences illustrate that going for a walk with a regular partner, instead of meeting indoors to minimise the risk of infection, carried its own risks for LGBTIQA+ people due to pandemic-specific modes of policing as well as the more general risk of harassment present in public space.

Men's dating strategies: Expanding the scope beyond social boundaries

Many cisgender heterosexual single men did not know how and where to meet new partners. In open-ended answers on dating, it became apparent that they often felt negatively affected by the restrictions. In our interview study, two men tried to connect with any available woman in their everyday lives. Their strategies not only involved approaching ex-partners or random people in public spaces, but also psychological and medical professionals, and academic researchers doing fieldwork, as one of the authors of this paper experienced personally during the qualitative interview study.

Daniel, for example, found a new partner during the pandemic. In interview, he explained he actually liked the lockdown because the lonely people he had met in public places such as at the Würstelstand (sausage booth) were very talkative and more approachable than before the pandemic, an experience which reminded him of his youth. Daniel said it was positive that the majority of people had to go for a walk to meet new people as it made everyone more equal in terms of social class.

> It makes everyone the same to go for a walk in the park. It doesn't matter if you have a big car or expensive restaurants, none of that counts anymore. You go for a walk in the park or in the forest or something [Interviewer: mhm] like in the old days, you put a beer can in your pocket like a teenager … Uh it's the same for the millionaire.
>
> (Daniel)

In a second male interviewee's narrative of dating transformations, we encountered a similar pattern of face-to-face flirting across a wide range of social settings. David, a 59-year-old man with a chronic illness, had experienced a difficult breakup at the start of the pandemic, leaving him depressed and alone during the first lockdown. He tried to find a new partner, with only temporary success. During a long interview lasting a total of two and a half hours with just a short break, he described in detail his pandemic dating routine.

David: I started doing certain things so that I wouldn't completely rot away, I started loving doctor's appointments because then I'm with people … . When I went shopping, I always tried to make sure I have eye contact with people because unfortunately half of the face is covered now, yes.

Interviewer: Yes, that's unfortunately the case, yes, mhm

David: And, I have been told that I am quite good with my eyes in conveying charisma, communication and facial expression … yes, that is also, communication, the facial expressions. And now, it is just the eyes, only half of it [the face], yet somehow something still comes across, and that feels helpful. I always try to do these things - in order to be with people again.

This interview sequence not only illustrates the heightened importance of visual cues and particularly the eyes in initiating contact when mask wearing. It also provides an explanation for the relatively extensive and somewhat exhausting time the interview took. David tries to get hold of people and keep their attention for as long as possible to distract him from the psychosocial stress and loneliness he might otherwise experience.

The expansion of dating spaces beyond conventional boundaries was a strategy that became particularly visible when directed towards professionals. In the interview, David performatively enacted the dating techniques he described. He remarked that after the experience of a 'happy ending' at a Thai massage salon during lockdown, he had invited the masseuse and her female friend to join him for a weekend away at his vacation home. He indicated that he similarly managed to become friends with his psychotherapist, and then tried to do the same with the female interviewer (one of the authors of this paper) during the interview, as illustrated in the following interaction:

David: No, I'm not doing that [online dating] at the moment, at the moment I'm just trying to do it in real life or rather, when I'm with, aw, there's a university study, yes, and there's a very nice woman sitting in front of me at the screen. And so, I'm trying it out.

Interviewer: Still in direct contact.

David: Yes, like now.

Interviewer: Yes, yes, I understand, yes.

David: And I say it explicitly [smiles], if I may take the liberty?

Interviewer: You can say anything, it's an interview situation and, it's just being recorded [smiles] but [laughs briefly]

David: Well, then it will be recorded that I am flirting a little, I will survive that too.

In the above interchange, the researcher did not initially respond to the interviewee's advances. As a result, he sought to address her more personally while sexualising the interview setting. The interchange signals embarrassment on the part of the interviewer who sought to reinforce the formality of the setting after the interviewee had crossed the boundaries.

Due to the lack of other dating options and social isolation, some of our male interviewees who were looking for a female partner approached a wide range of women with sexual and/or romantic intentions during lockdown. Such an 'expansion of dating efforts' extended to spaces, individuals and groups of women who likely would not have been approached in the absence of the pandemic.

Traditional patterns, new commitments: Discussion and conclusion

At the beginning of the spread of any unknown disease, anxieties and stigmatisation tend to be prevalent. A key lesson from past pandemics such as HIV as well as COVID-19 is that social factors are as important as medical interventions in successfully tackling a health crisis. In the case of COVID-19 in Austria and Germany, and based on the evidence contained in this chapter, our research indicates that sexual behaviour and dating practices changed until vaccination and testing justified a relaxation of social distancing. Yet, as we know from the case of HIV, the historical memory of past pandemic cannot be undone even after effective treatment is available and the advent of new forms of prevention such as pre-exposure prophylaxis (PrEP). What then, might we expect the COVID-19 pandemic to leave behind?

Pandemic times bring to light the social dimensions of human sexuality. People are able to navigate complex intimate arrangements and adapt their sexual practices to new health risks. Yet, public health policies have unintended and unanticipated consequences that nobody wants to be responsible for and are therefore easily forgotten, particularly in regards to the treatment of minorities. Acknowledging more openly in the future that pandemic mitigation policies' side effects and stressors are part of the everyday experiences of minorities as well as others will promote greater recognition and inclusion during the societal changes necessary during and after a pandemic.

Like all research, the studies described here had their limitations. Importantly, we did not collect longitudinal data and thus our analysis only provides glimpses into intimate transformations over time. The generalisability of our findings is also impacted by the limitation that two out of the three quantitative surveys did not assess attitudes and practices in the general population. However, data from the quasi-representative population sample provide limited evidence that social distancing has had a long-term impact on the sexual behaviour of different sections of the Austrian population.

Our qualitative data offer some insight into how the described transformations have unfolded over time and rendered meaningful by social agents. Pandemic lockdown allowed people to identify new values, new desires and embrace what they actually wanted and needed from relationships, including intimacy, cohabitation and emotional security. These results pointing to an intensification of intimacy during the pandemic are in line with those from other research emphasising that in times of crisis, people value emotional intimacy (Schröder et al. 2021, p. 236) and trusting relationships (Döring and Walter 2020, p. 68). Going through difficult times may bring couples, friends and family closer together, at least temporarily (Rothmüller 2021b; Estlein et al. 2022).

Yet, interventions that shut down societies for whole weeks at a time, while effective in public health terms, fail to engage with the importance of social contact at a time of crisis. Similar to other pandemics, mitigation imposed an additional stressor on already marginalised populations and negatively impacted their intimate relationships. Previous studies have highlighted how, during the HIV pandemic, social solidarity proved central to coping through collective networks of care (Logie and Turan 2020). Unfortunately, in the COVID-19 pandemic, policies promoted the value of the nuclear family at the expense of friends, peers and the wider community, resulting in the isolation of single people and a moralisation of casual sexual relationships (Rothmüller 2021a). Future pandemic management should seek to learn the lessons from this – and aim instead to provide solutions that engage with varying interests and needs, and which are available to all.

Ultimately, the effects of pandemics are uneven and exploit the faultlines present in an already unequal world. The narrative of COVID-19 being the great equaliser is first and foremost the product of a male heterosexual imagination informed by an unnoticed privilege that fails to recognise the experiences of women and non-binary, lesbian, gay and queer people. For the former, public settings provided opportunities to expand dating efforts and experience intimacy and closeness beyond normal social boundaries. For the latter, who encounter inequality on a daily basis, there were few safe spaces for intimacy and closeness during a global health crisis.

Note

1 Studies 1–3 were financially supported by *Wissenschafts- und Forschungsförderung der Stadt Wien Kulturabteilung*, and the *Netzwerk Wissenschaft der Arbeiterkammer*. Study 4 received funding from *Krone Verlag*, Austria. We thank Emelie Rack, Laura Wiesböck, Mascha Leskien, Sophie König, Anna Maria Diem and David Seistock for assistance with data collection, survey implementation and coding. Thanks also go to members of the Institute of Qualitative Social Research at Sigmund Freud University – Nora Ruck, Markus Brunner, Natalie Rodax, Katharina Hametner and Markus Wrbouschek – for their feedback on an earlier draft of this chapter.

References

Berlant, L., 1999. Intimacy: A special issue. *Critical Inquiry*, 24 (2), 281–288.

Dionne, K. and Turkmen, F., 2020. The politics of pandemic Othering: Putting COVID-19 in global and historical context. *International Organization*, 74 (1), E213–E230. doi:10.1017/S0020818320000405

Döring, N. and Walter, R., 2020. Wie verändert die Covid-19-Pandemie unsere Sexualitäten? Eine Übersicht medialer Narrative im Frühjahr 2020. *Zeitschrift für Sexualforschung*, 33 (2), 65–75.

Esacove, A.W., 2010. *Love matches: Heteronormativity, modernity, and AIDS prevention in Malawi*. Los Angeles: Sage.

Estlein, R., Gewirtz-Meydan, A., and Opuda, E., 2022. Love in the time of Covid-19: A systematic mapping review of empirical research on romantic relationships one year into the Covid-19 pandemic. *Family Process*, 61 (3), 1–21. doi:10.1111/famp.12775

Garcia, J., et al., 2015. Casual sex: Integrating social, behavioral, and sexual health research. In J. DeLamater and R. Plante, eds. *Handbook of the sociology of sexualities*. Cham: Springer, 203–222.

Herrmann, W.J., et al., 2022. Loneliness and depressive symptoms differ by sexual orientation and gender identity during physical distancing measures in response to COVID-19 pandemic in Germany. *Applied Psychology: Health and Well-Being*, 15 (1), 1–17.

Inman, E.M., et al., 2021. Discrimination and psychosocial engagement during the COVID-19 pandemic. *Stigma and Health*, 6 (4), 380–383. doi:10.1037/sah0000349

Joshi, B. and Swarnakar, P., 2021. Staying away, staying alive: Exploring risk and stigma of COVID-19 in the context of beliefs, actors and hierarchies in India. *Current Sociology*, 69 (4), 492–511. doi:10.1177/0011392121990023

Logie, C.H. and Turan, J.M., 2020. How do we balance tensions between COVID-19 public health responses and stigma mitigation? Learning from HIV research. *AIDS and Behavior*, 24 (7), 2003–2006. doi:10.1007/s10461-020-02856-8

Nelkin, D. and Gilman, S.L., 1988. Placing blame for devastating disease. *Social Research*, 55 (3), 361–378.

Panzeri, M., et al., 2020. Changes in sexuality and quality of couple relationship during the COVID-19 lockdown. *Frontiers in Psychology*, 11, 1–8. doi:10.3389/fpsyg.2020.565823

Roberto, K.J., Johnson, A.F., and Rauhaus, B.M., 2020. Stigmatization and prejudice during the COVID-19 pandemic. *Administrative Theory & Praxis*, 42 (3), 364–378. doi:10.1080/10841806.2020.1782128

Rothmüller, B., 2021a. The grip of pandemic mononormativity in Austria and Germany. *Culture, Health & Sexuality*, 23 (11), 1573–1590. doi:10.1080/13691058.2021.1943534

Rothmüller, B., 2021b. Aufblühen trotz Corona? Intimitätsgewinne und andere positive, unintendierte Nebeneffekte pandemiebedingter Gesellschaftsveränderungen. *Psychosozial*, 44 (4), 50–66. doi:10.30820/0171-3434-2021-4-50

Schröder, J., et al., 2021. Veränderungen sexueller Interessen und Erfahrungen während der Covid-19-Pandemie – Eine qualitative Inhaltsanalyse. *Psychotherapeut*, 66, 233–239. doi:10.1007/s00278-021-00506-5

Toldam, N., et al., 2022. Sexual health during COVID-19: A scoping review. *Sexual Medicine Review*, 10 (4), 714–753. doi:10.1016/j.sxmr.2022.06.005

Witzel, A., 1989. Das problemzentrierte Interview. In G. Jüttemann, ed. *Qualitative Forschung in der Psychologie, Grundfragen Verfahrensweisen, Anwendungsfelder*. Heidelberg: Asanger, 227–255.

3 75 loads in LA

Situating the 'queer mundane' in viral times

Chris Ashford and Gareth Longstaff

Introduction

HIV and AIDS have continued to cast a long cultural and legal shadow over the lives of gay, bisexual and other men who have sex with men. In multiple jurisdictions, including many US States and in England and Wales, HIV transmission laws continue despite the changed scientific landscape, most recently transformed with the increased availability of pre-exposure prophylaxis (PrEP). Whilst COVID-19 has seen a significant re-casting of law – as the science changed, the law changed, and with it, a cultural re-set of how desire and intimacy between men are expressed and practised – HIV continues to be held in a legal and cultural time bubble, out of sync with contemporary queer life and the everyday contours of how many queer sexual subjects form their intimacies around the politics of queer desire and pleasure. Ultimately, the pandemics remain linked by one substance and our reaction to it.

Cum, jizz, junk, spunk, semen and sperm are words that can arouse and trigger sexual shame, pleasure, excitement and discomfort in equal measure (see for example, Dean 2009; Ashford 2015; Gonzalez 2019; Tziallas 2019; Morris 2021). Each of these terms seeks to define and thus culturally signify the organic fluid created in the male sexual organs and ejaculated through a penis. They are also quotidian and mundane yet also speak to a power of visual and linguistic transformation; this secretion as an orgasmic point of pleasure, as a residue of desire, and simultaneously as a carrier of life or a cause of death, and the abject platitudes of power (Kristeva 1980) and visibility in between.

Like most sources of power, it is perhaps unsurprising that this substance and its complex and precarious layers of meaning have attracted the attention of both law and culture. This is notable in the visual representation both of this as a triumphant fluid ('the cum shot' and 'the money shot' – see Williams 1989; Attwood 2007) and also as part of a broader framework of desire and queer praxis, particularly in the context of how we understand the shifting field of pornography. The 'queer mundane' is part of a 'veritable explosion of sexually explicit materials that cry out for better understanding' in the context of virality and temporality (Williams 2004, p. 1).

DOI: 10.4324/9781003322788-4

The production and consumption of pornography – like the seminal fluid depicted – becomes both a mundane and powerful transmitter of viral desire. It can 'infect' change and, in the eyes of some, adversely affect the recipient. And just as with the seminal fluid itself, law and culture have sought to create and impose barriers to that transference, regulating, for example, HIV transmission and other sexually transmitted infections that meet a 'grievous bodily harm' threshold in English law, whilst Los Angeles County in California has one of the most restrictive pornography laws in the world, imposing a series of strict rules limiting the operation of bareback sex pornography.

These complex laws – cultural and statutory – may *prima facie* appear to create a rigorous norm in which queer celebration at disrupting these barriers can thrive, in which sex without barriers – bareback sex in this case – becomes an affirmational point of resistance. Yet in the context of dramatic scientific changes in recent years and with the increased availability of PrEP, bareback sex arguably forms part of what we term here a new 'queer mundane' (see more generally Ashford et al. 2020; Sandset 2021). In specific contexts and situations 'unprotected' bareback sex, whilst still desirable, excessive and 'authentic', simply *is*. The alternative – 'protected' sex with condoms – is rendered and signified as unusual, fetishised or deviant. To acclaim and participate in bareback sex, and revel in 'pig' identity (Florencio 2020) in which the abundance of bodily fluids and sexual promiscuity are embraced and celebrated, arguably becomes what we term the 'queer mundane'. In this ideological and cultural space, the pleasures of barebacking go against the acceptability of homo- and hetero-normativity and are arguably no longer an extreme or shameful counterpoint to that normativity. Rather, they form a situational and ordinary form of queer desire that empowers and affirms pleasure beyond the normative assumptions that mainstream hetero- and homo-sexual orthodoxy presupposes (see more generally Klesse 2007; Florencio 2020).

This chapter takes '75 Loads Guy' (hereafter 75LG) as an intersection amidst two pandemics – HIV and COVID-19 – to explore for the first time from a legal and cultural perspective how what we develop, situate and term the 'queer mundane' operates and navigates law and culture. In doing so, we hope that the analysis provides queer insights for future law and policy-makers alongside cultural curators and shapers to better understand queer mundanity as a vital element of society, sexuality, subjectivity and desire.

Pandemics and the queer mundane

The queer mundane strongly connects to conceptual modes of queer futurity and utopia (Muñoz 2009) and their potential to create a temporal horizon of queer transformation (pp. 19–32) in which 'multiple forms of belonging in difference adhere to a belonging in collectivity' (p. 20). The position of the 'queer mundane' also operates as 'something that is not yet here' (p. 22) and as a form of sexual desire and visuality 'beyond the limited vista of the here and now' (p. 22), having emerged amidst the intersection of two notable pandemics – the ongoing HIV and COVID-19 pandemics. The COVID-19 pandemic quickly created a set of reductively 'new' norms and assumptions in which people adjusted their sexual behaviour to navigate new forms of risk, for example through the – sometimes officially promoted – use of 'safer sex' measures such as gloryholes (Ashford and Longstaff 2021) whilst at other times and in other contexts most sexual behaviour became illegal.

Just as with the HIV pandemic, there was initially confusion and uncertainty about risk, but this evolved as people became informed by scientific knowledge and 'the everyday transaction of heteronormative capitalism' (Muñoz 2009, p. 22). So too, the appropriate boundaries of law were debated, and extraordinarily draconian legal measures were imposed around the world limiting, if not prohibiting, travel alongside human interaction. It was in this uncanny setting that the contours of queer mundanity were formed through an 'impulse that we see in everyday life' (Muñoz 2009, p. 22) and a quotidian way to capture queer desire through the resistance and affirmation of 'utopian bonds, affiliations, designs, and gestures that exist within the present moment' (p. 23). The practices that emerge between these lived elements of 'everyday queer' experience and the conceptual possibilities of a 'queer utopia' form this space of the 'queer mundane'. Here, the interplay between queer mundanity and queer utopia allows for the day-to-day contours of queer life to be reshaped as forms of resistance to heteronormative law and broader modes of cultural normativity. For example, just as using Grindr and other hook-up apps was not a criminal offence, for some 'locked-down' time periods during the pandemic, to meet up with someone using these apps (beyond your designated 'bubble' individual) was a criminal offence in England and Wales. Group sex or promiscuity became anathema to many legal jurisdictions, including English law. The enforced closure of hospitality venues encompassed saunas, gay bars and clubs, and also meant that vast swathes of the everyday elements of queer sexual existence along with the queer mundane were changed, prohibited and/or removed.

In turn, these levels of restriction and regulation formed a space where the potential for new and alternative queer utopias also emerged. One sex venue in Newcastle-upon-Tyne in the UK took to turning their steam room into a seating space for what became a cafe as they sought to navigate the oft-changing legal landscape in which some venues were allowed to re-open amidst new restrictions but not as a sauna. Their Twitter account promoting the new 'facilities' showed a photograph of newly installed tables and cushions positioned on the normally bare tiled benches. It was a time at which 'safer sex' became 'no sex' in commercial spaces, mirroring earlier HIV and AIDS debates in many global cities, notably San Francisco in the 1980s. These physical changes reflected a tangible shift in which elements of the queer mundane – in these cases sites of promiscuous intimacies in commercial public spaces – so much an 'everyday' yet still oft-hidden element of queer life, were extinguished. A steamy and intense dark space that once reverberated with the sound of joyful groans and walls occasionally splattered with cum became a well-lit and sanitised space in which people could sit and drink coffee. Their wet hard dicks, naked or towel-draped bodies now fully dressed and their cocks flaccid and safely hidden.

It was against this backdrop that in January 2022 a Twitter account rapidly gained traction in documenting a young Black American man engaging in anonymous sex with a large number of guys, principally as the receptive sexual partner. The account seemingly shocked a largely heterosexual – or at least heteronormative – audience with a guy taking '75 loads' in a Los Angeles hotel room quickly generating a series of viral memes and joking tweets about the volume of cum involved. This initial viral reaction in which the behaviour was viewed as 'extraordinary' was then followed by sustained popularity as men discovered they too could access the 'ordinary' as documented and presented as sexual pleasure. Here, the contours of the 'queer mundane' went viral. On the one hand, 75LG was something 'extraordinary' to those viewing scenes and behaviours they might not otherwise have encountered, and yet the scenes – particularly given the large number of men involved – were anything but extraordinary, rather they reflected a quite 'ordinary' and mundane experience of bareback multi-partner play for the men who engaged and consenting to these behaviours.

In May 2022, the account re-branded and transitioned to a Twitter handle that focused more on the individual persona of 75LG rather than his actions. By this time, the profile had attracted 49.3k followers and followed just 73 accounts, including collaborators and other high-profile promiscuous receptive partners (aka 'cumdumps') such as Ryan Cummings. Such would be the success of both the Twitter account and the subsequent OnlyFans profile, that '75 Loads Guy' would travel around the USA and also other parts of the world, including the UK as COVID-19 restrictions eased, continuing and documenting his sexual adventures. His London 'session' took place at a central hotel, advertised on a well-known global bareback hook-up site with party listings as well as on his social media accounts. The hotel site is noteworthy for being a regular site for similar non-commercial events promoted on social media and bareback sites, as well as being a popular central hotel for unsuspecting tourists and business visitors. At other times, 75LG visited commercial spaces such as a London cruise bar and also a sauna. These videos and tweets sharing his sexcapades served to document a re-queering of these spaces and their potential to frame sexual promiscuity and risk as affirmingly ordinary and mundane features of queer intimacy.

When 75LG went viral in 2022, he did so by capturing and articulating a form of intimacy that nurtured part of the 'queer mundane', but he also did so amidst a period of intense legal scrutiny in relation to COVID-19, as well as a legacy of legal measures shaped by the HIV pandemic. It was the authenticating visual documentation and content curation of a raw and well-fucked arse and churned up cum that would form a visceral rebuke to law and normative assumptions of desire. This was a sexcapade that took place in a

Los Angeles hotel, just off Hollywood Boulevard and was at the epicentre of a space where the law had sought to prevent the visual documentation of such things. The subsequent commercialisation of these images disrupted dominant conceptions and constructions of commercial and studio-based pornography (Mercer 2017) and during the COVID-19 pandemic constituted in many instances the only pornography that was being produced. In turn, it also energised a space where forms of sexual desire, pleasure and authenticity were transformed both within and by the 'queer mundane'.

Regulating safer sex

Leo Bersani once observed that 'queer intellectuals are curiously reticent about the sexuality they claim to celebrate' (2011, p. 91). In the same chapter, Bersani also noted that 'for the overwhelming majority of positive gay men, to acknowledge being infected [with HIV] amounts to a sexual confession: I have been fucked' (Bersani 2011, p. 92). These two observations speak to the shame that continues to inhabit not only a significant number of scholarly interventions but also our understanding of pandemics and their relationship to the regulation and realisation of desire. For law and culture alike, to acknowledge and affirm the desires allied to fucking, anal sex in particular, and the associated pleasures and complexities provided by bodily fluids, is to position front and centre that which remains largely hidden outside of the 'queer mundane'. The emergence of the homonormative frameworks of civil partnerships, same-sex marriage and concomitant social expectations has arguably further silenced discussion of sex rather than encouraged it; instead emphasising state-sanctioned relationships structures and (sex free) reproduction, although as Maine (2022) has noted, the reality of same-sex relationships is more complex than that outwardly projected or arguably understood by mainstream straight culture.

The HIV and COVID-19 pandemics have, in their own ways, played into these narratives and contributed to a range of 'queer domesticities' (see more generally Cook 2014), but have also often been in the forefront of legal and cultural attempts to regulate and limit the undesirable behaviours or intimacies which typically amount to queer sex. The UK COVID-19 sex ban – whether by accident or design (Wagner leans towards accident) – was serious, although Wagner also notes there was 'a lot of sniggering' (Wagner 2022, p. 86) about it. The ban was the practical effect of a series of regulations and the assumption that most people would live in a 'family' unit or, during some of the more lenient phases, be a 'linked' couple able to 'bubble' in two properties. Local regulations further added to the complexity, with Wagner noting Leicester as a particularly extreme example, observing that, 'for residents of Leicester who did not live together and were not part of a linked household, sex indoors was illegal for one year, one month and twenty-one days – 417 days in total' (Wagner 2022, p. 89). Many other jurisdictions – both in the UK and elsewhere – introduced similar legal restrictions between 2020 and 2022.

Recent years have seen a transformation in the biomedical landscape associated with HIV, specifically the increased availability of PrEP in addition to treatment as prevention (TasP) and post-exposure prophylaxis (PEP). The associated global messaging of U=U or undetectable = untransmittable is intended to highlight the evidence-based messaging that those who achieve an undetectable viral load following HIV treatment represent no risk of passing the virus on to another partner. Yet the law has arguably lagged behind in responding to this shift in science, still often being framed with a focus on condoms and a construction of HIV that owes more to the science and fears of the 1980s than the contemporary scientific and social landscape (see Ashford et al. 2020). In the USA, the AIDS Healthcare Foundation campaigns to strengthen the law in relation to the use of condoms in pornography. Most pornography in the USA is produced in California and most of that production has historically taken place in the greater Los Angeles area (Bergman 2014). Occupational health laws in California require a range of safer sex behaviours to be followed when producing porn, but these requirements only relate to employees under section 5193 of the California Code of Regulations and many porn performers do not operate as employees. Measure B – a California ballot measure (effectively a form of referendum) was successfully passed in 2012, entering into law as the County of Los Angeles Safer Sex in the Adult Film Industry Act. This new law applies to porn performers rather than employees and requires the use of condoms in all vaginal and anal sex scenes (see more generally Berg 2021).

Stadler (2021) has suggested that the COVID-19 pandemic was another inflection point for pornography just as the 2008 economic crash was. Whilst it had a direct impact in terms of the visual documentation of COVID-19, with the production of pornography featuring performers in hazmat suits, masks and other personal protective equipment, it also arguably contributed to both the value of pornography – not least for those places such as Leicester with strict sex ban regulations – but also the ease, through OnlyFans and similar profiles, of creating entrepreneurial and monetised platforms for pornographic content (see Downs 2020; van der Nagel 2021). With large commercial porn production stopped, amateur sites became all the more important as spaces to provide pleasure and document desire. In turn, these spaces cultivated communities of shared meaning and desire (Rodriguez-Amat and Belinskaya 2023) linked to those forms of the ordinary and authentic embedded in the 'queer mundane' and more specifically the persona of 75LG.

Pleasure, desire and the queer mundane

On platforms such as Twitter and OnlyFans, the reliance that sexual pleasure has upon authenticity, and the ways in which 'bodies are expected to spontaneously and sexually react in an authentic manner' (Rodriguez-Amat and Belinskaya 2023, p. 247) suggest that the closer we get to a 'claim for authenticity as a form of truth' the more aroused, intensified and absorbed we are. In these online spaces, the cultural and legal tensions which form and emerge between pleasure, authenticity and regulation allow us to map how that desire is articulated and mediated.

The legal and cultural context of 75LG is contoured by utopic (Muñoz 2009) approaches to queer desire and 'the understanding that utopia exists in the quotidian' (p. 9) and the banal forms of authenticity aligned to the 'queer mundane' where authentic traces of the sexual self can visually, emotionally or sexually trigger and fulfil an ordinary sense of queer credence. Authenticity is perfectly captured in the sexually charged content curation and tone of 75LG and the broader shifts in law and culture that were amplified by the 2020 COVID-19 pandemic. 75LG and his approach to the excess of sex with strangers and their 'loads' produces an authentic form of sexual self-representation that actuates the platitudes and fantasies of 'bareback porn' (Dean 2009; Longstaff 2019). Perhaps most tellingly, on 75LG's Twitter profile, we find narratives that oscillate between fantasy and authenticity, excess and banality, as well as self and other. These narratives are simultaneously self-presented as both a sexual persona and a quotidian one on platforms which provide 'a certain guarantee of authenticity, [so] that this authenticity becomes a process of self-expression, self-realisation, and self-validation' (Andrejevic 2002, p. 265). Here, the affirmation of excess and the scale of the loads received works to enhance and inform the tensions that emphasise 75LG's queer mundanity and the broader contexts of how authenticity is articulated and mediated.

Tensions between the politics of an authentic rawness (see Varghese 2019), the freedom to take excessive loads, the enjoyment of promiscuity and pleasure alongside the regulation and fear associated with risk, disease and shame also speak to the reality and legacy of AIDS. The AIDS Healthcare Foundation campaign to introduce the mandatory wearing of condoms in the production of pornography was in part rooted in the classic trope of anti-pornography campaigners, that if you stop depicting acts, these acts stop happening. Put simply, by showing only 'condom' mandated pornography, it was assumed that people would come to understand condoms as the 'norm' for sex. There has been limited research into this association although there exists some evidence of a link (Wright et al. 2022). Such an account failed to recognise that the ongoing Othering of 'raw' pornography might serve to underline the deviance, desire and pleasure of bareback sex so that the law paradoxically reinforces what McNamara (2013, p. 242) has called bareback power – by highlighting the failure of condom campaigns – to create a space in which better alternatives then fill this space, arguing that 'maybe bareback porn has the potential […] to save rather than harm us' through revealing true desire, the limits on control of that desire and, in turn, what practical cultural and legal interventions remain as workable interventions.

PrEP is arguably such a practical response. 75LG and his Twitter account serve to penetrate legal attempts at control but also to counter what Kagan (2018, p. 134) has termed 'the latex paradigm' and the moral *and* behavioural norms established around the use of condoms in response to the HIV pandemic. 75LG arguably highlights the absurdity of attempts to mandate condoms in commercial pornography when anyone can produce pornography and document the utopic habitus of the queer mundane. Here 75 loads in a banal and anonymous hotel room are just the beginning of 'an ideality that can be distilled from the past and used to imagine a future' (Muñoz 2009, p. 1) where desire precedes regulation. The authentic yet ordinary sight of cum dripping from a guy's anus, cum that acquires a foamy quality from the vigorous fucking and churning of many men and which 75LG seems to document without fear or exaggeration. This is not the extraordinary but the ordinary intimacies of the queer mundane and its embodied pleasures point towards a quotidian way of repositioning sex beyond the reductive binaries of bareback vs condomless and/or unprotected vs protected sex.

Importantly, bareback sex persists, arguably less as a symbol of sexual risk but more because of the pull of the associated acts and aesthetics for the men who enjoy and are involved in it. When we see these acts such as in the content of 75LG, we are arguably seeing liberationary depictions of men enjoying slutty promiscuous play with other men, the more men the better. Within them, it is not merely that the fucking is 'raw' or 'authentic' without the intervention of latex (see Dean 2009) that excites, but rather the excessive and available cum that is celebrated and vindicated as part of the sexual encounter. Whilst defining bareback sex arguably remains what Kagan has described as 'fraught and rarely free of moral adjudications' (2018, p. 136), PrEP has perhaps simplified some of the multiple definitions of bareback offered by Junge (2002) given that the assumptions of risk associated with it have been disrupted by the advent of PrEP, TasP and PEP.

The County of Los Angeles Safer Sex in the Adult Film Industry Act (more commonly known as Measure B) was seen by some healthcare professionals as 'taking on' the interests of the porn industry (Cohen et al. 2018), although Cohen's account was produced in collaboration with AIDS Healthcare Foundation allied researchers participated in the Measure B campaign. As Ferris (2017, p. 204) has argued, given the historic impact of HIV on the LGBTQ community, 'it is reasonable to assert that the choice to use or not use condoms represents a vibrant aspect of the transgressive nature of the community'. He goes on to note that 'the assimilationist sector of the LGBT community treats the adult entertainment industry and general sex work with the same disregard because it distracts from the streamlined agenda of a heteronormative living' (Ferris 2017, p. 205).

The advent of PrEP has triggered a major queering of gay sex post-AIDS. In the context of the early HIV epidemic, Dowsett (1996, p. 279) noted that 'where once male homosexual abandon was premised on a fearless exploration of flesh, fluids, and numerous fantastic permissions to transgress, now wariness is ever present'. The legal focus on condoms as a means of protection serves to preserve condom use as an identity in which 'wariness is ever present' in the moment of sex. PrEP removes this dimension from the sexual encounter, positioning the pill outside this moment, and instead alongside the equivalent of a daily vitamin pill. 75LG and his PrEP-enabled slutty power bottoming provide us with a utopic vision of post-pandemic queerness. Yet, legal challenges to Measure B are rooted in more orthodox areas of legal concern. Measure B was unsuccessfully challenged on freedom of expression (First Amendment) grounds with the Appellants arguing that the law was unconstitutional (see Shaffer 2015). In the 2014 case of *Vivid Entertainment v Fielding* (No. 13-56445), the US Court of Appeals for the Ninth Circuit deemed the law to be constitutional as whilst the law did target a specific form of speech, the law targeted the secondary effects of speech, i.e. the sexual transmission of sexually transmitted diseases. Yet as Wagner and Jones (2019) have argued, the arguments for the application of what is known as the secondary effects doctrine were broad, as often occurs in cases affecting Sexually Orientated Businesses, such as pornography. At a time when PrEP is widely available, it is questionable whether prescribing the precise ways that an industry must operate and exactly how sex workers in the porn industry must protect themselves is proportionate.

Conclusion

Dowsett (1996) has written that we could consider 'pornography as a lecture in technique, a fantastic adventure out of the mundane, a visitation to a pleasure dome' (p. 269), and 75LG arguably offers us a glimpse into the pleasure dome and the queer mundane habitus to be found within. It is within this 'everyday' and 'ordinary' that queers navigate pandemics and laws that seek to assert normativity in the name of 'good'. 75LG provides but one example of a disruption to the binaries of good and bad, risk and desire, and an alternative to how we think about law, culture, sex and sexuality.

Where the law has been used as an attempt to ban the production of bareback pornography, it has been to intrude into behaviour that is lawful and to prevent depictions which are, separate from the behaviour, lawful and protected by law (Shepard 2018). Yet 75LG highlights that this Californian law is but one small piece in the contemporary expression of the queer mundane and its potential for queer futurity. In both the COVID-19 and HIV pandemics there were cultural and legal responses that made normative assumptions about how society in general and gay, bisexual and other men who have sex with men should be controlled. Yet, the sexual practices that 75LG affirms seek to queer these forms of regulation, creating space for the subversion of legal and cultural assumptions and confronting the normative frameworks provided by legal framings and by culture. By so doing, however, they reveal the mundane 'ordinariness' of the practices for those who participate in them.

The visual documentation of affirmationally queer and mundane group sex goes some way towards troubling the notion that 'gay men's bodies have become untrustworthy' (Dowsett 1996, p. 279) which has been the legacy of the HIV and COVID-19 pandemics. In the liberationary space of the cum slut encounter, multi-partner encounters take place in the absence of condoms, but with the tacit assumption that PrEP, TasP or PEP are available and/or being utilised. Bareback simply is. Here new formations of how sexual consent, trust, risk, joy, hope and pleasure are performed and navigated signify 'a vast lifeworld of queer relationality, an encrypted sociality, and a utopian potentiality' (Muñoz 2009, p. 6) yet to be attained. Yet attempts to control these representations – as we can see in California with Measure B – are attempts to deny this utopia by inserting an alternative and artificial condom-only vision of gay sex. Whilst this *can* be gay sex, it is not the only form or even, we would suggest, the everyday experience. As Webber (2015) has noted, legal interventions such as Measure B, positioned as health measures, also exert moral pressure. Within them, the law is used to create an artificial truth about how gay men have sex while simultaneously seeking to extinguish efforts to document a queer desire that favours bareback sex.

Some 20 years ago, Crimp (2004, p. 98) observed that,

> unlike other oppressed groups, we gay people do not acquire our culture as a birthright. We have to create it after we find our way out of the hostile environments we grow up in [...]. Among our greatest achievements are the diverse possibilities we have invented for the expression and fulfilment of affectional and sexual relations.

75LG and the aspects of the queer mundane that he captures provide an example of this process of cultural creation. The original reaction to these encounters – and the ephemeral moment that ejaculated 75 loads into the cultural 'mainstream' – highlighted the disconnect between normative assumptions of sex in pandemics and the queer mundane experience of them. The challenge for law and lawmakers is to understand this culture in order to create workable and credible laws. Amidst the COVID-19 and HIV pandemics, our viral times highlight both of these tensions and also the possibilities that queer theory and praxis present to them.

References

Andrejevic, M., 2002. The kinder, gentler gaze of Big Brother: Reality TV in the era of digital capitalism. *New Media and Society*, 4 (2), 251–270. 10.1177/1461444022226361

Ashford, C., 2015. Bareback sex, queer legal theory, and evolving socio-legal contexts. *Sexualities*, 18 (1/2), 195–209. 10.1177/1363460715569130

Ashford, C., and Longstaff, G., 2021. (Re)regulating gay sex in viral times: COVID-19 and the impersonal intimacy of the glory hole. *Culture, Health & Sexuality*, 23 (1) 1559–1572. 10.1080/13691058.2021.1930173

Ashford, C., Morris, M., and Powell, A., 2020. Bareback sex in the age of preventative medication: Rethinking the 'harms' of HIV transmission. *The Journal of Criminal Law*, 84 (6), 596–614. 10.1177/0022018320974904

Attwood, F., 2007. No money shot? Commerce, pornography and new taste sex cultures. *Sexualities*, 10 (4), 441–456. 10.1177/1363460707080982

Berg, H., 2021. Porn work, independent contractor misclassification, and the limits of the law. *Columbia Human Rights Law Review*, 52 (3), 1159–1198.

Bergman, Z.R., 2014. Testing solutions for adult film performers. *Cornell Journal of Law and Public Policy*, 24, 183–208.

Bersani, L., 2011. Shame on you. In J. Halley, and A. Parker, eds. *After sex? On writing since queer theory*. Durham: Duke University Press, 91–109.

Cohen, A.C., Tavrow, P., and McGrath, M.R., 2018. Advocacy coalition for safer sex in the adult film industry: The case of Los Angeles County's Measure B. *Health Prevention Practice*, 19 (3) 400–419. 10.1177/1524839917713942

Cook, M., 2014. *Queer domesticities: Homosexuality and home life in twentieth-century London*. Houndmills: Palgrave Macmillan.

Crimp, D., 2004. *Melancholia and moralism: Essays on AIDS and queer politics*. Cambridge: The MIT Press.

Dean, T., 2009. *Unlimited intimacy: Reflections on the subculture of barebacking*. Chicago: Chicago University Press.

Downs, C., 2020. OnlyFans, influencers, and the politics of selling nudes during a pandemic. *Elle*, May 14. www.elle.com/culture/a32459935/onlyfans-sex-work-influencers

Dowsett, G.W., 1996. *Practicing desire: Homosexual sex in the era of AIDS*. Stanford: Stanford University Press.

Ferris, S., 2017. Sex panic and videotape. *Hastings Women's Law Journal*, 28 (2), 203–224.

Florencio, J., 2020. *Bareback porn, porous masculinities, queer futures: The ethics of becoming-pig*. London: Routledge. 10.4324/9781351123426

Gonzalez, O., 2019. HIV pre-exposure prophylaxis (PrEP) 'The Truvada Whore', and the new gay sexual revolution. In R. Varghese, ed. *Raw: PrEP, pedagogy, and the politics of barebacking*. Regina: University of Regina Press, 27–48.

Junge, B., 2002. Bareback sex, risk, and eroticism: Anthropological themes (re) surfacing in the post-AIDS era. In E. Lewin, and W.L. Leap, eds. *Out in theory: The emergence of lesbian and gay anthropology*. Chicago: University of Illinois Press, 186–221.

Kagan, D., 2018. *Positive images: Gay men & HIV/AIDS in the culture of 'post-crisis'*. London: IB Tauris.

Klesse, C., 2007. *The spectre of promiscuity: Gay male and bisexual non-monogamies and polymories*. Aldershot: Ashgate.

Kristeva, J., 1980. *Powers of horror: An essay on abjection*. New York: Columbia University Press.

Longstaff, G., 2019. 'Bodies that splutter' – theorizing jouissance in bareback and chemsex porn. *Porn Studies*, 6 (1), 74–86. 10.1080/23268743.2018.1559090

Maine, A., 2022. Queering marriage: The homoradical and anti-normativity. *Laws*, 11 (1). 10.3390/laws11010001

McNamara, M., 2013. Cumming to terms: Bareback pornography, homonormativity, and queer survival in the time of HIV/AIDS. In B. Fahs, M. Dudy, and S. Stage, eds. *The moral panics of sexuality*. London: Palgrave Macmillan, 226–244.

Mercer, J., 2017. *Gay pornography: Representations of sexuality and masculinity*. London and New York: I.B Tauris.

Morris, M., 2021. The politics of testing positive: An autoethnography of media (mis) representations at the 'start' and 'end' of different pandemics. *Culture, Health & Sexuality*, 23 (11), 1485–1499. 10.1080/13691058.2021.1930172

Muñoz, J.E., 2009. *Cruising utopia: The then and there of queer futurity*. New York and London: New York University Press.

Rodriguez-Amat, J.R., and Belinskaya, Y., 2023. 'No coronavirus can leave us without sex': Relations of complicity and solidarity on Pornhub. *Porn Studies*, 10 (3), 233–251. 10.1080/23268743.2022.2085161

Sandset, T., 2021. *'Ending AIDS' in the age of biopharmaceuticals: The individual, the state and the politics of prevention*. Abingdon: Routledge.

Shaffer, K., 2015. That's a wrap: Exploring Los Angeles County's adult film condom requirement. *Brooklyn Law Review*, 80 (4), 1579–1610.

Shepard, J.M., 2018. The First Amendment and mandatory condom laws: Rethinking the porn exception in strict scrutiny. *Nevada Law Journal*, 19 (1), 85–134.

Stadler, J.P., 2021. Pornographic altruism, or, How to have porn in a pandemic. *Synoptique*, 9 (2), 201–216.

Tziallas, E., 2019. The return of the repressed: Visualizing sex without condoms. In R. Varghese, ed. *Raw: PrEP, pedagogy, and the politics of barebacking*. Regina: University of Regina Press, 117–141.

van der Nagel, E., 2021. Competing platform imaginaries of NSFW content creation on OnlyFans. *Porn Studies*, 8 (4), 394–410. 10.1080/23268743.2021.1974927

Varghese, R., 2019. *Raw: PrEP, pedagogy, and the politics of barebacking*. Regina: University of Regina Press.

Wagner, A., 2022. *Emergency state: How we lost our freedoms in the pandemic and why it matters*. London: The Bodley Head.

Wagner, K.P.G., and Jones, R.L., 2019. Imbalance between speech and health: How unsubstantiated health claims in secondary effects regulations of sexually oriented businesses threaten free speech. *First Amendment Law Review*, 17, 213–236.

Webber, V., 2015. Public health versus performer privates: Measure B's failure to fix subjects. *Porn Studies*, 2 (4), 299–313. 10.1080/23268743.2015.1053094

Williams, L., 1989. *Hardcore: Power, pleasure and the 'frenzy of the visible'*. Berkeley and Los Angeles: University of California Press.

Williams, L., 2004. Porn studies: Proliferating pornographies on/scene: An introduction. In L. Williams, ed. *Porn Studies*. Durham and London: Duke University Press, 1–25.

Wright, P.J., Herbenick, D., and Paul, B., 2022. Casual condomless sex, range of pornography exposure, and perceived pornography realism. *Communication Research*, 49 (4), 547–566. 10.1177/00936502211003765

4 Narratives of pandemic lives

Everyday experiences of the plague, HIV and COVID-19 in literary fiction

Deborah Lupton

Introduction

Epidemics and pandemics confront us with life-changing or life-destroying challenges, forcing us to face our own and our loved ones' state of health and well-being, consider our mortality and reflect on profound questions about life's meaning and purpose. When new pathogens and illnesses emerge, they become invested with meaning, as people struggle to make sense of what is happening, how they should respond and who should take responsibility for the outbreak. In doing so, they build on pre-established ideas about the body, health and well-being: many of which have been in existence since ancient times (Lupton 2012; Martin 2022). As scholars in medical sociology, anthropology, history and cultural studies have demonstrated, social and cultural practices and discourses are inextricable from the biological dimensions of infectious disease outbreaks (Sontag 1990; Mack 1991; Douglas 1992; Brandt and Rozin 1997; Wald 2008; Lupton 2012). Embodied sensations and affective forces combine with discourses and practices from medicine and popular culture in complex and dynamic assemblages of sense-making and preventive action. Moral meanings are integral to lay concepts of illness and disease. Certain social groups are identified as 'risky' or threatening, portrayed as the Other and requiring surveillance and disciplining, even social exclusion.

The bubonic plague (Black Death) was one of the most stigmatised and feared infectious diseases globally, with an infamous legacy of centuries of high death tolls and horrifying suffering following continual outbreaks in medieval and early modern times. Marginalised social groups such as Jews were regularly identified as the source of the infection and persecuted or cast out from communities (Glatter and Finkelman 2021; Martin 2022). The cultural impact of the plague can be discerned across Western literature and popular culture, used metaphorically to denote a curse, an unwelcome event or divine retribution (Sontag 1990). Late last century, the period following the identification of the first cases of what came to be named AIDS was characterised by a plethora of literature seeking to cast light upon the sociocultural and political dimensions of the pandemic (Watney 1987; Carter and Watney 1989; Brandt 1991; Douglas 1992; Lupton 1994; Treichler 1999).

DOI: 10.4324/9781003322788-5

Social and cultural theory was applied to understanding the rhetoric of blame, shame, stigma and marginalisation as well as the moral judgements and Othering that pervaded news and popular media portrayals of HIV and AIDS and those people who were categorised in 'at risk' groups or who became ill. These analyses pointed out the homophobia that pervaded these accounts, based on the early strong association of gay men with HIV risk, part of a long trajectory in Western culture of associating 'deviant' or 'unnatural' sexual practices with punishment by disease and death. Racist discourses built on a similar history spanning centuries of the Othering of people of colour as less-than-human and inhabiting locations filled with rampant infection.

In her book *Contagious: Cultures, Carriers, and the Outbreak Narrative* (Wald 2008), the historian Priscilla Wald uses the term 'outbreak narratives' to describe the imaginaries, characterisation, figurative language, discourses and storylines that have featured in recent popular cultural portrayals of epidemics and pandemics. Wald identifies some key features in the outbreak narratives she describes, which include discussion of films, news stories, popular science books, genre fiction and literary fiction. These features include tropes of racism in representations of viruses emerging in African countries; victim-blaming of people who were presented as carriers of contagion or as not properly protecting themselves from infection; and the heroicising of expert figures such as virologists and epidemiologists as part of the mythic struggle of the human against the microbe. Other scholars have employed the term 'pandemic narratives' to encapsulate the forms of storytelling that have appeared in public and private accounts of major infectious disease outbreaks such as the 'swine flu' (H1N1) pandemic of 2009 (Davis and Lohm 2020) and the 2014 Ebola outbreak (Gerlach 2016). Recent analyses have begun to identify outbreak or pandemic narratives in popular cultural portrayals of the COVID-19 crisis (for example, Alexander and Smith 2020; Pascual Soler 2021; Pietrzak-Franger et al. 2022).

In this chapter, I build on these previous analyses of the cultural meanings of outbreak and pandemic narratives, presenting a cultural sociological analysis of works of literary fiction that describe people's experiences of infectious disease outbreaks: or what I term, 'narratives of pandemic lives'. Cultural sociology brings together studies of the shared meanings, symbols, categories, discourses, norms and values expressed in popular culture with a sociological interest in the broader social structures, social group membership, human relationships, belief systems and practices in which popular culture is produced and consumed (Spillman 2020). Literary fiction is one meaning-making medium that has received attention in cultural sociology analyses. When we are engrossed in reading literary fiction, we can learn not only about ourselves but also about how others think and feel. Novels can also stand as detailed accounts of what life was like during a momentous historical event, such as a pandemic. Literary fiction writers lyrically portray the depth of human experience: its materialities, its sensory and affective forces, its everyday contradictions and powerful motivations for action and reflection. From a cultural sociology perspective, analysis of literary fiction involves 'theorising the social' by exploring how these media portray social life, identities and structures with the use of aesthetic devices such as figurative language, narrative, theme and characterisation (Váňa 2020).

In what follows, I describe and compare the outbreak narratives and imaginaries that have been presented in selected works of literary fiction from the fourteenth century onwards, focusing on portrayals of the plague, HIV and COVID-19. I adopt a cultural sociology perspective in addressing the question of what we can learn about pandemic lives through these narratives. The discussion begins with *The Decameron* (Giovanni Boccaccio), *A Journal of the Plague Year* (Daniel Defoe) and *The Plague* (Albert Camus) and moves onto HIV narratives featuring in *The Line of Beauty* (Alan Hollinghurst) and *The Great Believers* (Sarah Makkai). The newly emerging body of literary fiction that has been published on COVID-19 is then analysed, focusing on four books that were among the first to be released: *The Fell* (Sarah Moss), *Life Without Children* (Roddy Doyle), *French Braid* (Anne Tyler) and *Our Country Friends* (Gary Shteyngart). The resonances and differences in the COVID-19 narratives with previous pandemic fiction are identified, as are the insights offered across this body of literature into human relationships and social responses to major infectious disease outbreaks.

Pandemic fiction prior to COVID-19: The plague and HIV

One of the best-known and influential fictional accounts of the mediaeval plague outbreaks is *The Decameron*, a collection of 100 short stories penned in the mid-fourteenth century by writer and poet Giovanni Boccaccio and published in English translation in 1620. The stories are presented as tales recounted to each other by a group of seven young women and three young men who are sheltering in an isolated villa outside Florence while the Black Death, which swept through Europe in 1348–9, rages in that city. The book's title translates to 'ten days': the period during which the tales are shared between the protagonists as a way of passing the time while they wait out the plague.

The Decameron collection is not only a major contribution to early Italian fiction, but also a valuable insight into what life was like for people living through the plague during this era. The book also offers a trenchant political critique, with the stories drawing attention to the moral degradation and loss of community occurring in the face of the epidemic. In his opening words, Boccaccio refers to the plague as either 'the action of heavenly bodies' or 'visited upon us mortals for our correction by the righteous anger of God'. He describes the signs of the pestilence – swellings developing into dark blotches on the skin, followed within three days by death. Boccaccio goes on to describe the actions of the citizens of Florence: closeting themselves in groups within their houses or the wealthy departing for their country estates, while the 'stench of corpses' filled the air in the city streets, with sick people left to fend for themselves.

English author Daniel Defoe's *A Journal of the Plague Year*, first published in 1722, is an account of living through the Great Plague in London in 1665. Categorised as historical fiction, the book is presented as an eyewitness account of the bubonic plague outbreak that decimated the city. Defoe presents the narrator as 'a citizen who continued all the while in London', according to the novel's title page. The affective and material dimensions of pandemic lives are compellingly described in this detailed narrative of 'the plague year'. Like Boccaccio, Defoe provides vivid descriptions of the lethal disease as it spreads throughout the city, and the accompanying distress and fear that pervades its residents. As the narrator remarks, the streets are empty, businesses are shuttered, and wealthy people have fled the city for the country. 'Sorrow and Sadness sat upon every Face' and 'London might well be said to be all in Tears' [sic] as the deaths mount for the unfortunate people left behind.

The novel details the measures put in place by the city authorities to contain the spread. Defoe describes the orders that heads of households must notify the authorities as soon as plague symptoms were noticed in any household member. Houses with infected residents inside were shut for at least one month, marked with a red cross on the front door and the words 'Lord have mercy on us'. Guards were posted to ensure that no-one could enter or leave. The dead were buried unceremoniously as soon as possible in crowded pits. The narrator observes that 'This shutting up of houses was at first counted a very cruel and Unchristian method, and the poor People so confin'd made bitter Lamentations' [sic].

A more contemporary account of an epidemic, Albert Camus' novel *The Plague* (*La Peste* in the original French) published in 1947 in the wake of World War II, offers equally dramatic storytelling. Written in an absurdist style with Camus' signature existentialist philosophical perspective framing the narrative, *The Plague* portrays humans as powerless in the face of their destinies. The novel is set in Oran, a French Algerian city in which a serious infectious disease (referred to only as 'the plague') is quickly spreading. In the novel, epidemic disease is a motif by which Camus demonstrates the human condition as subsumed to the force of nature. For example, one of the main characters in *The Plague*, Dr Bernard Rieux, a physician, attempts to warn authorities of the danger of the pestilence spreading, and that action should be taken immediately by health authorities to contain the outbreak. His words are initially unheeded, and he feels helpless to relieve the human suffering and death he sees around him. Another character, Father Paneloux, places his trust in God to save him, but perishes anyway.

In *The Plague*, there are many descriptions of the horror, panic and desperation felt by citizens of Oran as their city is locked down, with disease rapidly overwhelming them. Nonetheless, Camus' novel acknowledges that humankind can demonstrate admirable qualities such as kindness, compassion, courage, connection and concern for each other in the face of great suffering. It is these everyday acts of care and, as Dr Rieux puts it, 'common decency' rather than 'heroism' that are celebrated in *The Plague*, with the meaning and community found in such acts challenging the nihilism that can pervade existentialist thought. As Camus writes: 'What's true of all the evils in the world is true of plague as well. It helps men to rise above themselves'.

The rhetorical relationship between plague and AIDS narratives was established early in that pandemic. For example, in her essay 'AIDS and its metaphors', Susan Sontag (1990) drew attention to the common discursive manoeuvre of comparing AIDS with the plague. As she pointed out, given the history of the horror and fear incited by the plague, when used as a metaphor, this disease evokes the worst calamity or evil that can befall humans. The close association of plague outbreaks throughout history with God's punishment for human wickedness brought with it these longstanding meanings when societies were making sense of the new lethal contagion that was HIV infection.

One of the best-known novels centring on the early years of the HIV pandemic is British author Alan Hollinghurst's *The Line of Beauty* (2004). The book is both an elegy to the carefree hedonism of the mid-1980s for young gay men such as Nick and a disquisition on the morality of power and privilege as well as the fleeting nature of such attributes. It presents a cool yet scathing critique of the preoccupations of hedonistic seeking after beauty while forsaking loyalty and true intimacy. This work presents a tale of the life of Nick Guest, a naïve young gay white man living a sybaritic existence in London during an era characterised both by hedonism and Thatcherite individualism. As the book's title suggests, Nick is beguiled by beauty: including that of other young men. Much of the narrative and characterisation, which span the years 1983 to 1987, is concerned with aesthetic considerations, but in the background is the growing impact of the HIV epidemic among the gay community.

At the beginning of the novel, Nick enjoys the pleasures offered him in London: sex with other men, connections with the wealthy, glamorous parties, cocaine use, fine dining and grand houses in the city and the country. As the decade wends on, however, Nick's life begins to sour. By the book's end, he must confront the reality of the homophobia of the privileged class he has idolised and the effects of HIV infection on previously beautiful and healthy young men such as himself. There are subtle references throughout the novel of the growing threat of HIV infection (for example, men with illnesses they can't seem to 'shake off'). AIDS is finally mentioned by name around two-thirds into the book, referred to a few pages later as 'this bloody plague' by Nick's straight friend Toby, but also with repugnance by friends of Toby's parents as something that 'the homosexuals' had 'brought on' themselves, and 'had coming to them'. By 1987, the young men Nick knows in the gay London community are wasting away, and the death toll is mounting. A former lover, Leo, has already perished from AIDS: glimpsed by Nick in a bar months before his death, described with pathos as reduced to a 'little woolly-hatted figure'. The wealthy and glamorous Wani, his current lover, is dying. In the book's final pages, Nick is about to take a test to determine whether he too has contracted HIV. While he had previously cast aside any concerns, 'It came over him that the test result would be positive'. Nick suddenly feels physically and emotionally vulnerable as he realises how shallow his lifestyle and relationships have been.

Rebecca Makkai's novel *The Great Believers*, published in 2018, is similarly a work of social realism but provides a much more direct and detailed reflection on the early years of the HIV pandemic from the perspective of several decades on. The novel's themes repeatedly highlight not only the long-lasting devastation and grief wrought by the combined effects of HIV and the related Othering of gay men but also the impacts on the gay community of the politics surrounding the US government's neglect of HIV. Like Hollinghurst's book, Makkai's novel depicts a sense of a fin de siècle: the loss of 'golden age', as one of Makkai's characters puts it, that gay men briefly enjoyed before the horror of HIV struck. The novel opens with the 1985 wake in Chicago for a young gay man, Nico, who has died from AIDS. Nico's younger sister Fiona and Yale, Nico's close friend and fellow member of the Chicago gay community, are confronting their grief at Nico's death and the devastation they see around them.

The novel jumps back and forth between the period spanning 1985 to 1992 (told from Yale's perspective) and 30 years later, when Fiona travels to Paris. She stays with Richard, an old friend but now a famous photographer who documented the AIDS crisis as it was unfolding in Chicago in those early years. The scenes set in earlier times vividly describe Yale's experiences of seeing his partners and friends fall sick and die around him. There are also many descriptions of the support offered by the gay community and their activist efforts, including Yale's participation in an ACT UP protest. There are references throughout the book to the horrifying numbers of gay men from that community who were lost to HIV-related disease during this time. As Yale describes it, he kept a mental list of 'acquaintances already sick, hiding the lesions on their arms but not their faces, coughing horribly, growing thin, waiting to get worse'. In 2015, Fiona is looking at Richard's memorabilia of the time: his photos, obituaries about friends he has kept. She thinks about how the city of Chicago 'was a graveyard' and that people living there today 'were walking every day through streets where there had been a holocaust, a mass murder of neglect and antipathy'.

These works of fiction about the plague and HIV span six centuries: from medieval times to the present day. Across the outbreak narratives presented, there are familiar themes and tropes: heightened fear when contagion strikes, the visual horror of the diseases as they attacked people's bodies, moral judgement and the stigmatising of marginalised out-groups, the lack of decisive action by government and health authorities, and the tendency for humans to cast aside their care for others in their desire to flee the danger. The goodness of at least some people in the midst of this chaos also shines through in these accounts, however. The importance of banding together for companionship and support and the need for communal action against infection is highlighted.

COVID-19 fiction

The rapidly growing number of cases of new cases caused the World Health Organization to declare COVID-19 a pandemic on 11 March 2020. At this point in the outbreak, many governments were beginning to implement measures to 'slow the spread' of the disease: testing, contact tracing and quarantine requirements and publicising hygiene measures such as hand-washing and physical distancing. In some countries, lockdowns were activated, severely restricting people's movement outside their homes. Schools, universities and businesses were closed and most people (apart from 'essential workers') were either laid off or began to work from home (Lupton 2022). By the following year, a slew of novels and short story collections had begun to appear that presented people's experiences of coming to terms with both the disease and the ramifications of public health measures they were required to follow.

One of the first novels to be released, *The Fell*, by British author Sarah Moss, is written from the perspective of four neighbours living in a village in England's Peak District over the timespan of a single night in the winter of 2020. *The Fell* presents a dark, claustrophobic portrayal of these characters' lives during the pandemic. Presented as a stream-of-consciousness in the present tense, Moss charts their experiences and reflections on life as they struggle with boredom, loss of employment, having to work and learn from home and feelings of isolation and confinement. Two of the protagonists are Kate, a middle-aged woman and Matt, her teenage son. They have been unable to leave their house for the past ten days after being required to go into quarantine following Kate's exposure to a COVID-19 case at work.

To escape the overwhelming feelings of despair and being trapped, Kate decides to take a late-night walk on the nearby fell, all the time worrying about being 'caught' for the transgression of leaving her home and the moral judgement she would receive from the community should this happen. She remembers how police were 'hunting people off the hills with drones a few months ago … playing loud accusations at them from the sky. Go home, you are breaking the law'. Alice, Kate's elderly neighbour who lives alone, reflects on the impacts of having to maintain a physical distance from other people, 'acting as if everyone's unclean and dangerous, though the problem of course is that they are, or at least some of them are and there's no way of knowing'. Consequently, 'No one's touched her in months', and Alice wonders if she ever will be touched again. These characters care about and watch over each other as best they can. None of them has had COVID-19, but each is struggling with how to cope with the effects of the social and economic disruptions the pandemic has wrought, including to their relationships with their neighbours, friends and family.

Irish writer Roddy Doyle's collection of ten short stories, *Life Without Children*, has a similar tone: desolate, with glimpses of humour and acknowledgement of the importance of the relational connections between people who know each other well. The primary characters in his stories, set in Dublin, are nearly all middle-aged or older men who are going through their days either in quiet desperation, or in some cases, with outbursts of anger, as they attempt to come to terms with COVID-19 and lockdown. As one man remarks (in the story entitled 'Masks'), 'The lockdown has ripped away the padding. There's no schedule, no job, no commute'. Some of the stories also feature stark descriptions of COVID-19 illness and death. For example, in the story entitled 'Nurse', a young female healthcare worker arrives home to her empty apartment and contemplates the deaths of two COVID-19 patients, Joe and Marie, she has seen that day. She thinks about how she held a computer tablet to Joe's face so that his wife could say goodbye, distanced from his deathbed by COVID-19 rules. She remembers how she helped prepare the bodies as they were washed and placed in two body bags, and the distinctive sound of the body bag as it is zipped up: 'it's the last thing she'll hear when she closes her eyes. When she goes to bed'.

The male characters in Doyle's stories have lost their jobs, their sense of community and the opportunity to spend time with others in places such as pubs and the workplace. The relationships the men have with their partners are strained, as each person attempts to cope with feelings of loss; particularly their sense of purpose in life. However, there is hope too in Doyle's stories, to counter the despair. Some stories present positive moments of renewed connection and intimacy of men with their wives and adult children, as they share the experience of listening to a favourite song, reminisce about their lives together or exchange loving words.

The two novels by authors based in the USA considered here adopt a rather different approach. The tone of their depictions of pandemic life is less dark than that offered in the books by Moss and Doyle: perhaps because neither features the kinds of state-imposed extended lockdowns endured by people living in the UK and Ireland. The latest novel by Anne Tyler, who has had a long and successful career writing about the everyday lives of Americans living mostly in the city of Baltimore, includes references to COVID-19 in its final chapters. *French Braid*, her 24th novel, presents a history of the Garrett family that spans six decades: white, middle-class parents Robin and Mercy and their children Alice, Lily and David. The novel's final chapter is set in 2020, when COVID-19 has just begun to affect parts of the USA. David, now aged in his late 60s, agrees that his son Nicholas and five-year-old grandson Benny should come for an extended stay to his home while Benny's mother continues to work in New York City: she is a hospital physician and therefore on the COVID-19 frontline.

Consonant with Tyler's quiet, highly observant writing style, the family's experiences of COVID-19 are presented in a matter-of-fact way. Tyler depicts small, telling details of COVID-19 life: the fears and frustrations but mostly the pleasures of bunkering down and forming closer family relationships. David has recently retired from his high school teaching job, finding online instruction difficult: 'It turned out he wasn't much good at Zoom'. He discusses with his wife Greta how strange it feels to stay home ('sheltering in place') when prior to the pandemic they took their freedom of movement so much for granted. Yet it was 'shockingly easy' and 'a relief' for David and Greta to give up their social life, while they eagerly embrace the chance to spend more time with their son and grandson. The final lines of the book describe a poignant moment soon after Nicholas and Benny return home to New York City. David finds one of Benny's fabric face masks, worn to protect himself against COVID-19 on outings. Still missing his grandson's presence intensely, he presses the mask to his face to inhale the 'trace of Benny's little-boy scent, salty but clean'.

Our Country Friends, a tragicomic novel by Gary Shteyngart, offers yet another perspective on pandemic lives. Shteyngart's writing style is satirical, the characters bordering on caricatures. There are echoes of *The Decameron* but also Chekhov's writings in his wry account of a group of privileged, self-preoccupied middle-aged people of varied ethnic/racial backgrounds coming together in a remote rural location at the beginning of the pandemic. Five guests are hosted by Russian Americans Alexander Senderovsky, a writer, and his wife Masha Levin-Senderovsky, a psychiatrist, owners of a country estate ('the colony') with several guest houses. The guests are Ed Kim, Karen Cho, Vinod Mehta, Dee Cameron (her name is a direct reference to Boccaccio's novel) and 'the Actor'. As COVID-19 rages in nearby New York City, the group wait it out in the idyllic spring and summer surroundings. If they express worries, these concern their relationships with each other, questions of social status or their finances, with the occasional pang of guilt about the glory of their isolation.

There are references throughout the novel to horrific news stories of disease and death in New York City, but for most of this period, life in the colony is little changed: 'People were dying in the city. Some more than others. The virus had roamed the earth but had chosen to settle down there'. As the plot unfolds, the protagonists become aware of media coverage of the Black Lives Matter protests and clashes between activists and the police, but much of these political tensions remain remote. Gradually, however, the pandemic and its impacts creep closer. As the weeks progress, the virus spreads to different regions of the USA: 'The corpses were stacking up in other parts of the country'. The virus eventually enters the colony, with three guests becoming infected. One of them becomes seriously ill and dies at the end of the book. Summer has ended, and with it, the brief sense of blissful isolation that the colony's residents had enjoyed.

In these COVID-19 narratives, a common tone is that of despair and disquiet at the early months of the crisis unfold and people struggle to come to terms with the sudden changes in their quotidian routines. The narratives also vividly recount the socio-spatialities of COVID living: the feelings of suffocation but also safety and comfort felt by some people during quarantine and lockdown, the attempts to find ways to fill the long hours, the negotiation of living arrangements and relationships with others sharing domestic or neighbourhood spaces, the need for physical contact at a time when touching others or even standing too close to them is potentially deadly. Across these works of COVID-19 fiction, there is evidence too of major differences in experience: people's gender, age, socioeconomic status, living arrangements, connections to others and physical location all play a role in how badly affected they are by the local conditions of this global crisis.

Discussion

Beginning from early fictional accounts of deadly infectious disease outbreaks, narratives of pandemic lives have offered us descriptions of how disease manifests in the human body and the public health measures undertaken to contain its spread, together with critical reflections on societal responses. These stories operate as cautionary tales, holding humanity to account in seeking to find some meaning and make sense of both infectious disease outbreaks and societal responses to them. Across the narratives they contain, certain broad themes are repeated: the difficulty of individuals and communities in coming to terms with a deadly pandemic; the changes in everyday life and concepts of risk and safety as people respond to the threat; the moral judgements made about people's behaviour; the ways that the shallowness or depths of interpersonal connections are exposed by deadly viruses; and the social and political contexts in which medical and public health responses are developed and implemented (or abandoned).

Beliefs about the vicissitudes of fate and the threat of God's punishment for human transgressions were central to portrayals of infectious diseases in early fiction: they linger still in contemporary pandemic narratives. As Camus' novel shows, even in the mid-twentieth century, by which time the role of pathogens as the cause of epidemics was well understood, literary fiction still featured philosophical disquisitions concerning broader issues such as humanity's control over life in the face of fate. Written in a more secular age, novels about the early years of the HIV pandemic portray narratives of the effects of disease, death, loss and grief, principally among gay men. Themes of homophobic stigmatisation, moral judgement and blame are prominent in this fiction. Together with these descriptions are critical depictions of the broader sociocultural and political contexts of the HIV pandemic. So too are narratives identifying and questioning the socio-economic effects of the neoliberalist systems of government that were emerging in the Global North in this period. While the gay community and its allies came together to agitate for action and challenge their marginalised status, the dominant discourse that people were self-made individuals who should take responsibility for their health and well-being was intensifying in these political currents.

What is most noticeable across the COVID-19 narratives is the combination of mundanity and boredom with dread, loneliness and isolation. Scenes of extreme illness, dying and death are hinted at rather than explicitly described. Characters are often portrayed as (at least initially) repudiating the threat of disease as personally affecting them. Unlike the lurid imagery of the plague novels, in the contemporary pandemic narratives the death and dying are not piled up in the streets, smelling to high heaven; houses are not marked with red paint, boarded up and guarded. Death and dying are hidden largely from sight in private homes or hospitals, reflecting a tendency more generally in the Global North to deny the visceral realities of such experiences. Yet the invisibility of COVID-19 risk offers its own fears and dilemmas, as any person could be infected and must be avoided. Both the value and threat of human touch are therefore intensified.

While COVID-19 has been a universal experience globally, the sociocultural, economic and political contexts in which people have experienced the pandemic have differed wildly (Lupton 2022). These differences are evident in the COVID fiction. In *The Fell* and *Life Without Children*, feelings of confinement and being trapped, losing identity and a sense of purpose in life are particularly dominant. The space of the home is a refuge from the world outside that is rife with invisible pathogens. However, this domestic space is also described as a place of entrapment, intensifying despair, depression and anxiety, making people feel crowded together if they are sharing the house with others from whom they cannot easily escape, or else as a place of severe loneliness. In *Our Country Friends*, the protagonists have more freedom, being able to live in their own domiciles as part of the colony and come together to eat and socialise. The family in *French Braid* finds pleasure and comfort in living closer together and sharing the stresses of the pandemic. These four works of COVID-19 fiction share similarities with the tone of the plague novels in recounting in realist and sometime absurdist terms the details of life in quarantine or lockdown. These include descriptions of almost magical thinking about how best to protect oneself against risk together with panicked apocalyptic visions and expectations that life will never be the same, combined with accounts of the importance of the small mercies that can emerge during these dark days.

While there are shared motifs, COVID-19 novels differ from HIV fiction in obvious ways. The HIV narratives centred around the upheavals to gay men's lives, their loss of newfound freedoms, the renewed stigma and pathologising of male-to-male sexuality that occurred in the wake of that pandemic. Feelings of difference, of being Othered, and the trauma and pain of losing loved one, as well as the fear of the same fate, were integral in the HIV fiction. In these novels – particularly *The Great Believers* – the sense of solidarity and community felt by gay men is often described: often in the face of shunning and shaming by members of their families and society in general. By contrast, as depicted in the COVID-19 fiction (and similar to the plague narratives), the COVID-19 pandemic and associated preventive measures affected people in every walk of life. As public health messages put it in the first year of the pandemic, 'everyone needs to play their part' to contain the spread. This message was often accompanied by disciplinary and moralising practices. In some countries, overt surveillance by authorities and consequences such as fines were implemented for those who were considered to break the rules. News and social media made reference to 'Covidiots', who were shamed for selfish behaviour such as not adhering to quarantine, failing to wear masks or distance themselves appropriately from others (Lupton 2022). Resonances of these messages were evident in the COVID novels, when characters expressed their struggles with ensuring that they engaged in the recommended preventive practices, their fear of going out in public and their concerns about others not behaving in appropriately 'safe' ways or being themselves disciplined or condemned for failing to follow the rules. While there are descriptions of feelings of grief and loss, these are mostly in relation to the loss of 'normal' life and the loneliness and fear – indeed anomie – experienced by people who are living through stay-at-home restrictions.

At the heart of each of these literary works, regardless of the pathogens and diseases that are portrayed, is the question of how to live with others in intimate relationships and the domestic space, when the outside world is fraught with danger and policed by both official and vernacular surveillance and censure. Across all the books, the nature of intimacy and how best to negotiate personal relationships in times of crisis involving separation from most other people but also close confinement with friends or family members are examined. The small details of quotidian life are held up to examination as the conditions of the health crisis probe for weaknesses – but also uncover strengths that may not have been anticipated.

Concluding comments

Across all these works of pandemic fiction, intense feelings of grief, loss and fear are evident. Indeed, the sheer covertness of disease spread – its invisibility and the need to treat others are potentially infected and to distance one's body from theirs – is part of the dread and shock that characters in these narratives endure. Fragmentation of community ties and family relationships are also highlighted. But so too are the 'small acts as kindness' (in Tyler's words) offered by family members, neighbours and friends that signal the 'common decency' described by Camus and provide comfort and connection in terrifying times. While we have the benefit of hindsight in knowing what the long-lasting effects of the plague and the HIV pandemic have been, we are still in the initial stages of the COVID-19 pandemic, with little knowledge of what future developments await us.

The conditions of COVID-19 life, even in the few years of the pandemic endured thus far, have been volatile. COVID-19 experiences have been extremely variable across the world as well as within nations, with people living with socioeconomic disadvantage suffering far more than those who are affluent from the health and economic impacts of the crisis (McGowan and Bambra 2022). SARS-CoV-2, we have learned, is dynamic and shape-shifting. Medicine and public health policy have floundered to keep up. A growing body of literature evaluating the effectiveness of governments' and public health authorities' COVID-19 responses across the years of the crisis has pointed to the significant failures in many nations (including the USA, Ireland and the UK) in allowing the virus to spread unchecked, instituting restrictive measures too late or loosening them too early, inefficiently implementing COVID-19 vaccination programmes, or not providing enough accurate information to the public about the long-term effects of COVID-19 infection for survivors (The Independent Panel for Pandemic Preparedness & Response 2021; Sachs et al. 2022).

The COVID-19 narratives discussed here articulate experiences during the early phase of the pandemic, when people across the world were coming to terms with what this new virus and disease meant for their lives, still shocked by the realities of a novel threat emerging apparently from nowhere and the restrictions that were brought in by governments to contain it. Readers are both reminded of how they might have felt during the early months of COVID-19 and offered glimpses into how others did so, in different socioeconomic and geographical settings. What all these fictional accounts of pandemic lives present is the sense of the world as we know it as changing, perhaps forever. It is inevitable that as the pandemic progresses, a new tranche of COVID-19 fiction will emerge to document these uncertain lives. While it is important to acknowledge the skill of the accomplished writers who have crafted these narratives, these works can only cast light on the experiences and feelings of relatively privileged protagonists in corners of a handful of nations in the Global North. Literary fiction that portrays the thoughts, feelings and experiences of those who are less privileged, living in countries other than the UK, USA and Ireland – and especially the nations of the Global South – would add further important insights into the diversity and situated contexts of pandemic lives across the world.

Works of fiction (in order of mention)

Boccaccio, G., 1998. *The Decameron*. Trans. G. Waldman. Edited and with an introduction and notes by Jonathan Usher. Oxford: Oxford University Press.

Defoe, D., 1886. *A Journal of the Plague Year*. 2nd ed. London: George Routledge and Sons.

Camus, A., 2002. *The Plague*. Trans. R. Buss. London: Penguin.

Hollinghurst, A., 2004. *The Line of Beauty*. London: Picador.

Makkai, R., 2018. *The Great Believers*. London: Fleet.

Moss, S., 2021. *The Fell*. London: Picador.

Doyle, R., 2021. *Life Without Children*. London: Vintage.

Tyler, A., 2022. *French Braid*. London: Vintage.

Shteyngart, G., 2021. *Our Country Friends*. New York: Random House.

References

Alexander, J.C. and Smith, P., 2020. COVID-19 and symbolic action: Global pandemic as code, narrative, and cultural performance. *American Journal of Cultural Sociology*, 8 (3), 263–269. 10.1057/s41290-020-00123-w

Brandt, A., 1991. AIDS and metaphor: Toward the social meaning of epidemic disease. In A. Mack, ed. *In time of plague: The history and social consequences of lethal epidemic disease*. New York: New York University Press, 91–110.

Brandt, A. and Rozin, P., 1997. Introduction. In A. Brandt and P. Rozin, eds. *Morality and health*. New York: Routledge, 1–11.

Carter, E. and Watney, S., 1989. *Taking liberties: AIDS and cultural politics*. London: Serpent's Tail.

Davis, M.D. and Lohm, D., 2020. *Pandemics, publics, and narrative*. Oxford: Oxford University Press.

Douglas, M., 1992. *Risk and blame: Essays in cultural theory*. London: Routledge.

Gerlach, N.A., 2016. From outbreak to pandemic narrative: Reading newspaper coverage of the 2014 Ebola epidemic. *Canadian Journal of Communication*, 41 (4), 611–630. 10.22230/cjc.2016v41n4a3098

Glatter, K.A. and Finkelman, P., 2021. History of the plague: An ancient pandemic for the age of COVID-19. *The American Journal of Medicine*, 134 (2), 176–181. 10.1016/j.amjmed.2020.08.019

Lupton, D., 1994. *Moral threats and dangerous desires: AIDS in the news media*. London: Taylor & Francis.

Lupton, D., 2012. *Medicine as culture: Illness, disease and the body*. London: SAGE.

Lupton, D., 2022. *COVID societies: Theorising the coronavirus crisis*. Abingdon: Routledge.

Mack, A., 1991. *In time of plague: The history and social consequences of lethal epidemic disease*. New York: NYU Press.

Martin, S., 2022. *A short history of disease: Plagues, poxes and civilizations*. Harpenden: Oldcastle Books.

McGowan, V.J. and Bambra, C., 2022. COVID-19 mortality and deprivation: Pandemic, syndemic, and endemic health inequalities. *The Lancet Public Health*, 7. 10.1016/S2468-2667(22)00223-7

Pascual Soler, N., 2021. Repetition and recognition in YouTube narratives of COVID-19 survival. *Prose Studies*, 42 (1), 68–84. 10.1080/01440357.2021.1995293

Pietrzak-Franger, M., Lange, A. and Söregi, R., 2022. Narrating the pandemic: COVID-19, China and blame allocation strategies in Western European popular press. *European Journal of Cultural Studies*, 25 (5), 1286–1306. 10.1177/13675494221077291

Sachs, J.D., et al., 2022. The Lancet Commission on lessons for the future from the COVID-19 pandemic. *The Lancet*, 400 (10359), 1224–1280. 10.1016/S0140-6736(22)01585-9

Sontag, S., 1990. *Illness as metaphor and AIDS and its metaphors*. New York: Anchor Books.

Spillman, L., 2020. *What is cultural sociology?* Cambridge: Polity.

The Independent Panel for Pandemic Preparedness & Response. 2021. *COVID-19: Make it the last pandemic*. Available from: https://theindependentpanel.org/wp-content/uploads/2021/05/COVID-19-Make-it-the-Last-Pandemic_final.pdf [Accessed 23 December 2022].

Treichler, P.A., 1999. *How to have theory in an epidemic: Cultural chronicles of AIDS*. Durham, NC: Duke University Press.

Váňa, J., 2020. Theorizing the social through literary fiction: for a new sociology of literature. *Cultural Sociology*, 14 (2), 180–200. 10.1177/1749975520922469

Wald, P., 2008. *Contagious: Cultures, carriers, and the outbreak narrative*. Durham, NC: Duke University Press.

Watney, S., 1987. *Policing desire: Pornography, AIDS and the media*. Minneapolis: University of Minnesota Press.

5 The politics of epidemics

From the local to the global

Dennis Altman

Carmel Bird has written that 'the term "pandemic", sinister as it is, carries echoes of pandemonium – a word invented by John Milton and used in Paradise Lost as the name of the capital of Hell' (Bird 2022, p. 14). The history of every epidemic is a combination of millions of personal stories and larger macro shifts in the political, social and cultural environment, so that to fully grasp their impact one needs creative writers and anthropologists as much as experts in public health and immunology. To write about two ongoing epidemics can be only an incomplete attempt to capture some aspects of the moment. But to view COVID-19 through the lens of our experiences of the HIV epidemic is to recognise how imperfectly governments have grasped the implications of pandemic diseases for national and global security. Sadly, there are many more examples of government failures to meet the challenges of the two epidemics than there are of successes.

My story

I know no-one well who died from COVID-19; in the terrible period between the early 1980s and 1996, when antiretrovirals appeared, death seemed everywhere. When I wrote a memoir (*Unrequited Love: Diary of an Accidental Activist*, Altman 2019), I remember pondering whose deaths would I choose to write about, as parts of my earlier life seemed to have been hollowed out by the AIDS epidemic. I lived in Paris for most of 1979: literally no-one I knew well there has survived.

My own loss from COVID-19 has been of a different order and involved the collapse of an intercontinental romance. Had the epidemic not happened we would have been together at a conference in Honolulu, marking two years since we first met at a similar conference in San Francisco. We'd stayed close ever since, and spent 18 weeks together, in the USA, in Melbourne and, most romantically, on a cruise up the coast of Norway. For the first time since we met, we could no longer make plans to see each other again, and Australia then closed its borders for almost two years.

For Juan Carlos, who teaches at a university in Ecuador, the epidemic meant enforced isolation and a massive workload as he struggled with an inadequate

DOI: 10.4324/9781003322788-6

laptop and students who don't always have good Internet access. I'm semi-retired and work from home: 'So what', Juan Carlos asked, 'is different for you?'

The difference, it turned out, was the end of the affair. Long-distance romances are kept alive by anticipation, they die when there is no realistic prospect for meeting again. Ours was a melancholic, not a tragic separation. It does not compare with the awful, enforced separations that terror, war, expatriation and incarceration forced on millions of people, separations that will only be intensified by COVID-inspired lockdowns. After all, as a wise friend pointed out, ours had been a virtual relationship for most of the previous two years.

Global lockdowns have disrupted relationships in all sorts of ways, either forcing people apart or ironically forcing them too much together. There are reports of Coronavirus divorces, pregnancies, break-ups and new romances. Marilyn Monroe allegedly said that 'It's better to be unhappy alone than to be unhappy with someone else', and the epidemic has tested this in unpredictable ways. Domestic violence reached new levels and in most countries support services have reached saturation point.

What COVID-19 came to signify for me was that there was no fixed point where the virtual might become real. The epidemic has upset our very notion of the future. As I write this, gay men are queuing for vaccines against mpox, in images that bring back the dark days of the 1980s.

Forty years ago

There was a similar feeling in those first decades after AIDS – briefly termed Gay Related Immune Deficiency Syndrome – first appeared. Those who were most affected, and those who were associated with the disease – men with haemophilia, homosexual men, sex workers, people who share needles – also felt the loss of faith in a predictable future. After combination therapies arrived, we heard stories of men who were destitute, having spent all their resources on the assumption they were about to die. Despite extraordinary efforts in the early part of this century by groups such as the Global Fund to Fight AIDS, Tuberculosis and Malaria to make treatments more readily available, HIV is by no means a manageable condition for most people who will be infected in poorer parts of the world.

It is an illusion to think that we are living in what someone once termed a post-AIDS world. A colleague recently wrote of the death of a friend in Indonesia who was cared for by his family. But as Beau wrote:

> It's confronting to see firsthand that young people are still passing away from AIDS, it's another thing entirely to know that so many of them are still dying ostracised from their loved ones. Their last moments in hospital wards far from the places they were born. Their last human touch from a nurse with hands covered by two pairs of gloves 'just in case'.
>
> (Newham 2022)

The stories we heard in Western cities in the 1980s are replicated as we write in cities across the world.

There are echoes of those stories in accounts of patients dying from COVID-19 in isolation, cut off from visitors, and in some countries, such as Brazil and South Africa which have experienced major death rates from both, there are real resonances. But while there are apparent similarities, the impact of the two epidemics has been very different. The global death toll from AIDS has been far higher, but COVID-19 has caused far greater disruption to global society. Unlike AIDS it has been universal in its impact, affecting both rich and poor countries, even though its impact has exacerbated already existing global inequities.

For those of us living in countries such as Japan, Australia and New Zealand, the personal impact has been very different. COVID-19 created a national emergency, whereas HIV created a disaster for specific and largely marginalised groups. In many cases, this has increased stigma and discrimination, as AIDS was identified as 'a gay disease'. Elsewhere, initial scapegoating gave way to a far greater acceptance of homosexuality, which I have referred to elsewhere as 'legitimation through disaster' (Altman 1988). But after some initial hesitation, COVID-19 was quickly perceived as a universal threat and therefore demanded a rather different response.

COVID-19 is far more easily transmitted and has a far lower death rate than did AIDS before the development of antiretroviral therapies, though AIDS deaths came more slowly, as HIV destroyed the immune system and laid bodies open to myriads of infections. Most important COVID-19 is not associated with stigmatised behaviours around sex and drugs, although it has produced its own share of stigma, particularly in the early years. As with AIDS, COVID-19 produced a search for culprits: in Ecuador, one woman, who had arrived in Guayaquil on a plane from Spain at the onset of the epidemic, was targeted as the source of the city's epidemic. The then President of the USA was determined to blame China for the epidemic, shifting attention away from his deliberate reduction of the country's ability to respond to new epidemic diseases, and attacks on people of Chinese descent were common.

Once HIV was identified as the cause of AIDS, it also became clear that the retrovirus could only be transmitted through what was coyly termed the 'exchange of bodily fluids', so that semen and blood were identified as the routes of infection. The greatest death toll in those early years was among young men with haemophilia, who had received infected blood products, but preventing the transmission of HIV required far less interference with daily life than does Coronavirus. Despite this, there were occasional calls to quarantine people with HIV, and Cuba did this between 1986 and 1997, isolating up to 10,000 HIV-positive people in sanatoria. And while no other country followed suit, travel restrictions became common: the USA only lifted this ban on allowing people with HIV to enter the country in 2009. Many countries not only retain the ban but mandate deporting anyone with HIV who is not a citizen.

The restrictions imposed by COVID-19 were more draconian and involved literally shutting down many parts of the economy for long periods during 2020 and 2021. Two years ago, I wrote about Juan Carlos's experience during the first year of the pandemic in Ecuador, where there was a curfew that extended from 2.00 pm to 6.00 am and outdoor exercise was forbidden (Altman and Valarezo 2020). The only social contact he had for many weeks was to buy food and take it to his mother, leaving it outside her door. When I wrote this, I did not imagine that Melbourne, where I live, would eventually have the distinction of experiencing the longest continuous lockdown in the world, when for a total of 245 days our movements were restricted, though never as severely as those he experienced. As I write now – in late 2022 – there are still severe lockdowns in some Chinese cities, although they have largely been abandoned by health officials elsewhere. A new epidemic is forecast to hit Australia over the coming summer.

At various points over the past few years, we have been told to avoid any close contact in ways that disrupt vast swathes of what we had taken for granted as part of everyday life. For much of two winters, my social life consisted of long walks with friends, restricted to five kilometres from the home. Across Melbourne, as elsewhere around the world, small businesses collapsed as movement, once taken for granted, was increasingly curtailed.

I experienced lockdowns as a privileged citizen in a largely well-governed polity. Obeying lockdown orders was literally impossible for millions of people without adequate income or shelter, and restrictions exacerbated already existing class and racial divides. The first stages of lockdowns in Melbourne saw unnecessarily harsh restrictions imposed on a major housing estate which is the home of many recent immigrants (Zevallos 2020). As late as mid-2022, there were stories out of China of considerable dislocations and distress as the government sought to impose further lockdowns in major cities.

Globally, there were massive abuses in the name of public health, including police brutality and excessive force:

> Kenyan police fired tear gas on hundreds of ferry commuters ahead of an overnight curfew and arrested many … In South Africa, the military raided a hostel for workers in a township where residents had ignored the lockdown, and citizens have reported police use of rubber bullets on a crowd of shoppers.
>
> (Trenkov-Wermuth 2020)

Steven Thrasher (2022) has dramatically demonstrated the ways in which both epidemics reinforced already existing racial and class inequalities, although his book deals overwhelmingly with the USA.

The travel bans imposed by COVID-19 created extraordinary hardship for hundreds of thousands of people, cut off from family and employment. These restrictions have had a direct impact upon HIV-related services; UNAIDS estimates COVID-19 lockdowns and restrictions have badly disrupted HIV testing, with many countries showing steep drops in HIV diagnoses, referrals to care services and HIV treatment initiations (UNAIDS 2021). There is a tragic irony in the reality that one pandemic is reversing many of the gains made in fighting another.

The political impact

The political impact of the responses to COVID-19 has some resemblances to that of the AIDS epidemic, but on a much greater scale. The two epidemics have their own national and regional particularities, and it is difficult to generalise. But there are few countries where COVID-19 has not weakened social ties, affected livelihoods and disrupted communities, in ways only experienced in sub-Saharan Africa and parts of the Caribbean during the worst years of the AIDS epidemic.

In some ways, COVID-19 undermined the dominance of neo-liberal economics, both increasing demands on the state and inflaming opposition to government regulations. Government spending on relief measures exploded, at least in countries with the resources to provide them, while governments simultaneously introduced unprecedented restrictions on freedom of movement. As I write there are major reactions against both developments, but it is probable that COVID-19 has marked a significant turning point in dominant perceptions of the role of government. In 1996, Bill Clinton proclaimed that 'the era of big government is over'. The 2020s have seen the return of the centrality of government. Even right-wing governments massively increased social spending to meet the crisis of COVID-19, which has contributed to the global inflation that developed from mid-2022 onwards.

AIDS also demanded unprecedented interventions by governments, particularly in providing adequate information to protect people from infection, and it changed attitudes towards sexuality and injection drug use. Not surprisingly countries with a strong public sector have done better in managing both epidemics – the USA stands out in both cases for its failures, a product of weak and decentralised government, a lack of universal health coverage and rigid moralism. In countries with major outbreaks, AIDS, like COVID-19, stretched health and welfare services beyond their limits. But even in countries with huge HIV caseloads, it is hard to find examples of governments being toppled because of the epidemic. Certainly, there were substantial deaths among the political elites in certain countries and President Mbeki's scepticism about HIV was a factor in his losing support in South Africa.

At least in the English-speaking world, COVID-19 changed the political fortunes of right-wing governments; in rather different ways Donald Trump, Boris Johnson and Scott Morrison all lost office in part through their inability to sufficiently manage the epidemic. But the most dramatic political impact of COVID-19 came when Brazilian police sought to charge Jair Bolsonaro for failures to apply appropriate health measures, which was undoubtedly a factor in Bolsonaro's narrow loss in November 2022. In time we will have account of the impact of COVID-19 on electoral politics in other countries – there is already an exhaustive study of its impact on the number of elections postponed and changes in voter turnout during the epidemic (International IDEA 2022). While turnout declined in about two-thirds of countries since the onset of the epidemic it is difficult to assert that COVID-19 was the primary cause. Fear of COVID-19 prompted an increase in postal and absentee voting, which became the basis of many of Trump's complaints about the 2020 election being 'stolen' from him (e.g. Kaufman 2022).

But if COVID-19 meant greater claims on the state, it simultaneously produced an upsurge of right-wing rhetoric that defended 'freedom' against public health demands for isolation, masks and vaccines. AIDS had produced its share of conspiratorial theories, such as claims that it was a product of CIA experimentation – echoed in Trump's suggestions that Chinese laboratories were responsible for COVID-19 – but not to the extent of other right-wing anti-scientific conspiratorial politics. In an era of social media and politicians spouting nonsense about 'false news' conspiratorial rhetoric has become ubiquitous, with real political effect.[1]

There were many examples of hostility, discrimination, even violence towards people with – or associated with – AIDS, but whereas the major political responses we associate with it are demands for greater government and scientific responses, the opposite has been true of COVID-19. Some of the anti-vaccination demonstrations echoed the direct action associated with groups like ACT UP, although far more prone to violence. But ACT UP demanded more resources for medical research, not opposition to health regulations. Ironically, Anthony Fauci, who was an early target of AIDS demonstrations, then a significant ally, became the best-known global face of COVID-19 research during the Trump Administration, and an object of hatred for the conspiratorial right. In many countries across Europe, and most notably in the USA, anti-vaccination and anti-lockdown movements provided fuel for the extreme right (The Economist 2022).

Human security

How best can we move from a personal account of living through an epidemic to an understanding of the broader socio-political impacts? This is a question social scientists have sought to answer since the onset of AIDS, and it is disappointing to see the reversion to even greater emphasis on biomedical hegemony in the area. In 2023, the International AIDS Society is scheduled a 'research for prevention' conference in Lima, which is a city already scarred by a massive COVID-19 epidemic. The expertise of the five co-chairs of the conference is overwhelmingly biomedical, even though prevention is an area in which social, cultural and political analysis is crucial.

My sense of recent international AIDS conferences is that while politics are always acknowledged in the background, there is a remarkable absence of people who actually study the political. What the two epidemics have in common is the challenge to conventional notions of national security. Just as HIV-related biomedical research has been remarkably relevant to research on COVID-19, so too is the literature of public health and national security, though it has been far less acknowledged. Despite the disasters of climate change and new epidemics, wars in Ukraine and Gaza, and concerns about the rise of China have pushed consideration of non-military threats to security even further from the mainstream agenda of people concerned with security and international conflict.

The notion of human security became significant in the post-Cold War world, as fears of nuclear conflict subsided, and liberal democracy seemed to be increasing. In his writings on human security, former UN Secretary-General Kofi Annan wrote:

> Human security, in its broadest sense, embraces far more than the absence of violent conflict. It encompasses human rights, good governance, access to education and health care and ensuring that each individual has opportunities and choices to fulfill his or her potential. Every step in this direction is also a steep towards reducing poverty, achieving economic growth and preventing conflict. Freedom from want, freedom from fear, and the freedom of future generations to inherit a healthy natural environment – these are the interrelated building blocks of human – and therefore national – security.
>
> (United Nations 2001)

At the turn of the twenty-first century, there was a surge of writing which conceptualised HIV as a security risk, likely to destabilise the political and social order, most clearly in Sub-Saharan Africa (e.g. Garrett 2005; Elbe 2009; de Waal 2010). As the then Executive Director of UNAIDS, Peter Piot, wrote:

> AIDS and global insecurity coexist in a vicious cycle. Civil and international conflict help spread HIV, as populations are destabilized, and armies move across new territories. And AIDS contributes to national and international insecurity, from the highest levels of HIV experienced among military and peacekeeping personnel, to the instability of societies whose future has been thrown into doubt.[2]

The impact of AIDS, above all in sub-Saharan Africa, has been considerable. A 2004 United Nations report reported that:

> A survey in Zimbabwe found that agricultural output declined by nearly 50% among households affected by AIDS. The Food and Agriculture Organization of the United Nations has estimated that the ten most severely affected African countries will lose between 10 and 26% of their agricultural labour force by 2020.
>
> (UN Population Division 2004)

This projection was probably exaggerated but it is difficult to find accurate figures. The latest estimates of the number of children in Africa orphaned by AIDS range between 12 and 18 million (UNICEF 2022); one of the earlier studies showed that: 'Before the onset of AIDS, about 2% of all children in developing countries were orphans. By 1999, 10% and more were orphans in some African countries' (UNAIDS 2001). Even if the numbers have declined since then, as more prevention measures were developed, the ongoing impact on people who are now young adults has been enormous. How far this has contributed to ongoing civil strife and displacement is impossible to estimate, but it has certainly been significant.

A few researchers pointed to the interconnection between the AIDS epidemic and other issues of human security, in particular displacement and climate change. As Lieber et al. (2021, pp. 2273–2274) pointed out, HIV was responsible for 'increased food insecurity, increased prevalence of other infectious diseases, increased human migration, and erosion of public health and transportation infrastructure'. The death rate among members of the elites in some African countries undoubtedly had an impact on political stability, which seems to be a largely unresearched topic.

These grim warnings may now seem overexaggerated, but there are echoes of them in the impact of COVID-19 on growing civil disorder and public protests. Clearly, the impact of the epidemic on economic activity and the strains on already inadequate health systems have contributed to weakening political authority and increasing radical movements of both left and right. Across Latin America, COVID-19 certainly contributed to political instability, although it is difficult to separate its effects from other factors that have been involved (Mineo 2021). The figures are staggering: by mid-2022 at least 1.7 million people had died from COVID-19 in Latin America and the Caribbean. Far the highest death rates came in Peru, which may have had the highest per capita death rate in the world. (At the same time the vaccination rate in many of these countries, such as Chile and even Peru, exceeded that of the USA.) The collapse of tourism in 2020–2021 and the weaknesses of regional health systems meant that there was a clear connection between COVID-19 and socio-economic distress.

Similar conditions applied across some of sub-Saharan Africa and South Asia. It is impossible to know how far COVID-19 may have contributed to the collapse of political and economic order in Sri Lanka, but it clearly was a factor. In the same way, growing ethnic conflicts in India might well be linked to the impact of COVID-19. In a world that was already undergoing massive dislocations caused by climate change and massive numbers of displaced people, a global epidemic magnifies existing inequalities.

For a short period in the early 2000s, the global threat of HIV seemed to mobilise genuine attempts to meet the global inequities that were furthering the spread of the epidemic. The formation of the Global Fund to Fight AIDS, Tuberculosis and Malaria in 2002 and the commitment of the Bush,

Blair and Chirac governments were significant steps towards a genuine global response. Despite attempts by the World Health Organisation, there has been less consistent mobilisation around COVID-19, with rich countries hoarding vaccines despite the urgent need to make them universally available.

Analysing current events is always fraught, but it seems evident that the impact of COVID-19 on global politics has been considerable. Already in 2020 the energy economist Daniel Yergin saw COVID-19 as leading to a decline in globalisation: 'The world economy is now tormented by lives upended and tragedy, unemployment, small businesses fighting for survival, companies under severe pressure, countries impoverished, hope vanquished for many, governments stretched to the extreme by debt, and enormous loss of economic output' (Yergin 2020, p. 424). Several years later we can see that while some of this – most notably unemployment – has not occurred as predicted, the ongoing impact of the epidemic has disrupted supply lines, migration and productivity.

Both epidemics continue to develop, and even as new variants of COVID-19 appear it is likely that other viral epidemics will develop. However impressive our biomedical resources, the lesson from both epidemics is that without a global mobilisation of resources and a properly social and political response we face the prospect of increasing deaths and dislocation. The ongoing message from the HIV epidemic is that if rich countries ignore the majority of the world's population their security can only be illusionary.

A coda

I began this chapter with a personal note, and I end with one. I am writing this as the first vaccines against mpox have arrived in Australia and are being rolled out to those regarded as most vulnerable. But the reality that the epidemic seems to be spreading fastest among men who have sex with men has already produced a new wave of homophobia that will inevitably mean more infections and a bigger epidemic (Kay 2022). I read the article just cited while waiting on hold for 20 minutes to book an appointment for a vaccine, only to discover stocks are already running out. Of course, in time I gained access, as will other gay men in rich countries. The prospect for homosexual men in Latin America, where mpox is also spreading, is less hopeful. Like AIDS and COVID-19, this is another reminder that for millions of people the greatest threat to their security comes not from bombs and bullets but from microbes and the failures of national and international authorities to develop satisfactory global health programmes.

Notes

1 For an Australian analysis see Lewis (2022).
2 Speech by Peter Piot, UN, University of Tokyo, 2 October 2001.

References

Altman, D., 1988. Legitimacy through disaster. In D. Fox and E. Fee, eds. *AIDS: The burdens of history*. Berkeley: University of California Press, 301–315.

Altman, D., 2019. *Unrequited love: Diary of an accidental activist*. Melbourne: Monash University.

Altman, D. and Valarezo, J.C., 2020. Deaths and desperation mount in Ecuador, epicenter of coronavirus pandemic in Latin America. *The Conversation*, 24 April. https://theconversation.com/deaths-and-desperation-mount-in-ecuador-epicenter-of-coronavirus-pandemic-in-latin-america-137015

Bird, C., 2022. *Telltale*. Melbourne: Transit Lounge.

de Waal, A., 2010. Reframing governance, security and conflict in the light of HIV/AIDS: A synthesis of findings from the AIDS, security and conflict initiative. *Social Science & Medicine*, 70, 114–120. 10.1016/j.socscimed.2009.09.031

Elbe, S., 2009. *Virus alert*. New York: Columbia University Press.

Garrett, L., 2005. *HIV and National Security: Where are the links?* New York: Council on Foreign Relations.

International IDEA, 2022. Global overview of COVID-19: Impact on elections. *International IDEA* [online], 1 December. Available from: www.idea.int/news-media/multimedia-reports/global-overview-covid-19-impact-elections [Accessed 22 December 2022].

Kaufman, D., 2022. The takeover. *New Yorker*, 1 August.

Kay, C., 2022. Monkeypox cases driven 'underground' by anti-gay stigma in India: Report. *ndtv.com* (Bloomberg) [online], 9 August. Available from: www.ndtv.com/india-news/monkeypox-cases-driven-underground-by-anti-gay-stigma-in-india-3238187 [Accessed 22 December 2022].

Lewis, D., 2022. *Unvaxxed*. Melbourne: Hardie Grant.

Lieber, M., et al., 2021. The synergistic relationship between climate change and the HIV/AIDS epidemic: A conceptual framework. *AIDS and Behavior*, 25 (7), 2266–2277. 10.1007/s10461-020-03155-y

Mineo, L., 2021. From bad to worse in Latin America. *Harvard Gazette*, 27 July.

Newham, B., 2022. HIV in Indonesia: On shared trauma, global solidarity and grief. *Archer Magazine*, 29 September.

The Economist, 2022. Extreme goes mainstream: The insurrection failed. What now for America's far right? *The Economist*, 13 August.

Thrasher, S., 2022. *The viral underclass*. New York: Celadon Books.

Trenkov-Wermuth, C., 2020. How to put human security at the center of the response to coronavirus. *United States Institute of Peace* [online], 16 April. Available from: https://www.usip.org/publications/2020/04/how-put-human-security-center-response-coronavirus [Accessed 22 December 2022].

United Nations, 2001. Secretary-General salutes international workshop on human security in Mongolia. SG/SM/7382. *United Nations* [online], 8 May. Available from: https://press.un.org/en/2000/20000508.sgsm7382.doc.html [Accessed 22 December 2022].

UN Population Division, 2004. The impact of AIDS. New York: UN Department of Economic and Social Affairs. Available from: https://digitallibrary.un.org/record/532245?ln=en [Accessed 22 December 2022].

UNAIDS, 2001. *Children and young people in a world of AIDS*. Factsheet for UN Special Session on AIDS. Geneva: UNAIDS.

UNAIDS, 2021. Global AIDS update: Confronting inequalities – Lessons for pandemic responses from 40 years of AIDS. Geneva: UNAIDS. Available from: https://www.unaids.org/en/resources/documents/2021/2021-global-aids-update [Accessed 22 December 2022].

UNICEF, 2022. Global and Regional Trends: UNICEF Data Sheets. *UNICEF* [online], July. Available from: https://data.unicef.org/topic/hivaids/global-regional-trends/ [Accessed 22 December 2022].

Yergin, D., 2020. *The new map*. London: Allen Lane.

Zevallos, Z., 2020. Pandemic, race and moral panic. *Other Sociologist*, 5 July. Available from: https://othersociologist.com/2020/07/05/pandemic-race-and-moral-panic [Accessed 22 December 2022].

6 An unlimited intimacy of the air

Pandemic fantasy, COVID-19 and the biopolitics of respiration[1]

Tim Dean

to the memory of Leo Bersani

Preamble

This chapter explores the basic proposition that human coexistence with viruses depends, to a greater degree than is usually acknowledged, on the language used to think about them. If we treat viruses as essentially enemies of human health and flourishing, then we will be perpetually at war with the virosphere that surrounds and, indeed, pervades us. Here I consider how counternarratives of viral intimacy that emerged from the HIV pandemic might spark different ways of talking and thinking about living with viruses in the age of COVID-19. Pursuing this inquiry, I ask after the role that psychical fantasy plays in thinking about virality beyond the bioscientific rationalities that often regard the virosphere in militaristic terms, as enemy territory to be conquered. How, in short, might humans inhabit the virosphere otherwise? Such questions grow out of my ongoing work on HIV and AIDS, which has been sharpened and renewed by the COVID-19 pandemic. The key difference in transmission routes between the human immunodeficiency virus and the novel coronavirus prompts reflection on the biopolitics of respiration: what is at stake in our sharing of the air? COVID-19 revealed the extent to which we are intertwined by virtue of our constantly inhaling each other – intertwined with viral processes and with all those, human and otherwise, who breathe the same air. This chapter endeavours to think through the multiple and often conflicting implications of getting inside one another without physically touching.

Misinformation versus fantasy

In March 2022, a friend who had avoided indoor restaurant dining for two years – her elderly mother is immunocompromised – drove to an academic conference in the state of Indiana, where she ended up, unmasked, eating inside a restaurant ('it was more like a sports bar') with a group of conference-goers. She told me this tale in a tone of horrified glee. For readers outside the USA, it may be worth underscoring that my friend travelled from the 'blue' state of Illinois, where strict COVID-19 protocols were in place, to

DOI: 10.4324/9781003322788-7

an adjacent 'red' state that had been comparatively lax about masking, social distancing and vaccination. When I inquired further about the experience, she likened her otherwise unremarkable dinner to 'being at an orgy.' 'Next thing you know, you're barebacking in restaurants,' I said. 'Exactly!' she replied. The group dining that often punctuates academic conferences – and, indeed, constitutes one of their greatest pleasures – suddenly feels like group sex. At that moment, taking off your mask to dine in a restaurant with people you've just met would be akin to dispensing with the condom when having sex with strangers. All bets are off, with the usual precautions suspended, as one experiences a pleasure that is intensified by consciousness of risk. The phrase 'barebacking in restaurants' offers a fantasy image, something that gives form to unexpected sensations of transgression in an ordinary public place.

What made dinner at a midwestern sports bar feel like 'being at an orgy' was the spectre of SARS-CoV-2, the microscopic causal agent of COVID-19. The super-saturated sociability of restaurant dining after the isolation of social distancing; the possibility of sharing food, air and, hence, oral exchange with a host of others; even the fact that, early in the pandemic, some referred to masks as 'face condoms': these elements all inform the phantasm of 'barebacking in restaurants.' Here my concern is less with the statistical risks of indoor dining from an epidemiological perspective (or the wearying calculations they entail) than our fantasies about risk. Viruses are an exemplary object of these fantasies. We have fantasies about viruses – and not merely notions or incomplete information about them – because viruses so readily traverse what we imagine as our bodily borders.

A virus may move from outside to inside 'me' without my knowledge or control, thereby making evident how unself-contained I am. This is especially true of airborne viruses such as SARS-CoV-2. It is the virus as a sign of corporeal porosity or borderlessness that provokes paranoid fantasies of invasion, penetration and foreign occupation. One might say that an airborne virus, in testifying to the human body's penetrability, threatens to make bottoms of us all. Whatever else they do, viruses remind their human hosts of our physical vulnerability: virality rouses the terror of human helplessness. Almost by definition, the viral stands for that which has escaped human control. These kinds of threats, imaginary and real, help to account for the extreme reactions witnessed during the COVID-19 pandemic, as well as the narratives devised to explain its origin. The 'lab-leak' hypothesis, for example, dramatises a fantasy that the novel coronavirus, whether bioengineered or otherwise, escaped the control of scientists who were working on it. Even the primary hypothesis of a zoonotic 'spillover' – in which the virus migrated from its natural host into humans, possibly via the intermediary of a non-human animal such as the heavily trafficked pangolin – encodes the spectre of losing control through failures of containment.[2] Indeed, the phrase 'failures of containment' sums up practically everything that has happened with the pandemic since SARS-CoV-2 first emerged. It would be something of a redundancy to observe that it is in the nature of viruses to 'go viral.'

Fantasy frequently functions as a psychical defence against microbial challenges to myths of bodily integrity, subjective omnipotence and human exceptionalism. The more we learn about viruses, the more of them we discover there are and, concomitantly, how poorly human knowledge comprehends the virosphere. As David Quammen (2022, p. 108) puts it,

> We live in a world of viruses – viruses that are unfathomably diverse, immeasurably abundant, and ambivalent in their effects, even upon human health and welfare. The oceans alone may contain more virions than there are stars in the observable universe. Mammals may carry at least 320,000 different viruses. [...] And beyond the big numbers are big consequences of a sort we wouldn't expect: many of those viruses bring adaptive benefits, not harms to life on Earth, including human life.

Virology apprises us of the mixed news that we are, in fact, crawling with viruses; no human body is virus-free. Not only do we not control them, but they are already inside 'us' and outnumber us by several orders of magnitude. Psychical fantasy responds vigorously to this image of ourselves as always already contaminated by the 'not-me.'

Yet psychical fantasy may also function in a less defensive, more creative fashion. In my research on HIV and AIDS over the past several decades, I have tried to make space for considering the suprarational ways that people think about viruses. It should come as no surprise that popular thinking about a disease regarded as sexually transmitted would be inflected by unconscious fantasies (Bersani 1987; Watney 1987). What has been striking about responses to the COVID-19 pandemic is how prone virtually everyone appears to non-rational thinking about a virus whose primary mode of transmission has little to do with sex. COVID-19 laid bare not only the deteriorated condition of societal infrastructures, but also how virally intimate we are with the people around us, whether friends, neighbours, co-workers or strangers. Fantasy responds to the discovery, or the reminder, that these folks can leave traces of themselves inside us more readily than we knew. This is viral intimacy without the pleasures of sex. It is disturbing to intuit that we may be tangled up in each other with barely any awareness of the fact.

If viral fantasies are fuelled by misinformation, nevertheless they cannot be dispelled simply by accurate (or more complete) data. The sciences of virology, immunology, microbiology and epidemiology, while crucial, remain insufficient in this context because they cannot account for how most people actually think about the novel coronavirus. Indeed, the wish *not* to think about it – to imagine that the pandemic is a hoax or that it is already over and we can 'go back to normal' – is, from the point of view of psychoanalysis, just one more sign of unconscious thinking about this virus. The primary psychological response to an unwelcome reality is to reject it. Although scientists have been warning for decades that a new global pandemic may be on the horizon (Garrett 1994) – and that it might well come from a novel coronavirus (Quammen 2022, pp. 27–70) – SARS-CoV-2 caught even the wealthiest and most powerful societies off-guard. The misleading results of global exercises in 'pandemic preparedness,' from which the USA emerged as most prepared (Wright 2021, p. 16), suggest that a more accurate descriptor would be 'pandemic *un*preparedness': as Freud (1919, p. 245) observed a century earlier, 'the prefix "*un*" is the token of repression.' Scientific knowledge, even when recognised as necessarily incomplete, remains radically insufficient thanks to the chasm between what is cognitively known and what can be psychologically accepted. As with climate change, we 'knew' a pandemic was coming but collectively we preferred not to know.

From the gap between what is known and what is psychically tolerable spring fantasies that often rely on archaic stereotypes. With COVID-19, orientalist fantasies about racial difference played an especially insidious role. Designating SARS-CoV-2 as 'the China virus' (as Trump and his allies did) promoted a dangerous fantasy that the epidemic would be curbed via border lockdowns, racial segregation or anti-Asian violence.[3] It was akin to describing HIV as 'the gay virus' and calling for the tattooing, quarantining and segregation of gay men – as reactionaries did during the 1980s. Of course, racialising a virus contains it in fantasy only; no virus respects our manufactured identity categories or imaginary boundaries. The racialising fantasy has had real effects – it led to Asian American people being attacked in the street – just not the containment effects stipulated. And yet, even as we insist that SARS-CoV-2 is not a Chinese virus, we also need to acknowledge that the clarification is not enough to defuse the fantasy. Othering that which is present never actually eliminates it.

More than ever, it has become imperative to grasp how we think about viruses – and how distant from empirically verified data our thinking about them can be. That gap between knowledge and fantasy is not an empty space waiting to be filled with greater or more refined knowledge. The cure for rampant misinformation can never be only valid scientific information, vital though that is, because fantasies are not merely errors or illusions. Instead, fantasies are modes of symbolisation at the level of the unconscious that we ignore at our peril. For human subjects, fantasy is neither trivial, secondary nor irrational but, rather, constitutive of our psychic lives. Moreover, fantasies are not simply products of individual psychology but structure group mentalities at various scales; as critics from Jacqueline Rose (1998) to Slavoj Žižek (1997) have demonstrated, fantasies are eminently political.[4] We think with and through our fantasies – and never more so than when confronting those pathogenic entities, invisible to the naked eye, that retain a capacity to enter human bodies seemingly at will.

However, it is because we think via fantasy, rather than solely through rational processes of cognition, that we can do unexpected things with viruses. This, at least, was my contention in *Unlimited Intimacy*, an informal ethnographic study of the particular subculture that emerged in the USA, towards the end of the twentieth century, around barebacking – deliberate unprotected sex among gay men (Dean 2009). The rational explanation at that time for what appeared as a disconcertingly widespread abandonment of condoms, including for anal sex with strangers, was that middle-class gay men now had access to an armature of effective pharmaceutical treatments for controlling HIV infection. Yet the availability of medications – highly active antiretroviral therapies (HAART) and pre-exposure prophylaxis (PrEP) – fails to completely explain the efflorescence of a specific sexual subculture, along with its own brand of pornography, based on viral transmission. For that, one needs an understanding of fantasy – and not only because pornography, including so-called documentary porn, inevitably involves fantasy.[5]

What I discovered while researching condomless sex at the millennium was that gay men had not simply forgotten about HIV. Instead, many had incorporated it into their sex lives quite intentionally. The development of fantasies of viral transmission – expressed in a vernacular of 'breeding,' 'seeding' and 'pozzing' as forms of initiation into 'the bug brotherhood' – testified to an inventive (not to say disturbing) approach to the human immunodeficiency virus. Men who identified as 'bugchasers' and 'giftgivers' were having sex with a virus, as well as with each other; at the level of fantasy they were using HIV to form kinship bonds, based on what anthropologists call shared substance (Dean 2008). One might say that, through a collective process of fetishisation, these men were transforming HIV from a phobic object into an object of desire – though even that characterisation strikes me as oversimplifying what was going on. Given how stridently pathologising the discourse about bareback was 20 years ago – and how unprotected anal sex had barely been acknowledged as the basis for a distinct subculture – I wanted to analyse it more dispassionately. Endeavouring to describe certain kinds of sexual activity as specifically subcultural practices, I aimed in *Unlimited Intimacy* to anatomise the fantasies fuelling those practices too.[6] Without the fantasies, none of it made sense; only by grasping the unconscious rationalities that organised the subculture could bareback be distinguished from self-destructive hedonism. For me, fantasy was the analytic category whereby an intensely stigmatised sexual practice could be depathologised.

My goal at that time was neither to defend nor to denounce bareback subculture, but instead to think alongside it; I tried to take its fantasies seriously rather than simply dismissing them. Because I refused the predictable route of critiquing condomless sex among gay men, some readers of *Unlimited Intimacy* believed I was celebrating the subculture as transgressive and queer. That is a misreading based on the methodological incomprehension borne of politicising complex phenomena too quickly. We need to be able to think about difficult material without either praising or condemning it, and no less so now than then. Particularly when it comes to viruses, we need to make space for thinking that eschews the blame/praise binary, without supposing that our thinking thereby escapes the mediation of fantasy. The idea of 'misinformation' tends to assume that people just need the right information – scientifically verified data – along with access to vaccines, medications, prophylactics such as masks or condoms, and the proper support. But that public-health approach, earnestly inclusive though it is, overlooks all the ways in which fantasy mediates people's thinking about virality. My claim is that 'misinformation' is itself a misleading idea.

The subculture I documented in *Unlimited Intimacy* has since been transformed thanks to PrEP, an antiviral treatment regime that prevents infection by inhibiting the reverse transcription HIV needs to replicate. Over the past decade or so, once-a-day pills marketed under the brand names Truvada and Descovy – and, more recently, long-acting antiviral injectables – have altered the sexual landscape dramatically (Mandavilli 2023). As a result, barebacking today is not what it once was. Indeed, condomless sex among men on PrEP can no longer be characterised simply as 'unprotected' sex; the risks have changed substantially, although the fantasies have not evaporated (Dean 2015; Varghese 2019; Florêncio 2020; García-Iglesias 2022). Bareback subculture may be worth considering in the era of COVID-19 because it offers an example – by no means definitive – of what it might mean to live with a virus, rather than only to die from it. The COVID-19 pandemic has furnished a parable about how we navigate, or fail to navigate, viral intimacy. How do we want to live with this coronavirus, with its proliferating variants and subvariants, which have colonised 'our' world faster and far more efficiently than could have been imagined?

From HIV to SARS-CoV-2 and the viral beyond

Despite the prominence of Anthony Fauci, longtime director of the National Institute of Allergy and Infectious Diseases, during not only COVID-19 but also the early years of AIDS, it often has felt as though US society learned nothing from the previous pandemic. For those involved in AIDS activism during the 1980s and 1990s who are still alive today, Fauci represents a striking point of continuity between then and now. In view of that continuity, it is disheartening to witness how many of the social reactions to SARS-CoV-2 – vehement denial, hysterical othering – along with the institutional bungling and failures of leadership all appear uncannily similar from one pandemic to the next. There has been, as Peter Hegarty and Joe Rollins (2021) demonstrate, a conspicuous 'viral forgetting' of the hard lessons learned during AIDS. This kind of amnesia is what Jacqueline Rose (2023) – ironically in a book about the COVID-19 pandemic that never mentions AIDS – designates as the 'historical forgetting against which the whole of psychoanalysis pitches itself' (p. 11). In order to properly remember, it may be necessary to analyse just what spurs and abets these historical amnesias.

Remarkably, even with mpox on the heels of COVID-19, it seemed the USA had failed to grasp the lessons of recent pandemic history: 'the response in the United States has been sluggish and timid, reminiscent of the early days of the Covid pandemic [...] raising troubling questions about the nation's preparedness for pandemic threats' (Mandavilli 2022). The gay community watched with disbelief as the same institutional mistakes were repeated during the mpox outbreak of 2022: viral forgetting at breakneck speed. Again and again, we have been confronted with the inadequacies of public-health infrastructure – inadequacies that new, emerging and long-established viruses quickly exploit. For this reason, one group of researchers has pointedly redescribed COVID-19 as a 'political pandemic,' arguing that 'there is no such thing as a *natural* pandemic,' since 'it is through the social production of vulnerability and political failure that viral outbreaks scale into pandemics, pandemics translate into disasters, and disasters escalate into catastrophes' (Boyle et al. 2022, p. 4). Although these researchers focus on COVID-19 in the UK, their cogent critique of the compound effects of neoliberal governance holds true for the USA too.

As a result of the neoliberal production of vulnerabilities, queer sexual culture faces not only a resurgence of homophobic discrimination ('Don't Say Gay') but also a 'tripledemic' or *syndemic* of HIV, COVID-19 and mpox, as viruses circulate and mutate.[7] The notion of syndemic (or synergistic epidemic) provides a framework for grasping how epidemics overlap and may be exacerbated by a population's pre-existing vulnerabilities. Since there is no shortage of parallels among these overlapping pandemics, targets for critique multiply almost as fast as viruses replicate. Even as recent epidemiological data have confirmed that the most socially disenfranchised groups suffer disproportionately in pandemics, we are hectored by calls to 'return to normal' – as if the normal were not a fundamental part of the problem in the first place. The queer critique of normalisation, which grew out of the HIV epidemic during the late 1990s, remains highly relevant to our current 'post-COVID-19' moment, since the normal to which we are urged to return is one of stark inequality, with some social groups persistently rendered more vulnerable than others. The 'normal' appears desirable only if it has not been the rubric under which one has already been stigmatised, marginalised and punished (Warner 1999).

The similarities, overlaps and compounding exacerbations among pandemics suggest that we stand only to lose by treating them in isolation, as if they were separate rather than complexly interwoven. Nevertheless, the fact that SARS-CoV-2 is airborne, and therefore exponentially more transmissible than HIV, constrains the parallels that may be drawn between these viruses and their respective pandemics, in my view. The persistent underestimation of the novel coronavirus's infectivity contrasts sharply with the general overestimation of how easy it is to get HIV. Those differences tend to be obscured by fantasies about purity and contamination, particularly fantasies about the contaminating properties of sex. When we apprehend COVID-19 primarily through the lens of our experiences with HIV, we risk erasing the specificity of both pandemics. It is not only ignorance and denial that defend against the novel and unknown, but also our established frames of reference, our knowingness. The widespread conviction during COVID-19, among gay men of my generation, that 'we've been here before' may make it harder to appreciate what is significantly new. Differences between mechanisms of viral transmission, and their implications for intimacy, thus remain crucial. Unpacking those differences here, I return in the chapter's postscript to some of the stakes of apprehending one pandemic in terms of another.

Although the illness subsequently named as 'acquired immune deficiency syndrome' first attracted medical notice in 1981, its viral cause was not identified until 1983 and not definitively named as HIV until 1986. Easy to forget, 40 years later, the social panic that once surrounded this new disease's uncertain mechanisms of transmission. During that early period, fear about AIDS spread more rapidly than HIV itself. Entrenched homophobia stoked anxieties that one could 'catch AIDS' from ordinary social interaction – by shaking hands or dining in restaurants, for example, or simply by being around queer people. Gay waiters became a distinct object of irrational terror at a time when homosexuality itself was regarded as contaminating. Once transmission mechanisms were known, however, it became politically imperative to emphasise that HIV could not be spread through ordinary social interaction. Gay men then realised that the pandemic driver of asymptomatic transmission need not pose an insuperable problem after all. You just had to approach every potential sex partner as if they were HIV-positive and avoid exchanging bodily fluids (Crimp 1987). Easier said than done, of course, especially if activities such as cum-swapping were integral to your sense of erotic intimacy.

Nevertheless, there emerged in gay sexual culture an ethos that insisted we were all living with HIV, regardless of anyone's actual serostatus. Early in the pandemic, we redescribed 'AIDS patients' as 'people with AIDS' (PWAs); as it gradually became evident that one could be HIV-positive for a decade or more without developing symptoms, we reframed the person 'dying from AIDS' as one 'living with HIV'; in a concerted effort to destigmatise the disease, we avowed that we were all living with HIV, albeit unequally. Phrases such as 'person with AIDS' foreground the person rather than the infection, condition or disability, while also highlighting the conjunction *with* as a potential sign of togetherness. If you are *with*, you are no longer isolate or alone; *with* implies a degree of intimacy, for better or worse. It is the status of living-with, or being-with (*Mitsein*), that we are now trying to conceive in the massively expanded context of the virosphere – the global totality of viruses, those identified and named, as well as the legions unknown.

Although four decades later there is still no vaccine or cure for HIV, people have learned to live with this virus in various ways. Bareback subculture remains among the least anticipated ways of living with HIV because it embraces the virus by eroticising its transmission. Hardly surprising, then, that survivors of the traumatic early years of AIDS – when there were no effective treatments, just stigma and terror and death – often become enraged at the very mention of organised barebacking. Gay elders such as Larry Kramer could see in bareback subculture only the reckless dissemination of illness and death.

What one self-identified barebacker described as an experience of 'unlimited intimacy' may be viewed conversely as manifesting unwanted intimacy. Recently, I have come to think that SARS-CoV-2, owing to its far greater infectivity, is the virus that better exemplifies unlimited – and unwanted – intimacy. Now we have an unlimited intimacy of the air.

As with HIV, the COVID-19 pandemic is driven by asymptomatic transmission. Unlike with HIV, however, ordinary social intercourse, including indoor restaurant dining, offers ample opportunity for SARS-CoV-2 to spread. If the most salient feature of this novel coronavirus is that it is airborne, nevertheless it took the World Health Organization, the US Centers for Disease Control and other national authorities too long to properly register the fact. Not until late in April 2021 did the WHO publicly acknowledge that this virus spreads via aerosols – tiny respiratory particles that remain suspended in the air – as well as via respiratory droplets, which stay airborne only momentarily and generate fomites when they land on surfaces (Greenhalgh et al. 2021; Tufekci 2021). In a compelling account of institutional reluctance to acknowledge the role of aerosols in viral spread, sociologist Zeynep Tufekci relates how the emergence of modern germ theory during the nineteenth century gradually displaced miasma theories of disease. It was not foul smells and bad air that caused illness, the thinking went, but pathogenic particles invisible to the naked eye: microbes replaced miasma. And yet this advance in scientific knowledge concerning infection subsequently made the significance of aerosol transmission harder to accept, insofar as it hearkens to outmoded theories about 'bad air.' Tufekci (2021) elaborates:

> If the importance of aerosol transmission had been accepted early, we would have been told from the beginning that it was much safer outdoors, where these small particles disperse more easily [...]. We would have tried to make sure indoor spaces were well ventilated, with air filtered as necessary. Instead of blanket rules on gatherings, we would have targeted conditions that can produce superspreading events: people in poorly ventilated indoor spaces, especially if engaged over time in activities that increase aerosol production, like shouting and singing. We would have started using masks more quickly, and we would have paid more attention to their fit, too. And we would have been less obsessed with cleaning surfaces.

Imagining that SARS-CoV-2 spreads primarily through direct physical contact, we underplayed its capacity to hang in the air that surrounds us, the air we inhale and exhale, constantly and involuntarily. For too long we apprehended this novel coronavirus through a phobic tropology of contaminating touch, as if, like Lady Macbeth, rigorous handwashing might save us. But a virus understood as fully airborne – present in aerosols as well as in droplets – redirects the focus from surfaces to orifices, displacing attention from touch to breath.

Breathing, a process of perpetual exchange between inside and outside, marks an original openness to the world beyond any organism's discrete bodily envelope. An aerosolised virus renders ordinary respiration a site of new vulnerability by disclosing how unself-contained we truly are. Now, more than ever, we are 'living with' whether we like it or not – indeed, whether we acknowledge it or not. Human respiration is an involuntary activity that nevertheless remains amenable to discipline (think yoga), politics (think 'I can't breathe') and fantasy. One key correlate of the psychoanalytic theory of embodiment is that autonomic systems such as respiration are no less subject to fantasy than the organs and systems of sexual reproduction. We need only consider the 'breath play' involved in certain BDSM rituals – or the phenomenon of heavy breathing in an anonymous telephone call – to see how readily the mundane activity of respiration may be eroticised. Over 60 years ago, Jacques Lacan (2006) alluded without elaboration to 'respiratory erogeneity' (p. 692). And long before COVID-19, *Instigator*, a gay porn magazine produced in West Hollywood for the kink community, regularly depicted men having sex in gasmasks. It is because breathing functions as a process of exchange between inside and outside – and thus marks a vital bodily threshold – that it lends itself to metaphor, overcoding and fetishisation. In human subjects, respiration is never an exclusively physiological process, despite what some biologists would like to believe.

We become intimate through the air we share. With SARS-CoV-2, one need mingle no bodily fluids, only breath: the atmosphere is our medium of intimacy. In the biopolitics of respiration, what we are sharing is effectively our insides. I take the image of 'shared insides' from the German philosopher Peter Sloterdijk (2014), whose *Spheres* trilogy redefines intimacy at multiple scales, including the atmospheric. 'Like every shared life,' he claims in a revision of Bismarck, 'politics is the art of the atmospherically possible' (Sloterdijk 2014, p. 697). If facemasks are but the most visible sign of this politics of the air, then we may need a 'spherological' critique of the virosphere. Notwithstanding Sloterdijk's own troubling politics, such a critique would need to begin by acknowledging that, as the sharing of air is unequally distributed, so is the atmospheric intimacy frequently unwanted. Social privilege tends to determine the quality and quantity of air you're compelled to share, how many others you must perforce inhale. *I can't breathe* – a rallying cry of the Black Lives Matter movement after the killing of Eric Garner – refers to not only African American citizens asphyxiated by the police but also the suffocating effects of anti-Black racism in the USA more generally. In this context, Ibram X. Kendi (2021) names racism as 'the original American virus.'

Not being able to breathe freely is both a metaphor and, too often, a material condition as well. During the summer of 2023, when Canadian wildfires polluted the atmosphere to such an extent that people living hundreds of miles downstream from the fires had to break out their N-95 masks in order simply to walk down the street, we were reminded of how climate change and pandemics of respiratory disease intersect – and how that intersection of ostensibly natural calamities is politically exacerbated. 'Breathing in unbreathable circumstances is what we do every day in the chokehold of racial gendered ableist capitalism' (Gumbs 2021, p. 21). As various critics have argued, it is the political atmosphere as much as what is airborne in the virosphere that compromises human respiration (DiCaglio 2021). My point is that the identification of SARS-CoV-2 with a respiratory illness (severe acute respiratory syndrome) helps to distinguish it from HIV (which gives rise to an immunodeficiency syndrome when left untreated). Emphasising the respiratory dimension differentiates COVID-19 from AIDS, while at the same time connecting COVID-19 with the epidemic of police violence that sparked protests worldwide following the murder of George Floyd on 25 May 2020. Although SARS-CoV-2, like all viruses, remains invisible to the naked eye, Floyd's death achieved global visibility during the first year of the pandemic, becoming an iconic image of suffocation. His death was the one whose cause we all could see. *I can't breathe* is the anguished cry that links COVID-19 with Black Lives Matter through the biopolitics of respiration.

Breathing intimacies

Akin to the rhythms of breathing, respirational biopolitics pushes in competing directions – negative and affirmative – at once. I advocate for considering the creative and erotic possibilities of this biopolitics, as well as its destructive side. If we take Michel Foucault's (2003) definition of biopolitics as involving the power to make live or let die (p. 241), then we may see the negative pole of respirational biopolitics in the unequal distribution of risk during the COVID-19 pandemic, which allowed the elderly, the poor and the disenfranchised to succumb more readily to respiratory illness. Older people may be more physically vulnerable to disease, but that vulnerability has been exacerbated by social attitudes that permit their segregation into badly ventilated and poorly monitored nursing homes, which quickly became *de facto* morgues during the pandemic's first wave. US culture's pervasive devaluing of its elders makes them a disposable population that may, in Foucault's words, be 'let die.' Respirational biopolitics hits home when the burden of risk in breathing is borne unequally – when we share the air but refuse to share its risks.

The negative pole of the biopolitics of respiration manifests also in those logics of social segregation that allow some people to breathe more easily by leaving others to bear the brunt of environmental pollution. The COVID-19 pandemic made clear how humans are universally vulnerable to airborne viruses – though some are rendered, by deliberate social policies and by neglect, as vastly more vulnerable than others. For example, the elevated incidence of asthma among African American populations, resulting from more frequent exposure to air pollution, intensified their vulnerability to this new respiratory virus (Johnson 2020). If the biopolitics of respiration contributed to Eric Garner's asthma in some unquantifiable way, then in his case biopower fatally intersected with a performance of sovereign power – the ancient right to take life – when a New York City police officer put him in a chokehold on 17 July 2014. Sovereign power (embodied in a monarch or ruler) involves the right to take life or let live, whereas biopower (diffused throughout social processes rather than embodied in individuals) involves the right to make live or let die. It was biopower that left Garner struggling to breathe with asthma, and then an illegitimate exercise of sovereign power by the police that asphyxiated him.

The Italian philosopher Franco 'Bifo' Berardi (2018) reports feeling 'asthmatic solidarity' (p. 15) when he watched the public cellphone recording of Garner's last, gasping breaths. I would suggest that Berardi's sense of solidarity stems not from national or racial identification, but from the elemental struggle to breathe shared by people with asthma. In this view of respiratory biopolitics, what is shared is less air or breath than the struggle for them – a struggle Berardi understands to be political as well as physiological. When George Floyd died after a Minneapolis police officer knelt on his neck for more than nine minutes, the sense of solidarity sparked around the world, in people of all races and nations, testified to a globally shared feeling of respiratory vulnerability, as well as to the abhorrence of racial injustice. At that moment in 2020, we were all, in different ways, struggling to breathe. Unimpeded respiration could no longer be taken for granted by anyone.

Since breathing is not a purely passive process, the power of respiration may be actively mobilised for intimacy, for community, for eros and for aesthetics. Struggling to breathe may become a basis for political solidarity. The affirmative pole of respirational biopolitics can be seen, for example, in projects of 'feminist breathing,' which are usually collective and draw on rich traditions of Black feminism (Tremblay 2019; Gumbs 2020). In such endeavours, women gather not only to talk, exchange information and strategise, but also to breathe intentionally together. Collective respiration begets inspiration. For one queer Black feminist, it inspires the acknowledgement that breathing is 'beyond species and sentience':

> Is the scale of breathing within one species? All animals participate in this exchange of release for continued life. But not without the plants. The plants, in their inverse process, release what we need, take what we give without being asked. And the planet, wrapped in ocean breathing, breathing into sky.
>
> (Gumbs 2021, p. 20)

Human respiration depends on an exchange of gases that involves – and thereby connects – all planetary life. In her lyrical meditation on breathing, Gumbs explores the fact that marine mammals process air similarly to land mammals (including us) as ammunition against human exceptionalism. Her analysis pushes so far beyond identity politics as to evoke 'trans-species communion' (Gumbs 2021, p. 24), a radically unlimited intimacy. Our mutual dependence on the earth's atmosphere means that the biopolitics of respiration must be acknowledged as a multispecies affair (see Kirksey and Helmreich 2010).

It is perhaps no coincidence that Gumbs, the Black feminist author of reflections on mammalian respiration, is also a poet, since poetry entails hyperawareness of breath, its rhythms, and of a performer's lung capacity. Poetry, in purposefully making art out of breath, contributes to the positive aesthetics of respiration, suggesting how to do things not only with words but also with air (Tremblay 2022). There is power in sharing and in shaping breath together; communities of the breath evoke what barebackers once called communities of the bug. Another poet, Jennifer Scappettone (2018), locates the issue of poetic breath in the context of air pollution: 'Seen not as an empty virtual space but as particulate, air makes for a democracy of harm that has had artists and authors strategizing for remedies for generations – remedies that are always necessarily incomplete' (p. 47). In air contaminated by particulate matter, whether from factories or wildfires, we now appreciate the additional threat of airborne viruses. Ironically, an in-person poetry reading, once a vital source of community, may serve in the age of COVID-19 as a 'super-spreader' event. If it has become harder to disentangle the negative from the affirmative poles of respiratory biopolitics, then this may be because the atmosphere we breathe intersects with what we are coming to understand as the virosphere. We inhabit – and are inhabited by – both spheres at once.

Healthy human beings carry approximately 174 different species of virus in their lungs alone, most of whose functions are still unknown (Willner et al. 2009). It is not only that millions of viral species remain unfathomed by science, but also that viruses equivocate standard biological definitions of life; we live with them, vastly outnumbered, while barely knowing them at all. The history of virology manifests successive instances of viruses escaping each and every category through which the scientific mind attempts to comprehend them. Part of 'us' – ancient viral DNA constitutes a significant percentage of the human genome – they are nevertheless thoroughly 'other.' And since viruses challenge fundamental human ways of knowing, including scientific epistemologies, it is extremely difficult to discuss them without using metaphors that help us to grasp what they represent even as we thereby misconstrue their nature. Here the distinction between psychical fantasy (understood as irremediably subjective) and the scientific language for describing viruses (understood as unimpeachably objective) becomes wafer-thin.

Given how scientific expertise became snarled up in the culture wars sparked by COVID-19, we need to affirm that acknowledging the extent to which scientists make mistakes does not automatically consign one's critique to the populist 'anti-science' position. Certainly, scientific consensus has always been more open to dispute – primarily by scientists themselves – than the COVID-19-era slogan of 'follow the science' would have us believe. Early in the pandemic, for example, a group of scientists in New Delhi claimed to have discovered through genetic analysis that the novel coronavirus had been bioengineered from HIV (Pradhan et al. 2020). That paper was quickly discredited as junk science, even as researchers in South Africa were registering the intense vulnerability to SARS-CoV-2 of people living with HIV, thanks to the latter's aptitude for compromising human immune systems (Quammen 2022, p. 177). Scientists make mistakes; they routinely revise their findings; and their ways of thinking about viruses may be subject to rigorous critique. Indeed, historian of science Stephan Guttinger (2022) argues that virologists have been working all along with a mistaken ontology, one in which viruses are understood as microscopic entities rather than as ineluctably dynamic processes. Regarding viruses as microscopic entities stabilises them for purposes of comprehension and research but also, Guttinger shows, fundamentally misconstrues them, with a myriad of scientific and social consequences. This 'entification' of complex, multi-dimensional processes cannot help but distort our understanding of the virosphere. The objective-seeming language of virology may turn out to have been hopelessly biased.

That nontrivial bias stems in part from the pervasive problem of anthropomorphism. A team of virologists in Brazil has observed how the science of virology tends to apprehend viruses from an anthropocentric point of view, which inevitably warps perspective (Rodrigues et al. 2017). When we consider the virosphere anthropocentrically, we naturally want to know, first and foremost, which viruses are likely to harm us. From the vantage point of human life, viruses tend to be regarded as potential enemies – as 'foreign invaders' against which we must defend ourselves by every means possible. This view of viruses as foreign to – rather than as part of – the human may be traced to assumptions about immunity as a biological property of individual bodies. Before it became a medical concept at the end of the nineteenth century, immunity was a longstanding legal and political concept that concerned an individual's rights of self-defence against the community. Roberto Esposito (2008, 2011), an Italian philosopher of biopolitics, argues that ancient political ideas about the foreigner and the enemy have been encoded into our biomedical concept of immunity, with profound consequences for understanding how biopower functions in modernity. Following Esposito and Foucault, the cultural historian Ed Cohen (2009) develops the connection between political and medical notions of immunity by showing how the idea of immunity-as-defence became naturalised in modern science. If what we take to be our biological immune systems operate by identifying and rejecting that which is deemed foreign, then the notion of immunity assumes an antagonistic stance towards the question of 'living with' from the outset. Our understanding of the virosphere is distorted by paranoid fantasies that viruses are always our enemy.

An antagonistic approach to the virosphere overlooks all the ways in which, as Eben Kirksey (2022a) says, 'viruses are us' (p. 186). Already among and inside every human body, viruses remain inseparable from Homo sapiens. Yet even those viruses unknown to science need not automatically be considered as foreign; that which is unknown is not inevitably hostile or threatening. The Brazilian virologists who registered the anthropocentric bias of their ostensibly objective discipline contend that 'a huge effort and change in perspective is necessary to see more than the tip of the iceberg when it comes to virology' (Rodrigues et al. 2017, p. 1). We need not only to learn more about viruses but also to fundamentally rethink the paradigms through which we approach them. The anthropologist Heather Paxson (2008) has proposed a notion of *microbiopolitics*, 'to call attention to the fact that dissent over how to live with microorganisms reflects disagreement about how humans ought to live with one another' (p. 16). The *bios* of biopolitics is replete with microbes, including viruses, just as our biosphere encompasses the virosphere. Perhaps, in the end, viruses may be useful for their capacity to confound the antagonistic us-versus-them mentality on which the concept of immunity is based. Viruses are us and not-us simultaneously.

The COVID-19 pandemic has made it plain that how we think about virality is shaped but not totally determined by scientific ways of knowing. I have suggested that viruses, in their equivocation of boundaries between inside and outside the human body (as well as their controverting the distinction between me and not-me), remain susceptible to the workings of psychical fantasy. Although fantasy frequently functions as a defence against unwelcome realities, it also bears the potential for creative thinking about phenomena that remain invisible to the naked eye: not all fantasies are paranoid. One example of that creative thinking would be those subcultural fantasies that treat the human immunodeficiency virus less as an enemy to be feared than as a friend to be embraced. Indeed, it is not only bugchasers but also distinguished researchers who aspire to invert the enemy-friend polarity when it comes to conceptualising human–virus relationships. In her work on HIV, for example, the French anthropologist Charlotte Brives (2017) advances a model of 'reciprocal domestication' to describe the ongoing symbiosis that may develop between virus and host. Picturing viruses 'as companion species,' Brives joins scholars who are trying to transcend the antagonistic us-versus-them mindset that otherwise constrains thinking about virality.

Unfortunately, however, the companion-species approach to viruses risks simply inverting the enemy-friend polarity without effectively dislodging its terms – terms we've inherited from classical political philosophy that have been the source of so many problems in our attempts at living with others, human and non-human. Derived from Donna Haraway's (2003) pioneering work, the companion-species approach has been extended to viruses by anthropologists such as Brives (2017) and Kirksey (2022a, 2022b), among others. The scientific conceptualisation of immunity has made it extremely challenging to conceive of viruses outside a friend-or-foe paradigm; and this is as true of SARS-CoV-2 as it has been of HIV. Even Kendi's characterisation of racism as 'the original American virus' relies on the metaphor of virus as an obstacle to human flourishing and racial justice: he keeps viruses in the 'enemy zone.'

If we cannot evade metaphorical conceptions of viruses, then perhaps we can creatively elaborate them beyond the binary friend-or-foe framework that currently dominates, as it distorts, our thinking. Guttinger (2022) warns that 'talk of "good" or "bad" viruses [...] should not tempt us to split the microbial world into two well-defined parts.' Counselling against such dualistic thinking, he insists that

> there is no essence of the pathogen, or the 'good' microbe for that matter. Microbes are constantly evolving entities that are shaped by their interactions with their host and their ecological context. Recognizing this empirical fact undermines any strict pathogen/nonpathogen distinction. Other dualities such as friend/foe, war/peace, or probiosis/antibiosis also turn out to be too narrow.

I would describe this as a psychoanalytic insight, insofar as it encapsulates how we may get a better handle on the virosphere by relinquishing our all-too-human tendency to apprehend it through the infantile duality of 'good' versus 'bad.' Despite the binary schemas with which we categorise in order to comprehend, the universe ultimately remains indivisible into good and bad breasts. Although poor consolation, it helps to bear in mind that virtually the sum total of those highly complex social and viral worlds we inhabit is neither our friend nor our enemy.

Postscript: Thinking analogically

This chapter has argued that the language we use to describe viruses determines how we think about them, and that how we think about viruses largely determines how we go about living with them: the ethics of *Mitsein* flows from our evolving epistemologies of the virosphere. Allow me to clarify that, by situating COVID-19 in the context of a sexual subculture that emerged from the HIV epidemic, I have not been suggesting we should go ahead and eroticise SARS-CoV-2 but, rather, that models of coexistence based on something like an ethics of hospitality may be relevant to thinking post-anthropocentric multispecies sustainability in the twenty-first century. For me, barebacking has always been significant above all as a *figure* for the ethics of openness or radical vulnerability to the other, including non-human alterity (Dean 2009, pp. 176–212). As an erotic practice in which a layer of protection is deliberately renounced, barebacking may serve as a metaphor for dismantling the barriers that divide us from each other. 'Unlimited intimacy,' in one sense a promiscuous fantasy, evokes on another level the ethics of being-with.

If we grant, at least provisionally, that the lasting significance of bareback sex lies in its metaphoricity, then this returns us to the meta-question of discussing one virus or pandemic in terms of another – the question, that is, of discerning similarities or kinship between ostensibly disparate phenomena. How does one thing – particularly when lived viscerally through human bodies in all their variation and frailty – become a metaphor, allegory or analogy for something else? The issue of how certain illnesses, notably cancer and AIDS, take on the burden of conveying invidious moral meanings has been treated at length by Susan Sontag (1978, 1989) and others. I am after something else. Having registered some of the intransigent problems of apprehending viruses metaphorically – by biomedical experts no less than by the lay public – I want to examine what's at stake, ethically and epistemologically, in analogical thinking.

When, in July 2022, another friend – this one a distinguished historian – read an earlier version of the present chapter alongside my recent book, *Hatred of Sex*, her summary verdict was: 'You do love an analogy, don't you?' It was clear from the drift of our discussion that the remark was not meant as a compliment. From her perspective, it appeared that my penchant for analogical thinking was a source of my work's limitations. The objection took me by surprise in part because my friend had just pointed out a likeness — between the mode of argumentation in *Hatred of Sex* and that in 'Barebacking in Restaurants' – of which I had been blithely unaware until that moment.[8] She opened our conversation by identifying an analogy between the two pieces of writing and then, paradoxically, specified analogical thinking as the root of the problem. At the time, I did not have the wherewithal to notice that she was engaged in analogical thinking even as she was objecting to it. And, of course, she was spot-on: I *do* love an analogy.

If we were to reframe this exchange slightly and say that I love sameness or 'homo-ness' – that I like how likenesses hold a capacity to equivocate the straitjacketing binarism of identity/difference – then we would glimpse the significance of analogical thinking for queer critique. There exists a substantial genealogy, in queer theory and criticism, of recuperating analogical thinking for counter-normative hermeneutic protocols and radical sexual politics. As Monique Wittig (1992) argued, mainstream culture's devaluing of similarity or likeness vis-à-vis difference – particularly the sexual difference that underwrites heterosexuality – stems from intransigently heteronormative assumptions (pp. 21–32). Indeed, same-sex kinship arrangements have always been derogated as poor imitations – or corrupt likenesses – of normative heterosexual formations that are predicated on recognisable axes of difference. As a marker of sameness, the 'homo' in homosexuality has been understood as a sign of failure: psychological maturity is believed to entail the capacity to engage with difference and diversity (Warner 1990). Even in our era of amplified social tolerance for homosexuality – at least in its sanitised versions – the mantra of 'difference' continues unabated; the revamped ideal of inclusivity depends on human variation being clearly demarcated via the segregating logics of difference and identity. Still hegemonic, difference is widely assumed to be politically and ethically superior to sameness.

In the face of a crushing consensus about the priorities of difference, one strand of queer critique has made the case for revaluing sameness. A key figure in the genealogy of analogical thinking is Leo Bersani, who, having excoriated AIDS discourses early in the epidemic (Bersani 1987), segued to developing an affirmative account of sameness based on the 'homo' in homosexuality (Bersani 1995).[9] The ethical value of what he called 'homo-ness' lay in its propensity for dissolving the distinction between identity and difference upon which so many antagonisms depend. This project of 'sameness without identity' (Dean 2002) entails discerning analogies that betoken inexact copies – what Bersani often referred to as 'inaccurate self-replications.'[10] *Homos* contends that 'we exist, in both time and space, in a vast network of *near-sameness*, a network characterized by relations of inaccurate replication' (Bersani 1995, p. 146; original emphasis). It is crucial that the replications be understood as inaccurate, since what distinguishes analogy from metaphor stems from how any likeness or resemblance remains irreducible to identity. Prioritising sameness makes evident that analogical thinking confounds the lures of psychological identification.

The present chapter's thesis depends on a series of analogies – between sex without condoms and socialising without masks, between sexual and respiratory forms of intimacy, between respiratory illness and sociopolitical predations on breathing, between various paradigms of coexistence – that aim to stimulate reflection on the connections between pandemics. Some of the analogies involve stressing the key difference between airborne and blood-borne viruses, thereby drawing attention to the limits of analogy. What I wish to underscore is how analogical thinking deepens our awareness of human interconnectedness. It is not just that we are connected through the air we share (according to a spherology of 'shared insides') or that the rapid spread of a novel coronavirus has reminded us of how closely linked we are with those who inhabit distant corners of the globe. We are connected not only to other humans, who may be more or less like us, but also to the radically other – the virosphere – whose features make us less like ourselves than we typically imagine. Thinking in terms of the virosphere has the salutary effect of defamiliarising our habits of perception, which almost invariably centralise the human.

To consider viruses as somehow resembling us would be to reinstate the anthropocentric perspective we have been trying to dislodge. The purpose of analogical thinking is not ultimately to notice similarities between entities – such as the echoes of one pandemic in another – but to intuit the manifold relations among superficially dissimilar phenomena. This is what the aesthetic theorist Kaja Silverman (2015) describes as 'the miracle of analogy': once we appreciate 'that each of us is a node in a vast constellation of analogies,' we may grasp how 'everything [bears] the same ontological weight' (p. 11). At bottom, analogical thinking is an ontological equaliser; it disrupts our familiar hierarchies. If respiration connects all planetary life through the medium of the atmosphere, then it also discloses our entwinement with viral being. The COVID-19 pandemic has made vitally apparent, for those who care to see it, the fact that 'unlimited intimacy' was never only for gay men.

Notes

1 An earlier version of this chapter appeared under the title 'Barebacking in restaurants and other fantasies of the virosphere' in *e-flux Journal* (Dean 2022). Thanks to the journal editors and Antoinette Burton, Lucinda Cole, Jaime García-Iglesias, Eben Kirksey and Ramón Soto-Crespo for feedback on various drafts. The previously published version has been substantially reworked and updated for this volume.

2 See Quammen (2022) for a judicious assessment of the diverse scientific explanations for the emergence of SARS-CoV-2, including strong evidence for two roughly simultaneous discrete sites of emergence.

3 On the complex role of racism and racialisation in COVID-19, see Garcia et al. (2021), Grey et al. (2023), Johnson (2020) and Kendi (2021).

4 Fantasy (or 'phantasy') remains a key category in the Freudian, Kleinian, Lacanian and Laplanchean psychoanalytic traditions, though each of them conceptualises it somewhat differently. Here I am concerned less with technical distinctions than with using 'fantasy' to designate the human mind's strategies for handling what may be unknowable and deflecting that which it would prefer not to know.

5 Treasure Island Media, the San Francisco-based porn company most closely associated with bareback subculture, originally represented its product as a documentary form (see Dean 2009, pp. 97–144).

6 In the decades since my initial research, as Jaime García-Iglesias (2022) and others have elaborated, the practice of unprotected anal sex among gay men has become less subcultural and more mainstream. García-Iglesias' research is especially valuable for insisting that, despite this mainstreaming, the fantasies animating bareback sex have not disappeared, even as infection risk has diminished. The notion of risk cannot be reduced to its epidemiological dimension without losing sight of what motivates 'unprotected' sex among men who have sex with men.

7 In 2023, the US Centers for Disease Control and Prevention announced guidelines for DoxyPEP, a new post-exposure prophylaxis to prevent non-viral STIs such as syphilis, gonorrhoea and Chlamydia. This new form of PEP repurposes doxycycline, a common antibiotic, as a 'morning-after pill' (Nirappil 2023).

8 The analogy that motivates *Hatred of Sex* is between Jacques Rancière's political philosophy of the constitutive disorder of democracy and Jean Laplanche's psychoanalytic account of a fundamental perturbation at the heart of human sexuality (Davis and Dean 2022).

9 The difference paradigm has been challenged by a generation of queer theorists after Bersani (Dean 2002; Tuhkanen 2014; Flatley 2017; Khalip and Ricco 2023), but also by a range of aesthetic theorists working independently of queer critique (Stafford 1999; Silverman 2009, 2015; Zhang 2020).

10 Bersani's insistence on the language of replication (rather than that of reproduction) appears prescient, since 'inaccurate self-replication' also describes how viruses multiply inside their hosts, mutating as they make copies of themselves replete with transcription errors.

References

Berardi, F., 2018. *Breathing: Chaos and poetry*. South Pasadena, CA: Semiotexte.

Bersani, L., 1987. Is the rectum a grave? *October*, 43, 197–222.

Bersani, L., 1995. *Homos*. Cambridge, MA: Harvard University Press.

Boyle, M., Hickson, J., and Ujhelyi Gomez, K., 2022. *COVID-19 and the case against neoliberalism: The United Kingdom's political pandemic*. Cham, Switzerland: Palgrave Macmillan.

Brives, C., 2017. From fighting against to becoming with: Viruses as companion species. *HAL: Open Science*, 1, June. Available from: https://hal.archives-ouvertes.fr/hal-01528933

Cohen, E., 2009. *A body worth defending: Immunity, biopolitics, and the apotheosis of the modern body*. Durham, NC: Duke University Press.

Crimp, D., 1987. How to have promiscuity in an epidemic. *October*, 43, 237–271.

Davis, O., and Dean, T., 2022. *Hatred of sex*. Lincoln: University of Nebraska Press.

Dean, T., 2002. Sameness without identity. *Umbr(a): A Journal of the Unconscious*, 1, 25–41.

Dean, T., 2008. Breeding culture: Barebacking, bugchasing, giftgiving. *Massachusetts Review*, 49 (1–2), 80–94.

Dean, T., 2009. *Unlimited intimacy: Reflections on the subculture of barebacking*. Chicago: University of Chicago Press.

Dean, T., 2015. Mediated intimacies: Raw sex, Truvada, and the biopolitics of chemoprophylaxis. *Sexualities*, 18 (1&2), 224–246.

Dean, T., 2022. Barebacking in restaurants and other fantasies of the virosphere. *e-flux Journal*, 130. www.e-flux.com/journal/130/491394/barebacking-in-restaurants-and-other-fantasies-of-the-virosphere/

DiCaglio, S., 2021. Breathing in a pandemic: Covid-19's atmospheric fictions. *Configurations*, 29 (4), 375–387.

Esposito, R., 2008. *Bios: Biopolitics and philosophy*. T. Campbell trans. Minneapolis: University of Minnesota Press.

Esposito, R., 2011. *Immunitas: The protection and negation of life*. Z. Hanafi trans. Cambridge: Polity Press.

Flatley, J., 2017. *Like Andy Warhol*. Chicago: University of Chicago Press.

Florêncio, J., 2020. *Bareback porn, porous masculinities, queer futures: The ethics of becoming-pig*. London: Routledge.

Foucault, M., 2003. *'Society must be defended': Lectures at the Collège de France, 1975–1976*. M. Bertani and A. Fontana, eds. D. Macey trans. New York: Picador.

Freud, S., 1919. The 'Uncanny'. *The standard edition of the complete psychological works of Sigmund Freud*. Vol. XVII. J. Strachey, ed. and trans. London: Hogarth Press, 217–252.

Garcia, M.A., et al., 2021. The color of Covid-19: Structural racism and the disproportionate impact of the pandemic on older Black and Latinx adults. *Journals of Gerontology, Series B*, 76 (3), 75–80. 10.1093/geronb/gbaa114

García-Iglesias, J., 2022. *The eroticizing of HIV: Viral fantasies*. Cham, Switzerland: Palgrave Macmillan.

Garrett, L., 1994. *The coming plague: Newly emerging diseases in a world out of balance*. New York: Penguin.

Greenhalgh, T., et al., 2021. Ten scientific reasons in support of airborne transmission of SARS-CoV-2. *The Lancet*, 397, 1603–1605.

Grey, C., et al., 2023. Unpacking racism during COVID-19: Narratives from racialized Canadian gay, bisexual, and queer men. *International Journal for Equity in Health*, 22 (152). 10.1186/s12939-023-01961-z

Gumbs, A.P., 2020. *Undrowned: Black feminist lessons from marine mammals*. Chico, CA: AK Press.

Gumbs, A.P., 2021. Undrowned: Black feminist lessons from marine mammals: Why we need to learn to listen, breathe and remember, across species, across extinctions and across harm. *Soundings: A Journal of Politics and Culture*, 78, 20–37.

Guttinger, S., 2022. Viral things: Twelve keywords. *e-flux Journal*, 130. www.e-flux.com/journal/130/491396/viral-things-twelve-keywords/

Haraway, D., 2003. *The companion species manifesto: Dogs, people, and significant otherness*. Chicago: Prickly Paradigm Press.

Hegarty, P., and Rollins, J., 2021. Viral forgetting, or how to have ignorance in a syndemic. *Culture, Health & Sexuality*, 23 (11), 1545–1558.

Johnson, A.S., 2020. From HIV-AIDS to Covid-19: Black vulnerability and medical uncertainty. *African American Intellectual History Society*, 15 June. www.aaihs.org/from-hiv-aids-to-covid-19-black-vulnerability-and-medical-uncertainty/

Kendi, I.X., 2021. We still don't know who the coronavirus's victims were. *The Atlantic*, 2 May. www.theatlantic.com/ideas/archive/2021/05/we-still-dont-know-who-the-coronaviruss-victims-were/618776/

Khalip, J., and Ricco, J.P., 2023. Homoverse. *Differences: A Journal of Feminist Cultural Studies*, 34 (1), 1–5.

Kirksey, S.E., and Helmreich, S., 2010. The emergence of multispecies ethnography. *Cultural Anthropology*, 25 (4), 545–576.

Kirksey, E., 2022a. Virology. In E. Coccia, ed. *Unknown unknowns: An introduction to mysteries*. Milan: Triennale Milano XXIII International Exhibition Catalogue, 178–194.

Kirksey, E., 2022b. Editorial: Welcome to the Virosphere. *e-flux Journal*, 130. www.e-flux.com/journal/130/491400/editorial-welcome-to-the-virosphere/

Lacan, J., 2006. The subversion of the subject and the dialectic of desire in the Freudian unconscious. *Écrits: The first complete edition in English*. B. Fink trans. New York: Norton, 671–702.

Mandavilli, A., 2022. The U.S. may be losing the fight against monkeypox, scientists say. *New York Times*, 8 July. www.nytimes.com/2022/07/08/health/monkeypox-vaccine-treatment.html

Mandavilli, A., 2023. Expert panel recommends new options for H.I.V. prevention. *New York Times*, 22 August. www.nytimes.com/2023/08/22/health/hiv-prep-truvada-descovy.html

Nirappil, N., 2023. A morning-after pill to stop STIs could also make the problem worse. *Washington Post*, 24 July. www.washingtonpost.com/politics/2023/07/24/morning-after-pill-stop-stis-could-also-make-problem-worse/

Paxson, H., 2008. Post-Pasteurian cultures: The microbiopolitics of raw-milk cheese in the United States. *Cultural Anthropology*, 23 (1) 15–47.

Pradhan, P., et al., 2020. Uncanny similarity of unique inserts in the 2019-nCoV spike protein to HIV-1 gp120 and Gag. Preprint, bioRxiv, posted 31 January.

Quammen, D., 2022. *Breathless: The scientific race to defeat a deadly virus*. New York: Simon and Schuster.

Rodrigues, R.A.L., et al., 2017. An anthropocentric view of the virosphere-host relationship. *Frontiers in Microbiology*, 8, 1673. 10.3389/fmicb.2017.01673.

Rose, J., 1998. *States of fantasy*. Oxford: Clarendon Press.

Rose, J., 2023. *The plague: Living death in our times*. New York: Farrar, Straus and Giroux.

Scappettone, J., 2018. Precarity shared: Breathing as tactic in air's uneven commons. In M.M. Kim and C. Miller, eds. *Poetics and precarity*. Albany: State University of New York Press, 41–58.

Silverman, K., 2009. *Flesh of my flesh*. Stanford, CA: Stanford University Press.

Silverman, K., 2015. *The miracle of analogy, or, the history of photography, part 1.* Stanford, CA: Stanford University Press.

Sloterdijk, P., 2014. *Spheres, vol. 2: Globes.* W. Hoban trans. South Pasadena, CA: Semiotexte.

Sontag, S., 1978. *Illness as metaphor.* New York: Farrar, Straus and Giroux.

Sontag, S., 1989. *AIDS and its metaphors.* New York: Farrar, Straus and Giroux.

Stafford, B.M., 1999. *Visual analogy: Consciousness as the art of connecting.* Cambridge, MA: MIT Press.

Tremblay, J.-T., 2019. Feminist breathing. *Differences: A Journal of Feminist Cultural Studies*, 30 (3), 92–117.

Tremblay, J.-T., 2022. *Breathing aesthetics.* Durham, NC: Duke University Press.

Tufekci, Z., 2021. Why did it take so long to accept the facts about Covid? *New York Times*, 7 May. www.nytimes.com/2021/05/07/opinion/coronavirus-airborne-transmission.html.

Tuhkanen, M., 2014. Homomonadology: Leo Bersani's essentialism. *Differences: A Journal of Feminist Cultural Studies*, 25 (2), 62–100.

Varghese, R., ed., 2019. *Raw: PrEP, pedagogy, and the politics of barebacking.* Saskatchewan: University of Regina Press.

Warner, M., 1990. Homo-narcissism; or, heterosexuality. In J.A. Boone and M. Cadden, eds. *Engendering men: The question of male feminist criticism.* New York: Routledge, 190–206.

Warner, M., 1999. *The trouble with normal: Sex, politics, and the ethics of queer life.* New York: Free Press.

Watney, S., 1987. *Policing desire: Pornography, AIDS and the media.* London: Methuen.

Willner, D., et al., 2009. Metagenomic analysis of respiratory tract DNA viral communities in cystic fibrosis and non-cystic fibrosis individuals. *PLoS ONE*, 4 (10), e7370. 10.1371/journal.pone.0007370.

Wittig, M., 1992. *The straight mind and other essays.* Boston: Beacon Press.

Wright, L., 2021. *The plague year: America in the time of Covid.* New York: Knopf.

Zhang, D., 2020. *Strange likeness: Description and the modernist novel.* Chicago: University of Chicago Press.

Žižek, S., 1997. *The plague of fantasies.* London: Verso.

Part II
Biomedicalisation

7 How to survive *another* plague

Autoethnographic reflections on antiviral medication, cultural memory and dystopian metaphor

Max Morris

Introduction

All of us have memories of defining moments during the early days of the COVID-19 pandemic. Sometimes these 'scenes' flash across my mind like the opening credits of a dystopian film. 'Multiple countries close their borders', a newsreader announced as I turned to my boyfriend and said, 'This looks like a clichéd apocalypse movie' (Notes, 26 February 2020). A few days later, the World Health Organization (WHO) officially declared that COVID-19 was a 'pandemic', and I wrote, 'The similarities with past events are familiar and frightening' (Notes, 11 March 2020). As the number of global deaths surpassed 250,000, I celebrated my 29th birthday during the first 'official lockdown' in the UK, having already been wary of leaving my London flat 'due to underlying health conditions – asthma, diabetes, and HIV' (Notes, 19 May 2020). Another vivid memory I have is of staring at the bathroom ceiling and saying to myself, 'If you survived *that*, then you can survive *this*' (Notes, 17 July 2020), reflecting on personal experiences of being marginalised and stigmatised after my HIV diagnosis (see Morris 2021 for a further discussion of this).

The title of this chapter draws inspiration from the documentary *How to Survive a Plague*, alongside a non-fiction book of the same title by David France (2016), which provided a first-hand account of how activists and scientists responded to 'a cataclysmic plague' in the 1980s and 1990s (p. 84). As a book of 640 pages (including photographs) and a documentary of 110 minutes, I do not have space here to comment on every metaphor or theme which these important works drew upon. Therefore, I focus my attention on how the term 'plague' situates this real-world narrative within a dystopian frame of modern anxieties and existential fears (Leavy 1992). For example, although it was not included in the book, a defining scene from the documentary (which perhaps inspired its title) was when Larry Kramer, a founder of ACT UP (the AIDS Coalition To Unleash Power), interrupted the group's factional divisions by shouting: 'Plague! We are in the middle of a fucking plague. And you behave like this. Plague! Forty million infected people is a fucking plague. And nobody acts as [if] it is … Nothing is working'. A decade after the first AIDS cases were reported in the USA, the

DOI: 10.4324/9781003322788-9

metaphor of plague was used here to emphasise the scale, duration and devastation of the virus. It would take another five years before highly effective antiretroviral medications became available, meaning 'that those who test positive for HIV can expect long and healthy lives' (Ashford et al. 2020, p. 600). By comparison, as we enter the fourth year of COVID-19, the number of daily deaths has been reduced dramatically by much earlier medical interventions.

Bringing together memories of AIDS from France (2016), experiences of COVID-19 from my own notes, and cultural texts which have relevance to the themes of 'plague' and 'dystopia', this chapter builds on an article (Morris 2021) I wrote for a special issue of the journal *Culture, Health and Sexuality* on 'Viral Times: Rethinking COVID-19 and HIV'. The editors of that issue suggested that throughout 'the entirety of the COVID-19 pandemic, there has always been a personal sense of memory' (García-Iglesias et al. 2021, p. 1466). My contribution adopted the method of autoethnography – an approach to storytelling which includes 'artistic and analytic demonstrations of how we come to know, name, and interpret personal and cultural experience' (Adams et al. 2015, p. 1) – to consider how the ideas of (queer) anthropologists in the 1980s (e.g. Rubin 1984) could be applied to the 2020s. In this sense, my research responded to Kagan's (2018) question about the role of (mis)remembering the past to (re)interpret current events:

> If we consider it axiomatic that cultural memory functions as a means of producing and negotiating a contemporary cultural presence, then what do the ways in which AIDS history is being told indicate about queer politics and culture in the present?
>
> (Kagan 2018, p. 208)

Alongside the cultural texts I draw on in the chapter, as an autoethnographer, my approach can be juxtaposed with modernist methods that have 'constructed metanarratives, in the form of big stories about the medical, social, technological "progress" of society' (Morris 2021, p. 1489). In short, I use autoethnography as a *postmodern* or *queer* method which aligns with the politics of activists who were a part of ACT UP.

Having previously examined the role of horror metaphors for making sense of viral pandemics (see Sontag 1988), one reason for writing this new chapter became clear when I was reading back over my digital diary – a 'patchwork of sources' (Morris 2021, p. 1491) including 'scattered conversations, posts on social media, and other reflections' (p. 1497) collected over recent years – when I noticed that while I had used the word *horror* only 15 times, the word *dystopia* appeared 45 times. For comparison, the words (post)*modern*, *modernist* and *modernity* appeared 50 times, the words *bureaucracy*, *bureaucrat* and *bureaucratic* appeared 58 times, and the words *vulnerable* and *vulnerability* appeared 75 times. As such, these terms form the major themes around which this chapter is structured, following a brief discussion of how the genres of horror and dystopia may help us to analyse AIDS and COVID-19 as 'plagues', whatever this much used metaphor may mean for the present moment.

The horror of plague(s)

The bubonic plague – which numerous metaphorical uses of the term tend to refer to – was significant for Foucault's (1978) theorisation of biopower. He suggested that the emerging methods of modernism, including population measurement and panoptic surveillance, could be seen in the seventeenth century when describing 'the measures to be taken when the plague appeared', including 'a prohibition to leave the town' which was 'under surveillance' and where 'everyone is ordered to stay indoors', adding that: 'Each individual is fixed in his place. And, if he moves, he does so at the risk of his life, contagion or punishment' (Foucault 1978, p. 195). I have noted elsewhere that there was a 'parallel' between this characterisation of the plague and lockdown measures introduced during COVID-19 which 'confined most of us to home' (Morris 2021, p. 1498). Although the punishment for leaving one's home was not necessarily death (for most people), the fear of contagion was felt more acutely amongst those of us who were instructed to 'stay at home' in the UK because we were designated as 'clinically extremely vulnerable patient[s]' by the Department of Health and Social Care (Email, 18 March 2021). Around this time, I wrote, 'This fills me with horror' (Notes, 16 April 2021) and 'I have been waking up every day this week with a sense of existential dread, precipitated by the pandemic, and confronted by my own mortality' (Notes, 23 April 2021).

In *How to Survive a Plague*, France's (2016) description of AIDS had a similar sense of foreboding horror, especially where the language of *plague* took precedence: 'the shadow of plague' (p. 80), 'the bloom of plague' (p. 90) and 'the world of the plague' (p. 150). Being based in New York City, 'the epicentre of the plague' (p. 61) or 'the heart of the epidemic' (France 2016, p. 316), it is perhaps unsurprising that France drew on the imagery of himself orbiting an ominous entity, 'the core of the plague' (p. 87), 'the middle of the gay plague was unfathomable and disastrous' (p. 136), something which he was glad to remain distant from: 'I stood on the sidewalks of the plague, grateful to not enter its tower' (p. 149). This metaphor made me think of Kafka's (1926) *The Castle*, whose protagonist circles around a village, unable to access or hold accountable the authority figures represented by the castle, providing a parable for the horror of modern faceless bureaucracies. As the epidemic expanded, France moved closer and closer to this sense of impending doom as friends and lovers began to die, eventually finding himself trapped within it: 'Life inside the plague's bubble left little time or inclination for mourning' (France 2016, p. 433). Although I do not have space to discuss military imagery in sufficient depth – something which Sontag (1988) critiqued for stigmatising those who tested positive – war was another metaphor repeatedly used by France (2016): 'On the battlefield, one cannot step over so many bodies without imagining one's own lifeless cheek on the ground' (p. 434). Focusing on my own experiences with HIV and COVID-19, three or four decades after the events documented by France, I nonetheless related to his senses of fear and fate.

Previously, I have drawn on a 'mix of horror metaphors ... alien, vampire, werewolf, zombie' (Morris 2021, p. 1493) to examine how viruses are often constructed as dystopian in the cultural imaginary (see Hart 2018). For example, both the former and latter monsters could easily be characterised as existing within worlds which have been distorted by a natural disaster or unnatural cataclysm. A related theme I mentioned here was 'body horror' which, alongside paranoia, provided part of the chilling effect found in films such as *Invasion of the Body Snatchers* (1978), *Dawn of the Dead* (1978), and *They Live* (1988), where aliens or zombies represent an existential threat to – or perhaps liberation from – the conventional social order (see Dendle 2007). Alongside the real-world body horrors of AIDS mentioned by France (2016) – including the 'misshapen purple blobs, some with deeply colored centers, sprouting against freckled white flesh' (p. 70) of Kaposi's sarcoma – he also mentioned feelings of paranoia early in the epidemic:

> I withdrew my hand and saw that it was red with blood, my heart pounded. I lurched for the kitchen sink and repeatedly splashed myself with antibacterial soap, wringing my hands like Macbeth's widow and scrutinizing my flesh for cuts and abrasions, weaknesses the virus might exploit.
>
> (France 2016, p. 285)

In the context of COVID-19, alongside government instructions to wash our hands and wear face masks, many of us took additional steps to ensure hygiene which, looking back, may seem delusional, including 'scrubbing supermarket deliveries with soap and water, which had next to no preventative purpose for a respiratory virus, but became a habit for the better part of two years' (Notes, 1 November 2022). Like France, I became fixated on changes in my own body and developed a form of paranoia around breathing the same air as other people. For example, I had to leave a pub lunch with my boyfriend 'because a small child was coughing nearby', adding, 'I think I will carry a form of post-traumatic stress about breathing the same air as people who are coughing for a long time. It makes me jump and search for the nearest exit' (Notes, 8 October 2022). Moving beyond individual expressions of disgust, fear and paranoia *about the virus*, however, France also highlights the wider cultural, economic and political effects *of the virus*.

As a genre closely related to horror and science-fiction, dystopia has several distinctive features which make it useful for making sense of global events such as pandemics. One of these features is the scale of the horror. While an individual alien or zombie can be scary, they take on a different form of menace as a collective horde, becoming a threat to civilisation itself. As I wrote, 'I'm reminded of the crushing horror of the pandemic' (Notes, 26 June 2021) in part due to its density and weight, something massive, global in scale and impact for our species. Another feature of dystopia is that the fear is not immediate (as with a jump scare) but builds gradually, growing exponentially, towards doom of a greater order of magnitude. It is for these reasons that I have chosen to focus on dystopia as a unique form of horror to elaborate on how recent viral epidemics and pandemics may help us to make sense of modernity and neoliberalism as dominant ideologies.

Dystopia and bureaucratic modernity

Another feature of dystopian fiction is its critique of the defining aspects of late modernity from corporate plate glass skyscrapers to pervasive surveillance systems to burgeoning state bureaucracies. These themes provide a different kind of chilling effect, as found in novels such as *The Trial* (1925), *Brave New World* (1932), and *1984* (1948), among the most famous dystopian worlds in which inescapable systems of modern bureaucracy, medicalisation, and surveillance (i.e. 'Big Brother is watching you') provide the context, alongside their screen adaptations and in other films such as *Brazil* (1985), whose protagonist tries to escape 'from a mindless state-sponsored bureaucracy that threatens creativity, innovation and original thought' (Melton and Sterling 2013, p. 66). As Kafka, Huxley, Orwell and Gilliam did with these cultural texts, I turn next to the role of modernity in responding to pandemics by viewing people's lives and deaths as 'data points', akin to Foucault's (1978) characterisation of biopower emerging in response to a new discursive construction of human beings: 'One of the great innovations in the techniques of power in the 18th century was the emergence of "population" as an economic and political problem … birth and death rates, life expectancy, fertility, state of health, frequency of illness' (p. 25). To measure populations the state required vast bureaux to collect, manage and interpret information, becoming one of the main mechanisms by which biopower replaced sovereign power.

This modernist power provided another distinctively dystopian form of horror: the all-pervasive, genocidal and totalitarian state. The connection between modernism and such forms of governmentality (in the real world) was something Bauman (1988) captured well in his critique of the conventional view that 'the Holocaust was a *failure*, not a *product*, of modernity' (p. 473, original emphasis). It is also worth mentioning here that the Holocaust was another metaphor adopted by ACT UP activists. For example, France (2016) described the first 'SILENCE=DEATH' posters in which the pink triangle was 'inverted – no longer pointing downward like a yield sign' (p. 244), alongside Michael Callen who declared 'AIDS is our Holocaust' (p. 314) during New York City's gay pride rally in 1988, with the AIDS Memorial Quilt on display in Central Park.

Many activists and scientists loom large in France's (2016) account, either as heroes or anti-heroes (Larry Kramer, Joseph Sonnabend, Mark Harrington and Peter Staley among them), but one figure represented the flaws of the modernist state more than any other: Anthony Fauci. Described as 'the most powerful man in the epidemic' (France 2016, p. 181) who 'proved exceptionally adept at … seizing all the ceremonial trappings of authority' (p. 462), Fauci's demeanour and mannerisms characterised him as the personification of the scientific method: cold, rational and utilitarian. For example, he had 'the patronizing smile of a bureaucrat' (France 2016, p. 262) and replied to the demands of activists 'in a tone that was both officious and condescending' (p. 426) or 'with diplomatic obfuscation' (p. 472). Contrasted with the countercultural appearance and performative strategies of queer activists, Fauci was also described as 'ACT UP's chief nemesis' (France 2016, p. 302). Many dystopian texts have been concerned with such figureheads of scientific respectability and state authority as menacing or, perhaps more chillingly, indifferent symbols of modernist power.

The consequences of this bureaucratic approach to 'managing' AIDS were starkly illustrated by the way in which activists were ignored or sidelined by the scientific establishment. Given that one of ACT UP's main mantras was 'drugs into bodies', much of the direct action was aimed at scientists, whether working for governments or pharmaceutical companies. There was an urgency to get as many people onto study trials as possible, anger at the exclusion criteria of some – including 'the near-total exclusion of women, people of color, drug users, and children from the federal trials' (France 2016, p. 327) – and above all dismay at how slow the conventional scientific method was. In 1989, with lukewarm support from Fauci and outright hostility from other members, some activists gained access to a meeting of the AIDS Clinical Trials Group. However, as Mark Harrington reported to an ACT UP meeting (8 January 1990): 'They're not going to be able to start any new trials. They're not doing any opportunistic infection studies. They're at a standstill, *because they're changing their data center!*' France (2016) added, '*Who will be held accountable for these unnecessary deaths*, Harrington wondered, *this slaughter by unaccountable bureaucracy?*' (p. 389, original emphasis). As I have noted elsewhere, in the context of COVID-19 we became familiar with politicians being 'flanked by medical experts' (Morris 2021, p. 1486) and the sense of urgency surrounding behavioural change, national lockdowns and developing antiviral treatments to 'combat' the virus was in stark contrast to how AIDS had been ignored by political and scientific leaders for many years.

Even where Fauci was not singled out, the bureaucracy of the drug administration system and scientific research community were characterised as antithetical to the humanity of those experiencing AIDS by France (2016). For example, in one protest, ACT UP surrounded the Presidential AIDS Commission's meeting hall 'with bullhorns and leaflets while tying themselves together with miles of red tape to protest the bureaucratic morass that mired the epidemic' (France 2016, p. 316), and the government was characterised as a system of 'endless rules, regulations and red tape that are killing thousands … an unresponsive and destructive bureaucracy' (p. 332). Although I do not have space here to recount all of my own fraught experiences with modernist bureaucracy during COVID-19, it was something which I similarly described as 'systems upon systems upon systems of *structural stupidity*' (Notes, 22 April 2021, emphasis added) within the neoliberal economic model of privatised healthcare and welfare. This phrase was borrowed from Graeber's (2015) argument that bureaucratic systems make everyone involved act unintelligently, irrationally and often cruelly. For example, when I had an occupational health assessment to determine whether it was safe for me to return to in-person teaching after 18 months of shielding from COVID-19:

> The assessor said, 'You can't avoid going into work forever, people on the front line have to,' and I replied, 'You mean people working in hospitals, where I spend a lot of time given my health conditions? They're nothing like my workplace! Mask wearing is mandatory, for example.' At another point, the assessor said, 'There's nothing I can do, the government has ended shielding,' so I asked, 'Then what was the point of this assessment?' There was no answer.
>
> (Notes, 10 November 2021)

The 'cost' of this structural stupidity is often 'counted' in human lives, but the unquantifiable misery of it could be considered an emergent property of bureaucratic modernity.

These examples contribute further to my own critique of the 'religion of modernism, which held that science and reason are superior' (Morris 2021, p. 1490), by highlighting their thoughtlessness in response to life and death decision making. Finally, however, it is worth noting that as the bureaucrat-in-chief, Fauci had something of a redemption arc once he began to acknowledge limitations to the scientific method, particularly when it excluded HIV activists (or, as many of them later became, trial subjects). Indeed, in the context of COVID-19, Fauci became something of a hero for confronting President Trump's conspiratorial tendencies surrounding viral transmission and prevention, and he was a prominent voice, positively portrayed in two of France's documentaries, *How to Survive a Plague* (2012) and *How to Survive a Pandemic* (2021). The latter (like this edited collection) explored some of the key similarities and differences between HIV and COVID-19. Despite Fauci being heavily criticised by activist and community groups for his inaction, early on, his interventions in response to COVID-19 have been applauded by many on the political left, while being vilified by many on the political right who were deafeningly silent or virulently homophobic throughout the early years of the HIV epidemic in the USA. Ultimately, for all my critiques of bureaucracy, modernism and utilitarianism, it was scientific advisors and researchers who developed highly effective antiviral treatments in both cases.

Age, vulnerability and neoliberalism

The disaster genre also frequently contains elements of political dystopia and, when some form of global catastrophe provides the justification for an authoritarian regime, vice versa. Both set in eerily familiar near-futures, in *The Handmaid's Tale* (1985) and *Children of Men* (1992), it is the collapse of the world's birth rate which provides context for the cruelty and violence humans inflict on one another, in addition to extremist beliefs and strictly enforced policies around gender and migration. As noted above, this focus on the concept of *population*, including how to measure and control it, is what Foucault (1978) characterised as a distinctively modernist, biopolitical concern. Set in a more distant future, the film version of *Logan's Run* (1976) also centred around the problem of population control, where citizens of a seemingly utopian city encased within a geodesic dome are ritualistically killed ('renewed') when they reach the age of 30 (21 in the novel). The justification for this violent regime, however, is to maintain an equilibrium of resources in response to overpopulation rather than underpopulation. Part of the chilling effect such stories have is related to the social construction of life as a 'natural' and 'normal' process – birth, infancy, childhood, adolescence, adulthood, elderliness and death – where the state's intervention in this stage model is seen as 'unnatural' and 'abnormal'. This can be contrasted with attitudes expressed during COVID-19, where people's vulnerability to the virus due to age or disability was often viewed as a normal feature of risk assessment (Outka 2020).

Throughout *How to Survive a Plague* France (2016) draws attention to the youthfulness of those who died as a result of AIDS: 'He was twenty-eight when he died' (p. 277), 'He died at age thirty-one' (p. 87) and 'On one of the coldest days of the frigid winter, a fungus swept into [his] lungs and claimed his life at age thirty-three' (p. 335). As a queer person around the same age, it is difficult not to connect with the heartache France felt at the 'untimely death' of these men (France 2016, p. 519). There is, however, also a troubling if implicit logic at work in the discursive construction of young people as 'innocents'. As I have argued elsewhere, associations between HIV and 'lost youth' continue to shape stigmatising tropes that construct those of us living with the virus: 'the journalist adopted a melancholic tone when saying, "At the age of just twenty-four, Max's world came crashing down" – invoking a sense of lost innocence' (Morris, 2021, p. 1488). The problem with such a construction, in the context of COVID-19, is that it has made the loss of older people's lives seem less worthy of being grieved. As Butler (2016) has argued, in certain contexts (i.e. war), some human lives come to be normatively constructed in an instrumental and utilitarian manner as non-grievable; 'specific lives cannot be apprehended as injured or lost if they are not first apprehended as living' (p. 22). Others have drawn on Butler's concept of grievability to characterise how members of the public, alongside governments, made 'calculations' to reassure themselves that they did not belong to an 'at risk' category during COVID-19, adding that this 'fear may morph into victim blaming, into assumptions that health and even age are somehow a matter of personal responsibility' (Outka 2020). As with HIV, the tendency to blame individuals for characteristics such as age, disability and sexuality can be seen to closely align with neoliberal politics.

The body horror of AIDS (mentioned above) also seemed to 'age' those who France (2016) interacted with – 'in his twenties, but his hair had thinned, his skin had shrunk around his eyes, his chalky knuckle trembled atop the cane' (p. 188) – alongside the city in which he lived, 'where AIDS was now the leading cause of death for all men aged twenty-five to forty-four' (p. 316). It may be useful to draw attention to the dystopian realities of AIDS for certain groups, especially younger gay, bisexual and queer men in urban settings during this period. In addition to the physical markers, there was a change in the geographic landscape which also gave France's (2016) account a dystopian feel: 'There was now a permanent line of wheelchairs outside the Village Nursing Home, where bony young men napped in the sun. The gay bars, which had been the teeming hub of gay society … were now lifeless and ghostly places' (France 2016, p. 286). Images of deserted spaces, often juxtaposed with bustling cosmopolitan cities, are a common motif in dystopian films such as *Escape from New York* (1981) and *Blade Runner* (1982), alongside almost every natural or supernatural disaster film.

Classified as 'clinically extremely vulnerable' by the government, I often found myself surrounded by people four, five or six decades older than me, among the first to be offered vaccines for COVID-19. Occasionally, I encountered forms of resistance on the basis of my youth. For example, at my most recent booster vaccination (offered mainly to people over 50), I was treated with scepticism and 'interrogated' by a queue marshal who 'asked all kinds of questions about whether I was eligible or not … which would not be good for anyone who was less open about their health conditions' (Notes, 6 October 2022). Returning to the theme of age and responsibilisation, it is worth noting that young people were often blamed for the 'spread' of COVID-19 and contrasted with the 'innocence' of elderly people, such as those in care homes. There was significantly less sympathy for the younger people impacted by AIDS during the 1980s and 1990s as detailed by France (2016).

Despite these wider issues of being recognised as 'vulnerable', and therefore 'worthy' of protection, there has also been a difference in timescale for the availability of antiviral treatments for HIV and COVID-19. It took 15 years for highly effective combination therapies to become available for the former, compared with just one year for highly effective mRNA vaccines for the latter, something which was only possible due to ongoing HIV vaccination research. This lag had profound cultural impacts on sexual behaviour and ideology. As France (2016) recounted, people had 'sworn off sex' (p. 44) and the condom code became entrenched as a safe sex message. Adopting a similar level of caution to COVID-19 due to my vulnerability, I have often found myself 'the only person still wearing a mask' in public spaces

(Notes, 29 January 2023). In both cases, however, it has been antiviral medications which provided the 'freedom' to 'return to normal', whether that meant bareback sex or maskless social mixing (Ashford et al. 2020).

These observations led me to reflect on some of my frustrations with the way in which COVID-19 lockdowns were constructed by the government, media, members of the public and even some sexualities scholars who seemed to embrace a more neoliberal ('freedom loving' or 'libertarian') attitude. As I posted: 'I'm really fucking angry. No one needed a haircut. No one needed a pint [of beer]. I needed to see my dying grandmother … I'm not blaming any individual for what's happening, but fuck your economy and fuck your government' (Twitter, 5 July 2020). The following day, I drew attention to queer and feminist scholarship that had problematised the framing of gay men as 'reckless' or 'irresponsible' (e.g. Rubin 1984), when they were the ones who had invented and implemented safe(r) sex in the absence of government interventions, adding:

> Re-reading literature on misplaced fears about another pandemic which 'destroyed' parts of the 1980s queer culture and economy (e.g. sex clubs where transmission was unlikely). Adds to bitterness of normative venues reopening now, when fear is well-placed and transmission likely.
>
> (Twitter, 6 July 2020)

Often it seemed as if cultural memories of this period have tended to focus on government inaction, rather than community action (i.e. changing behaviours to avoid transmission). A key difference between the first few years of AIDS and COVID-19, however, has been which groups were constructed as 'blameworthy' or 'responsible' and 'at risk' or 'vulnerable', but each of these designations has a neoliberal, normative and dystopian dimension to it.

Conclusion

Another book I read in conjunction with France's (2016) *How to Survive a Plague* was Camus's *The Plague* (1947). There are many similarities between the two narratives, including scepticism towards religious authorities who (like neoliberal politicians) sought to blame individuals for their moral 'failures' or 'sins', alongside people's struggle to survive in the midst of a catastrophe. As I wrote, 'In both of these works, the tensions between religious superstition and scientific modernity plays a central role. The very term "plague" conjures up biblical imagery and ideas of divine retribution' (Notes, 5 July 2022). Relatedly, Leavy (1992) has noted that 'it is the word *plague* that, again, has raised specters of a world of sin and damnation, so that the word itself may seem inappropriate today' (p. 4, original emphasis), adding that:

> What constitutes the self and how much importance is given to the individual person (as opposed to the 'idea' of 'man' rejected in Camus's

The Plague) varies from age to age, writer to writer, but consistent in plague literature is the 'I' who strives to survive a deadly danger.

(Leavy 1992, p. 7)

This chapter has drawn on autoethnographic reflections to centre an 'I' who strove to survive COVID-19, placed into conversation with those who strove to survive AIDS. Some of the similarities in these stories include the neoliberal politics of blame, the construction of certain identities as vulnerable or risky and the transformative role of antiviral medications.

Illustrating this last point, while working on revisions to this chapter, the thing I had feared all along happened: I tested positive for COVID-19. Yet, as with access to antiretroviral treatments for HIV, my status as a clinically extremely vulnerable person meant that I had access to antiviral treatments for COVID-19. For the former, a combination of two drugs taken daily (Dovato) means that I can live a long and healthy life and cannot pass HIV on. For the latter, a combination of two drugs taken for five days (Paxlovid) meant that I fully recovered from what was a potentially fatal virus in less than a week. It is important to highlight the significance of *access* in both cases. As I have noted elsewhere, a 'form of chauvinism has emerged around the UK (and other wealthy nations) hoarding COVID-19 vaccinations', and regarding acute antivirals, 'the distribution of medicines is uneven, meaning that people (less privileged than … I) continue to die' (Morris 2021, p. 1495). Our location in time and space is therefore central to our ability to survive.

Another aspect of neoliberalism which warrants further discussion is that we live in a time of unprecedented environmental destruction due to the economic and technological innovations of modernity. Humans have increasingly altered, exploited and encroached on the habitats of other species, something that will make viral outbreaks ever more likely to occur (Ranger et al. 2021). As I said when presenting a preliminary version of this chapter online to the International Symposium on Autoethnography and Narrative:

> I think it is worth nothing that all of this is happening within a context which might be considered dystopian in a broader sense. You know, we are living with the reality of climate change, we are living with global pandemics, alongside other existential fears. And that's the kind of lens through which many of us are trying to interpret our own experiences.
>
> (Morris 2022)

I concluded by suggesting that 'although dystopia is a form of fiction, much of its appeal to audiences lies in identifying real-world injustices, developing empathy with characters as they attempt to "escape" or "survive" inhuman circumstances', adding that, 'such narratives may be used to exist in, but also make sense of, a world where disabled people are treated as lesser beings' within systems of bureaucratic dystopia (Morris 2022).

Finally, it is important to highlight a critique of the dystopia genre itself: namely, that it tends to centre the narratives of characters who belong to socially privileged groups, who are often placed into fictional circumstances which may be more aligned with the real-world experiences of marginalised groups. As I and others have noted, 'these forms of media usually have privileged protagonists, experiencing things which are not uncommon for disabled people, trans and non-binary people, queer people, people of colour, and women to experience daily' (Notes, 17 October 2022). This may be reflective of authorship inequalities and power imbalances in the media industries, given that almost all of the twentieth-century dystopian texts I have drawn on in this chapter were written or directed by abled, cisgender, straight, white men. It is my hope, however, that the dystopia genre has begun to diversify in the twenty-first century, incorporating a wider range of experiences, alongside existential threats which neoliberal bureaucracy poses. Some examples of this include Joon-ho's *Snowpiercer* (2013) and *Parasite* (2019) or Peele's *Get Out* (2017) and *Us* (2019), capturing the classed and racialised dimensions of modernity through dystopian science-fiction horrors, or McKay's *Don't Look Up* (2021), in which an apocalyptic comet serves as a metaphor for politicians and journalists ignoring the threats of climate change. Given that human impacts on the environment are likely to lead to further 'plagues', we may find the narratives of those deemed 'vulnerable', yet who somehow manage to 'survive' useful and uplifting at times, or a sombre warning at others. Although France's book and documentaries used the word *survive*, it is worth remembering that these narratives were not told and could not be heard by those who died. Therefore, as clichéd dystopias sometimes do, I will end on a weary but hopeful thought: 'At the very least we survived it, and if you're reading this, so did you' (Notes, 14 July 2021).

References

Adams, T., Jones, S., and Ellis, C., 2015. *Autoethnography: Understanding qualitative research.* Oxford: Oxford University Press.

Ashford, C., Morris, M., and Powell, A., 2020. Bareback sex in the age of preventative medication: Rethinking the 'harms' of HIV transmission. *The Journal of Criminal Law*, 84 (6), 596–614. 10.1177/0022018320974904

Bauman, Z., 1988. Sociology after the Holocaust. *British Journal of Sociology*, 39 (4), 469–497.

Butler, J., 2016. *Frames of war: When is life grievable?* New York: Verso Books.

Dendle, P., 2007. The zombie as barometer of cultural anxiety. In N. Scott, ed. *Monsters and the monstrous.* Amsterdam: Rodopi, 45–57.

Foucault, M., 1978. *The history of sexuality. Vol. 1.* R. Hurley trans. New York: Pantheon.

France, D., 2016. *How to survive a plague: The story of how activists and scientists tamed AIDS.* London: Picador.

García-Iglesias, J., Nagington, M., and Aggleton, P., 2021. Viral times, viral memories, viral questions. *Culture, Health & Sexuality*, 23 (11), 1465–1469. 10.1080/13691058.2021.1976564

Graeber, D. 2015. *The utopia of rules: On technology, stupidity, and the secret joys of bureaucracy.* Brooklyn: Melville House.

Hart, K., 2018. Ideologically charged urban and rural places in American movies about HIV/AIDS: Social constructionism and the cultural imaginary in the late twentieth century. In S. Allen, and K. Møllegaard, eds. *Narratives of place in literature and film.* Abingdon: Routledge, 171–184.

Kagan, D., 2018. *Positive images: Gay men and HIV/AIDS in the culture of 'post crisis'.* London: Bloomsbury Publishing.

Leavy, B.F., 1992. *To blight with plague: Studies in a literary theme.* New York: NYU Press.

Melton, J., and Sterling, E., 2013. 5: The subversion of happy endings in Terry Gilliam's Brazil. In J. Birkenstein, A. Froula, and K. Rendell, eds. *The cinema of Terry Gilliam.* New York: Columbia University Press, 66–78.

Morris, M., 2021. The politics of testing positive: An autoethnography of media (mis) representations at the 'start' and 'end' of different pandemics. *Culture, Health & Sexuality*, 23 (11), 1485–1499. 10.1080/13691058.2021.1930172

Morris, M., 2022. ISAN 2022 The economics of exclusion. Available from: www.youtube.com/watch?v=75WPTOlwnrI [Accessed 5 June 2023].

Outka, E., 2020. Grievability, COVID-19, and the modernists' pandemic. *Modernism/modernity*, 5 (1). Online article. https://modernismmodernity.org/forums/posts/outka-grievability-covid

Ranger, N., Mahul, O., and Monasterolo, I., 2021. Managing the financial risks of climate change and pandemics: What we know (and don't know). *One Earth*, 4 (10), 1375–1385. 10.1016/j.oneear.2021.09.017

Rubin, G., 1984. Thinking sex: Notes for a radical theory of the politics of sexuality. In C. Vance, ed. *Pleasure and danger: Exploring female sexuality.* London: Pandora Press, 267–319.

Sontag, S., 1988. *AIDS and its metaphors.* New York: Farrar, Straus and Giroux.

8 Thinking with HIV in pandemic times

A diffractive reading of COVID-19 and mpox

Kiran Pienaar and Dean Murphy

Introduction

Discussions of the impacts of infectious disease outbreaks such as COVID-19 and mpox (formerly monkeypox) have been shaped by the pernicious legacies of the HIV epidemic. Despite widespread recognition of the need to avoid exclusionary depictions of 'at-risk' populations and negative tropes such as 'patient zero' and 'covidiots', some public discourses have drawn on responsibilising framings that class certain groups as risky disease vectors who threaten the health of the 'general' public. In this chapter, we consider what lessons can be drawn from the HIV pandemic to understand responses to COVID-19 and mpox. We ask, how can the deleterious effects of stigmatising responses be avoided? Before we address this question and introduce the theoretical work that has guided our thinking, we present some background on COVID-19 and mpox to contextualise the discussion that follows.

At the beginning of 2020, a novel coronavirus, SARS-CoV-2 was identified in China and was soon documented in other settings. Epidemiologists and disease modellers warned that widespread transmission of the new virus was inevitable. In line with this warning, the World Health Organization (WHO) declared COVID-19 a pandemic on 11 March 2020. In Australia, where we are based, physical distancing measures were introduced in mid-March. Within two weeks, the international border had been closed and Australian federal and state governments pursued aggressive viral containment measures. In addition to border closures, these included widespread PCR testing and intensive contract-tracing regimes. Some jurisdictions, notably Melbourne and Sydney, endured strict lockdowns in this early period under a forceful regulatory approach and a policy of viral suppression. This strategy initially appeared successful and in June 2020 state governments began to ease restrictions. However, in late June, a rapid surge in infections prompted the State Premier of Victoria to announce a lockdown for metropolitan Melbourne. Then just over a month later, a state of disaster was declared, imposing tighter restrictions across the state, including confining people to their homes except for essential activities, and imposing a nightly curfew and a five-kilometre radius limit on movement. Importantly, these restrictions had significant implications for

DOI: 10.4324/9781003322788-10

single people living alone and non-heteronormative family configurations as authorities promoted the discrete household or nuclear family as the sole site of safe social contact (Pienaar et al. 2021).

The second phase of the pandemic comprised the rollout of COVID-19 vaccines in early 2021. By December of that year, Australian officials began to acknowledge that suppressing COVID-19 with the goal of no community transmission was no longer feasible and that people should learn to 'live with the virus' (Bennett 2021). By this time, Australia had achieved its double-vaccination target of 90% for people over 16 years, prompting the federal government to initiate a staged reopening plan involving minimal ongoing restrictions and mass home-based self-testing using Rapid Antigen Tests. Daily case numbers in Australia at the time of writing (March 2023) have reduced by approximately 50% since the previous year (March 2022), and experts report higher levels of community immunity through people having been infected, vaccinated or both, with many of those now infected experiencing only mild symptoms (Davey 2022).

Just as COVID-19 vaccinations and infection control measures were building momentum globally, another infectious disease outbreak was declared. On 23 July 2022, the WHO declared mpox (formerly monkeypox) a 'public health emergency of international concern' after infections had rapidly spread since May of that same year (WHO 2023). While many had not heard of mpox before the outbreak, it was not a new virus, having first been identified in 1970. Until 2022, outbreaks had mostly been confined to West and Central Africa with the few cases elsewhere being associated with import- and travel-related spread from endemic countries (Bunge et al. 2022). However, in the short period between May and July 2022, more than 16,000 cases were reported from 75 countries, the majority among gay, bisexual and other men who have sex with men (United Nations News 2022). The prevalence of the outbreak in this population differs from mpox's usual epidemiology, being the first outbreak with no clear links to endemic African countries (Zumla et al. 2022). At the time of writing (20 March 2023), 86,601 confirmed cases have been reported across 110 countries, mostly in Europe and the Americas (WHO 2023). Mpox is mostly spread through close, prolonged skin-to-skin contact and the epidemiology of the current outbreak in non-endemic countries has led some scholars to argue for treating the virus as a sexually transmitted infection (STI) among gay, bisexual and men who have sex with men (García-Iglesias et al. 2022). They suggest that doing so would have clear benefits in terms of developing targeted public health messaging and a nuanced understanding of the sexuality-related stigma imbricated in the current outbreak (García-Iglesias et al. 2022).

How to have theory in a pandemic age

In her groundbreaking book, *How to Have Theory in an Epidemic: Cultural Chronicles of AIDS,* feminist theorist Paula Treichler charts the 'cultural evolution of the AIDS epidemic' (Treichler 1999, p. 1) by drawing attention to the social meanings embedded in scientific discourses about HIV and AIDS. Treichler's formulation of the book's title was an intentional play on Douglas Crimp's (1987) earlier provocation, *How to Have Promiscuity in an Epidemic*, where he suggested AIDS presented an ethical juncture for a 'critical rethinking of all of culture: of language and representation, of science and medicine, of health and illness, of sex and death, of the public and private realms' (Crimp 1987, p. 15). Like Crimp, Treichler recognised the HIV epidemic as an opportunity for critical reflection and social change, characterising it as an 'epidemic of signification' that generated an explosion of media reporting and massive social transformations. Bridging the tension between theory and practice, Treichler presents a compelling case for careful, theoretically informed analysis, even in the midst of an epidemic:

> The AIDS epidemic is cultural and linguistic as well as biological and biomedical. To understand the epidemic's history, address its future, and learn its lessons, we must take this assertion seriously. Moreover, it is the careful examination of language and culture that enables us [...] to think carefully about ideas in the midst of a crisis [...] even as we acknowledge the urgency of the AIDS crisis and try to satisfy its relentless demand for immediate action.
>
> (Treichler 1999, pp. 1–2)

Lest she be misread as arguing for the pursuit of theory as a purely academic exercise divorced from the often tragic realities of the HIV epidemic, Treichler emphasises that the exigencies of the epidemic put 'theory stringently to the test, serving as a useful and often dramatic corrective for inadequate theoretical formulations' (1999, p. 2). In this respect, far from being irrelevant to practice, the theoretical engagements for which she argues are deeply embedded in the embodied experiences of HIV. As she stresses, 'theory *is* about "people's lives"' and we need to critically examine the sociocultural dimensions of the epidemic if we are to develop culturally informed, socially responsive interventions (Treichler 1999, p. 4, emphasis added).

Treichler's work has inspired a range of contemporary analyses of the COVID-19 pandemic, some riffing off her original book title (see e.g. Anderson 2021, *The Model Crisis, or How to Have Critical Promiscuity in the Time of COVID-19*; and Brown et al. 2021, *How to Have Theory in a Pandemic: A Critical Reflection on the Discourses of COVID-19*). Like this work, we draw on Treichler's influential account to chart the legacies of history, particularly the history of HIV, that have shaped responses to COVID-19 and the recent outbreak of mpox. We suggest that historically grounded engagements with HIV have the potential to inform more nuanced responses to contemporary disease outbreaks, responses that are alive to the social and cultural logics of epidemiological conceptions of disease.

Theoretical approach: A diffractive reading of viral outbreaks

To make our argument, we draw on the concept of 'diffraction' introduced by Donna Haraway in 1992 to theorise relations of difference beyond narrow binary oppositions. In rethinking difference beyond absolute oppositions (e.g. self/other, discourse/matter), diffraction offers a non-binary understanding of difference, one that recognises relations between particular phenomena as mutually constituted. The notion of 'diffraction' was later elaborated by feminist science studies scholar Karen Barad in her 'diffractive methodology' which she describes, following Haraway's original formulation, as a 'commitment to understanding which differences matter, how they matter, and for whom. It is a critical practice of engagement, not a distance-learning practice from afar' (Barad 2007, p. 90). Implicit here is a critique of the optics of reflection that underpin traditional realist epistemologies with their assumption that representations accurately reflect an anterior, fixed reality. As distinct from the metaphors of reflection and reflexivity, which focus on mimesis and mirroring, diffraction shifts the focus to differences, in particular the difference that knowledge practices make in the world. Haraway captures this distinction thus: where the metaphor of reflection 'repeat[s] the Sacred Image of the Same [...] diffraction patterns record the history of interaction, interference, reinforcement, difference' (Haraway 1997, p. 273). Barad elaborates this point in terms of the practice of reflexivity, noting that 'reflexivity is based on the belief that practices of representing have no effect on the objects of investigation and that we have a kind of access to representations that we don't have to the objects themselves. Reflexivity, like reflection, still holds the world at a distance' (Barad 2007, p. 87). In other words, the practice of reflexivity relies on conventional empiricist methods that seek to examine and describe a singular, stable reality. By contrast, a diffractive approach recognises that practices of knowing actively help to (re) shape realities (in the plural to capture their multiplicity). It therefore calls for careful attention to the material effects of knowledge practices, including those associated with research.

As an approach to social inquiry, diffraction prompts attention to the constitutive action of research, or the ways in which research methods and practices interfere with and help to create the realities they investigate. Importantly, the concept of diffraction is not an attempt to collapse difference but rather treat it as the effect of specific 'agential cuts', cuts that delimit ontological boundaries and thus produce ontologically distinct objects (Barad 2007). Understood this way, differences such as those articulated in binary oppositions are not inherent, they are produced in practice through the divisions we draw in acts of differentiation. Dichotomies are one such act of differentiation: far from simply indexing conceptual differences, they perform an agential cut that separates phenomena into seemingly distinct domains, enacting the boundary between them as determinate. In other words, unlike traditional Cartesian cuts (conceptual divisions), agential cuts are ontological divisions with far-reaching effects in terms of materialising certain realities and foreclosing the existence of others.

The notion of diffraction has been productively applied to analyse 'addiction' experiences in terms of how the polarising divisions of addiction discourses (e.g. volition/compulsion, health/disease and order/disorder) fail to capture people's diverse experiences of drug consumption, suggesting that common assumptions about addiction and its opposites are untenable, and serve to stigmatise people who use drugs as disordered subjects in need of treatment (Pienaar et al. 2017). Reflecting on the practical applications of their analysis, the authors highlight the need for an alternative range of narratives capable of articulating regular drug use in less pathologising ways, one that recognises the benefits that it can afford. This recognition, they suggest, could prompt drug policy responses oriented to promoting health and reducing harm, rather than preventing or stopping drug consumption. Such research is part of a broader intellectual shift in critical drug studies that takes inspiration from the 'ontological turn' to rethink dominant understandings of drugs and their effects. In a 2020 article, Fraser (2020) synthesises this shift as 'ontopolitically-oriented research' and defines its key features with reference to two research projects that generated new knowledge and practical outcomes for people who consume drugs, policymakers and service providers, including a public website and safer injecting resources.[1]

Here, we build on this work and apply its insights to another health-related domain, namely, the knowledge practices at work in contemporary disease outbreaks. We pursue a diffractive reading of the HIV epidemic to trace the 'diffraction patterns' or specific material entanglements through which HIV, COVID-19 and mpox emerge. In doing so, we identify the assumptions underpinning particular accounts of these diseases and their ontological implications, i.e. the specific realities they produce and their consequences for communities identified as at risk of infection.

Analysis

In what follows, we focus on two dominant concepts on which infectious disease discourses rely, namely, 'risk' and 'crisis'. Because these concepts surface repeatedly in our analysis of public discourses on HIV, COVID-19 and mpox, we identify them as central to contemporary accounts of disease. As we go on to show, they play an important role in governing populations, determining the urgency and scale of public health responses, and justifying the distribution of limited healthcare resources.

Risk profiling and public health as a tool of governance

Key to epidemiological accounts of disease is the notion of 'risk' and the profiling of populations based on assessments of their relative risk of infection. Yet, despite its centrality to the epidemiological enterprise, the concept of risk is often taken as given and thus largely evades analytic scrutiny in epidemiological discourses. However, it has been subject to close attention in the sociology of risk literature, notably in Beck's classic 'risk society' thesis where he defines risk as 'a systematic way of dealing with hazards and insecurities' that have emerged through the technoscientific advances of late modernity (1992, p. 12). Beck later elaborated on his original formulation, adding that '[r]isks are social constructions and definitions' and are therefore open to contestation and change' (2009, p. 30). Importantly, this formulation recognises that risks are not self-evident facts, but are based on consensual social definitions of what constitutes a 'hazard'. In the case of infectious disease control, understandings of epidemiological risk are the 'calculative basis on which the health status of a population is determined or rendered visible' and therefore assessments of risk are an important basis for public health interventions (Brown et al. 2012, p. 1185). As such, they play a crucial role in governing populations by, for example, classifying 'at risk' groups and guiding the allocation of limited healthcare resources.

In the early years of the HIV epidemic, scholars and activists expressed concern that the epidemiological identification of 'HIV risk groups' singled out marginalised populations (including gay men, sex workers and people who inject drugs), which could reinforce stigma and the dangerous misconception that the 'general' public was not at risk (Holt 2022, cited in Razzhigaeva 2022). Activists responded by arguing that HIV education programmes should prioritise risky practices or acts over identities. This understandable response to the stigmatising effects of HIV risk profiling seeks to emphasise that anyone is at risk of infection if they engage in 'risky' practices or activities. Gender and cultural studies scholar Kane Race calls this the 'anyone can get it rebuttal' (Race 2022, para 10), a well-intentioned, universalising strategy designed to counter the homophobic nature of early constructions of HIV as a 'gay disease'. However, as Race goes on to argue in reflecting on the lessons of HIV for contemporary disease responses:

> The most egregious, homophobic aspect of early governmental responses to AIDS was not the identification of risk groups per se, but the systematic inaction and shameful neglect of the health crisis under the US Reagan administration and in Thatcher's UK. The epidemiological identification of gay men and other marginalized, despised groups as 'HIV risk groups' was used to justify this murderous neglect: these lives were expendable, these deaths could be ignored, no crisis necessary.
>
> (2022, para 19)

Diffracting the history of HIV through responses to COVID-19 and mpox reveals how these legacies of stigma and moralising responses to HIV are imbricated in recent disease outbreaks. For example, when the WHO identified gay, bisexual and other men who have sex with men as a risk group for mpox, critics voiced concern that the focus on gay men was bound up with 'a homophobic refusal to acknowledge that *anyone* can get monkeypox, by virtue of its various modes of transmission … Why should vaccine programmes single out MSM [men who have sex with men] and not them they ask, presumably on behalf of the "general public"' (Race 2022, paras 10 and 17, original emphasis). Writing in the early years of the HIV epidemic, activist and historian Simon Watney offered a cogent critique of the exclusionary assumptions implicit in dominant imaginaries of the 'general public':

> Indeed, the relentless monotony and sadism of AIDS commentary in the West only serve to manifest a sense of profound cultural uneasiness concerning the fragility of the nationalistic fantasy of an undifferentiated 'general public,' supposedly united above all divisions of class, region, and gender, yet totally excluding everyone who stands outside the institution of marriage.
>
> (Watney 1987, p. 73)

We suggest that this observation remains relevant to discourses surrounding contemporary viral outbreaks: even as public health discourses are at pains to stress that a virus does not discriminate and 'anyone can get it', we are forced to reckon with the disproportionate impacts of the disease on marginalised groups. In the case of mpox, commonplace assertions in health outlets that 'anyone can get it' do not align with the epidemiology of the current outbreak among gay, bisexual and other men who have sex with men. If public health messaging neglects the role of sex between men in routes of transmission, there is a risk that accurate, empirically grounded information may not reach affected populations, eroding the effectiveness of prevention and containment measures. Even more insidiously, combining the 'anyone can get it' rebuttal with a coy elision of the role of sex may actually reinforce homophobic assumptions and stigma insofar as 'incomplete information about actual transmission routes and settings may lead to the assumption that gay men, based on the simple fact of being gay, are vectors of disease' (García- Iglesias et al. 2022, p. 4).

As these examples suggest, public health responses, however well-intentioned, can help to reinforce an uneven disease burden and associated patterns of disadvantage: rather than simply addressing the needs of a pre-existing health public, disease containment measures produce stratified health publics that entrench the privilege of some groups while disadvantaging others. In Barad's terms, such measures produce agential cuts, dividing populations into privileged communities (the imagined 'public' of public health) and excluding already marginalised groups. For example, in relation to COVID-19 responses in the first waves of the pandemic, stay-at-home directives relied on an idealised notion of home as a place of refuge and safety, housing a nuclear family in a large, suburban dwelling with private space to self-isolate (Lewis 2020). They also implied a normative definition of 'family', one that privileged the middle-class, heterosexual couple or nuclear family as the basic social unit. In doing so, 'the directive to "stay home" as the undifferentiated, dominant prophylactic response [to COVID-19] [...] reinforced the precarity of marginalised communities' and social groups (Pienaar et al. 2021, p. 251). Such groups include those experiencing domestic violence, homeless people, multi-generation extended family households, single people living alone, those in residential care facilities and HIV-positive queer migrants 'who live at the intersection of two pandemics' (Hegarty 2020, para 3).

Moreover, injunctions to stay home to protect one's family materialise the family as especially vulnerable and thus work to sanction protectionist measures aimed at safeguarding this foundational institution. For example, in Australia, the Premier of Victoria warned of COVID-19 mortality risks and exhorted people living in the state to 'Stay home. Save Lives', adding 'Saving lives is everyone's job [...] This is about all of us and *unless you want to be burying an elderly relative or your best mate or your parents* [...] *then do the right thing*' (Andrews 2020, emphasis added). The appeals to 'do the right thing' (an oft-repeated slogan in Australian public messaging campaigns), combined with the emphasis on the life-and-death stakes add a moralising imperative and an incontrovertible urgency to the public health injunctions. The exceptional status granted to the family in public health discourses owes much to the role of the family as the 'privileged instrument for the government of the population' (Foucault 1979, p. 17).

Our analysis suggests that pandemic containment measures and related public health strategies are not socially neutral interventions. Rather, as part of a constellation of practices centred on heteronormative, middle-class families, they are embedded in existing social structures and freighted with normative assumptions. Indeed, a diffractive reading of viral control measures reveals that they enact what medical sociologist Des Fitzgerald calls 'the reproductive legacy of epidemiology, a discipline centred on the health and viability of a certain idea of population' (Fitzgerald 2020, para. 10), one that is normative and exclusionary. Because such measures are made in the name of safeguarding public health and 'saving lives', their exigency tends to inoculate them from critique. However, diffracting accounts of COVID-19 and mpox through the history of HIV reveals the importance of critical, historically grounded responses to contemporary disease outbreaks.

Beyond 'crisis' discourses

Our second area of concern in thinking diffractively with HIV is the role of crisis discourses in pandemic responses. We suggest that the framing of disease outbreaks as 'crises' requires scrutiny in terms of the work that 'crisis' discourses do in constructing new objects of knowledge and insisting on urgent, decisive responses. As Janet Roitman argues: 'The point is to observe crisis as a blind spot, and hence to apprehend the ways in which it regulates narrative constructions, the ways in which it allows certain questions to be asked while others are foreclosed' (Roitman 2014, p. 94). In earlier work with collaborator Achille Mbembe, both scholars note that the 'structuring idiom' of crisis dramatises particular forms of subjectivity, legitimises appeals to urgency and authorises immediate, and sometimes ill-conceived, interventions (Mbembe and Roitman 1995, p. 325). In the process, critical questions are dismissed, and alternative responses displaced. As Anderson asks in his critique of crisis modelling in pandemic times, 'how to make time for [...] nuanced inquiry in a crisis? This is, of course, the regulatory question that framing an event as a crisis will generate' (Anderson 2021, p. 175).

The articulation of COVID-19 as a crisis was invoked from the earliest days of the pandemic. This framing made extraordinary measures possible, for example the closure of the international border by the Australian federal government. Ashford and Longstaff (2021, p. 1559) argue that COVID-19 also facilitated the (re)regulation of gay male sex 'with intimacy outside of the heteronormative framework of domestic coupledom at best discouraged and, at worst, made into a criminal offence'. Some public health researchers suggested that reductions in sexual encounters among gay men may even contribute to decreases in new HIV infections (Hammoud et al. 2020). However, as Ledin and Weil (2021, p. 1470) argue, the linking of COVID-19 with the goal of HIV's elimination 'reinscribes historical perceptions of abstinence and quarantine as idealised HIV prevention strategies' and supports a fantasy of quarantine as the 'end of HIV'. Also relevant here is the strategic mobilisation of the history of HIV to invoke the urgency and apparent exceptionalism of COVID-19. For example, in the first months of COVID-19, many HIV and LGBTQ health organisations advised queer communities to abstain from casual sex – the very strategy that they had expressly challenged during the first decade of the HIV epidemic was now being now endorsed on the basis of the unprecedented 'crisis' that COVID-19 posed (ACON 2020a; Thorne Harbour Health 2020). In this way, the logic of crisis – and its appeals to an unprecedented situation demanding urgent, decisive action – supports the regulation of queer sexuality via the public policing of queer people's private lives.

In terms of a broader politics of sexual inclusion, these examples are evidence of an inclusionary agential cut in which LGBTQ communities (and their representative organisations) were seeking membership of the category of the 'general public' from which gay and bisexual men had historically been excluded during the first decades of the HIV epidemic. Notably, advice from leading community agencies emphasised that while COVID-19 is 'not a sexually transmitted infection', sex demands physical contact, which is 'not in keeping with the important public health measures everyone in the general community are [*sic*] being asked to observe' (ACON 2020a). Importantly, community groups appealed to a sense of solidarity and civic duty, emphasising that LGBTQ communities were not being targeted specifically and the advice was consistent with that for 'the general population', adding that '[w]e all need to play our part' (ACON 2020a). In late June 2020, LGBTQ community organisations began actively promoting strategies to reduce the risk of COVID-19 while having casual sex (ACON 2020b). However, gay and bisexual men had already been developing risk-reduction strategies since the early months of the COVID-19 pandemic (Murphy et al. 2023). The development of these strategies can be understood as 'cultural responses to the pandemic, some of which have particular resonances with responses to HIV, including the development of care practices such as "safe sex"' (Murphy et al. 2023, p. 12).

Notwithstanding these solidaristic queer cultural responses, dividing practices were also at work within queer communities. As noted earlier, pandemic policies presumed a heteronormative domestic unit, most commonly referred to in public health messaging as the 'household'. While some LGBTQ community members – for example, cohabiting couples, either with or without children – were able to imagine themselves within such definitions, many fell outside. As a result, tensions emerged within queer communities between those who were seen as 'responsible' versus those presumed to be recklessly engaging in casual sex (notably gay and bisexual men). Such tensions were also evident in the USA with some male porn actors publicly called out for allegedly flouting restrictions (Instinct Magazine 2020). Reading these accounts diffractively, we suggest that efforts to police queer sex draws on cultural and political histories of HIV, and as Ashford and Longstaff (2021, p. 1559) note, 'provides a temporal praxis in which [some] gay men experience sex in the shadows once more, an echo of a historic legal and cultural regulation of desire'.

To return to the performative work of crisis framings in shaping realities, we turn now to the forms of subjectivity they generate. Scholars have observed that appeals to crisis discourses not only authorise modes of exceptionalism, but they also support the production of 'panic icons', i.e. the construction of particular social groups as sites of contagion, and 'patient zero' figures who are seen as the cause of the problem (González 2019, p. 33). In the early years of HIV, a period characterised by anxious, phobic responses and lurid spectacles of diseased or dying Others, the register of panic icons included homosexuals, Haitians, people who consume heroin and people with haemophilia (the '4-H' risk groups). As Kagan notes in an analysis of 'post-crisis' HIV discourse, the personification of AIDS via these panic icons 'was a means of symbolically and psychically cordoning it off from the white, middle-class, suburban, sexually decorous heterosexual "general population"' (Kagan 2018, p. 26). One might call this strategy a kind of discursive quarantining in that it performs an agential cut separating the purportedly healthy majority from 'diseased' minorities, groups already classed as 'Others'. In later decades, when HIV's modes of transmission were better understood, the focus shifted from 'risk groups' to 'risky practices' such as condomless sex or unsafe injecting practices (e.g. sharing injecting equipment). However, the association of HIV with gay men in the first decade of the epidemic has proved hard to shake and we live with the pernicious legacies of the conflation of HIV with the 'disease of gayness' (Miller 1993, cited in Kagan 2018, p. 9). Even in the era of lifesaving antiretroviral treatment when HIV has been transformed into a manageable illness, new moral panics have emerged (e.g. recurrent sex panics about barebacking [condomless anal sex] and chemsex) (Kagan 2018). These sites of moral panic resurrect the logics of crisis discourse and reinstall gay men at the centre of what we might call 'panic iconography'. Such panic icons serve as targets for apportioning blame for the spread of disease, attracting moral opprobrium, prurient fascination, fear and stigma.

In the first wave of COVID-19, the figure of the 'covidiot' was one such panic icon to emerge. The term was coined to describe people who flouted pandemic restrictions, in the process allegedly helping to spread the virus (Hoffower 2020). The hashtag #covidiot soon began to trend on social media, used to publicly shame those ignoring COVID-19 restrictions. Levelled at COVID-19 denialists, anti-vaxxers, those 'panic buying' or hoarding essential supplies and anyone flagrantly flouting lockdown rules, the panic icon of the covidiot performed an 'agential cut' between an informed, rational public with a sense of civic duty and an uninformed, irrational counter-public whose actions were selfish and irresponsible. Seen as threatening the health of the 'general public' or wider community, these counter-public figures or panic icons emerge out of crisis discourses and are singled out as disease vectors whose actions must be controlled to prevent the spread of disease.

As our diffractive approach implies, thinking *with* HIV may generate new insights into responses to COVID-19 and mpox, as well as future epidemics. It also offers new ways of understanding community responses, most notably within communities historically affected by HIV. Whereas in the early period of the COVID-19 pandemic (in 2020), LGBTQ community responses included dividing practices that marked some people as 'irresponsible' and counter-actions to ensure inclusion within the 'general public', the advent of effective vaccinations has seen even greater emphasis on the latter, with high vaccination rates in LGBTQ communities and the linking of sexual freedoms to vaccination (Prestage et al. 2022). Finally, while politicians and policy-makers are advised to 'never waste a good crisis', our analysis suggests that framing an event *as* a crisis authorises particular actions and even has a diffractive effect on time, contracting the temporal frame to justify the urgency of decisive action.

Concluding reflections: Forging new futures in pandemic times

In the epilogue of her influential book, Treichler notes her reluctance to offer a tidy 'conclusion' in the face of a still unfolding epidemic, the effects of which continue to be felt some 25 years later. Indeed, as the enduring legacy of HIV has starkly demonstrated, 'An epidemic, like a war, marks us for decades' (Treichler 1999, p. 315). We too hesitate before the impulse to neatly conclude and instead reflect on some key insights that thinking HIV diffractively affords for understanding disease outbreaks.

A diffractive, historical reading illuminates how the legacies of HIV ramify and become enfolded in future disease outbreaks. Thus, even as COVID-19 and mpox are 'new' viral outbreaks, they are, as Treichler observed in relation to HIV, 'already peopled' (1999, p. 316): these new viruses are conceptually and materially freighted, intimately connected to existing disease concepts, origin stories, notions of risk, unfolding epidemiological understandings, public health responses and myriad other phenomena. Treichler puts it thus in her analysis: 'At the same time that "AIDS" is new, however, it is always already occupied, peopled with discourse that predated it and establishing precedents for language not yet invented' (1999, pp. 323–324). As we have argued here, the histories and legacies of previous disease outbreaks (often framed as 'crises') are enfolded in current ones. In keeping with the ambit of this edited collection, our focus has been on the entanglement of HIV, COVID-19 and mpox, but one could equally expand or shift the analytic lens to map the diffraction patterns of other historic and contemporary infectious disease outbreaks, tracing how they are deeply imbricated. Applied to HIV, this observation echoes what Møller and Ledin (2020, p. 148) call 'viral hauntologies', the ways in which historic ideas, meanings, and interventions based on fear of HIV continue to 'haunt' contemporary cultural imaginaries of disease. Haunting is a productive metaphor here as it suggests a disturbing spectre from the past, a ghost-like presence that casts a shadow over the present and 'that many would prefer to ignore, prevent or exorcise' (Kagan 2018, p. 7).

While the focus of Møller and Ledin's viral hauntology is on HIV and the ways in which ingrained fear of the virus pervades current understandings, we suggest that their insights about the affective 'haunting' of disease concepts apply more broadly to COVID-19 and mpox, and the public reactions they have engendered. For example, scholars have been quick to caution that responses to mpox should guard against the kind of moralising rhetoric that circulated in the early years of the HIV epidemic: 'With monkeypox, we must avoid a moralising reaction like in the 1980s when HIV and AIDS were first recognised. Using the knowledge we have gained from handling the HIV and COVID-19 pandemics, we must guard against stigma and harmful rhetoric that may inhibit a public health response' (Holt 2022, cited in Razzhigaeva 2022, para 5). Conversely, responses to COVID-19 reshaped contemporary approaches to HIV in a range of ways. For example, as noted above, the social isolation measures employed in the first wave of COVID-19 sparked idealised notions of quarantine as facilitating a possible end to HIV. For a time, some public health officials in London posed social isolation as presenting a 'unique opportunity' to 'break the chain' in HIV transmission, reinstalling historical fantasies of HIV's elimination and promoting idealised HIV prevention strategies of abstinence and quarantine at the expense of more pragmatic safer sex strategies in the context of COVID-19 (Ledin and Weil 2021). Research with people living with HIV found the identification of COVID-19 risk groups prompted reflection on whether the concept of 'at-risk' populations could apply equally to COVID-19 (as a generalised pandemic) and to HIV as one that was understood to disproportionately affect marginalised communities (e.g. gay and bisexual men, people who inject drugs, sex workers) (Murphy et al. 2021). In this sense, COVID-19 risk profiling and the mobilisation of risk categories via COVID-19 surveillance systems have arguably contributed to denaturalising HIV risk groups.

Diffracting historical accounts of HIV through contemporary discourses of COVID-19 and mpox reveals the implicit, often stigmatising, assumptions enfolded into epidemiological accounts of infection risk. Our analysis therefore suggests a need for tailored, contextually contingent responses capable of registering the range of diffraction patterns (or specific material entanglements) that shape experiences of infectious disease outbreaks. These include the sedimented meanings and cultural imaginaries of past epidemics that fold into contemporary and future disease concepts, inciting deep-seated fears, moralising reactions and exclusionary practices that divide communities, reinforcing stigma and social marginalisation. Finally, a diffractive reading disrupts received wisdom and settled scientific 'truths' about disease. It makes visible the contingent and provisional nature of 'truth' claims and reveals scientific knowledge as contested and open to change. On this view, disease concepts are not simply representations of an objective, pre-existing reality; rather they have ontological power as key sites through which the realities of illness, suffering and death take shape.

Note

1 For more detail on these studies and the practical applications of ontopolitically oriented research, see Fraser (2013), Fraser et al. (2017), Moore et al. (2017) and Pienaar and Dilkes-Frayne (2017).

References

ACON, 2020a. COVID-19 update: Casual sex and social distancing. *ACON* [online], 20 March. Available from: www.acon.org.au/about-acon/latest-news/media-releases [Accessed 10 September 2020]

ACON, 2020b. COVID-19 update: Easing of restrictions, physical distancing and casual sex. *ACON* [online], 12 June. Available from: www.acon.org.au/about-acon/latest-news/media-releases [Accessed 10 September 2020]

Anderson, W., 2021. The model crisis, or how to have critical promiscuity in the time of COVID-19. *Social Studies of Science*, 51 (2), 167–188. 10.1177/0306312721996053

Andrews, D., 2020. Stay home, save lives. *Dan Andrews* [Facebook], 30 March. Available from: www.facebook.com/DanielAndrewsMP/videos/218306979422749/ [Accessed 13 March 2023]

Ashford, C. and Longstaff, G., 2021. (Re)regulating gay sex in viral times: COVID-19 and the impersonal intimacy of the glory hole. *Culture, Health & Sexuality*, 23 (11), 1559–1572. 10.1080/13691058.2021.1930173

Barad, K., 2007. *Meeting the universe halfway: Quantum physics and the entanglement of matter and meaning*. Durham, NC: Duke University Press.

Beck, U., 1992. *Risk society: Towards a new modernity*. London: Sage.

Beck, U., 2009. *World at risk*. Cambridge: Polity.

Bennett, C.M., 2021. Learning to live with COVID-19 in Australia: Time for a new approach. *Public Health Research and Practice*, 31 (3), 3132110. 10.17061/phrp3132110

Brown, T., Craddock, S., and Ingram, A., 2012. Critical interventions in global health: Governmentality, risk, and assemblage. *Annals of the Association of American Geographers*, 102 (5), 1182–1189. 10.1080/00045608.2012.659960

Brown, T. et al., 2021. How to have theory in a pandemic: A critical reflection on the discourses of COVID-19. In G.J. Andrews et al., eds. *COVID-19 and similar futures. Global perspectives on health geography*. London and New York: Springer, 93–99. 10.1007/978-3-030-70179-6_11

Bunge, E.M., et al., 2022. The changing epidemiology of human monkeypox – A potential threat? A systematic review. *PLoS Neglected Tropical Diseases*, 16, e0010141. 10.1371/journal.pntd.0010141

Crimp, D., 1987. How to have promiscuity in an epidemic. *October*, 43, 237–271.

Davey, M., 2022. Was 2022 the year that Australia came to terms with Covid? And what does 2023 hold? *The Guardian*, 19 December. www.theguardian.com/culture/2022/dec/19/was-2022-the-year-that-australia-came-to-terms-with-covid-and-what-does-2023-hold [Accessed 20 March 2023]

Fitzgerald, D., 2020. Stay the fuck at home. *Somatosphere* (Dispatches from the pandemic), 13 April. Available from: http://somatosphere.net/2020/stay-the-fuck-at-home.html/ [Accessed 13 March 2023]

Fraser, S., 2013. The missing mass of morality: A new fitpack design for hepatitis C prevention in sexual partnerships. *International Journal of Drug Policy*, 24 (3), 212–219. 10.1016/j.drugpo.2013.03.009

Fraser, S., 2020. Doing ontopolitically-oriented research: Synthesising concepts from the ontological turn for alcohol and other drug research and other social sciences. *International Journal of Drug Policy*, 82, 102610. 10.1016/j.drugpo.2019.102610

Fraser, S., et al., 2017. 'Affording' new approaches to couples who inject drugs: A novel fitpack design for hepatitis C prevention. *International Journal of Drug Policy*, 50, 19–35. 10.1016/j.drugpo.2017.07.001

Foucault, M., 1979. Governmentality. *Ideology & Consciousness*, 6, 17.

García-Iglesias, J., et al., 2022. Is monkeypox an STI? The societal aspects and healthcare implications of a key question. *Wellcome Open Research*, 7, 252. 10.12688/wellcomeopenres.18436.1

González, O.R., 2019. Pre-exposure prophylaxis (PrEP), 'The Truvada Whore,' and the new gay sexual revolution. In R. Varghese, ed. *Raw: PrEP, paedagogy, and the politics of barebacking*. Regina: University of Regina Press, 47–70.

Hammoud, M., et al., 2020. Physical distancing due to COVID-19 disrupts sexual behaviors among gay and bisexual men in Australia: Implications for trends in HIV and other sexually transmissible infections. *JAIDS*, 85 (3), 309–315. 10.1097/QAI.0000000000002462

Haraway, D., 1992. The promises of monsters: A regenerative politics for inappropriate/d others. In L. Grossberg, C. Nelson, and P. Treichler, eds. *Cultural Studies*. New York: Routledge, 295–337.

Haraway, D., 1997. *Modest_Witness@Second_Millenium. FemaleMan_Meets_OncoMouse™*. New York and London: Routledge.

Hegarty, B., 2020. A place apart. *Somatosphere* (Dispatches from the pandemic), 15 July. Available from: http://somatosphere.net/2020/a-place-apart.html/ [Accessed 13 February 2023]

Hoffower, H., 2020. COVIDIOT: The latest slang people are using to describe spring breakers, toilet-paper hoarders, and politicians during the coronavirus pandemic. *Business Insider*, 27 March. Available from: www.businessinsider.com/what-is-a-covidiot-coronavirus-pandemic-meme-2020-3 [Accessed 13 March 2023]

Instinct Magazine, 2020. Ty Mitchell in hot seat for post about Fire Island parties. 17 August. Available from: https://instinctmagazine.com/ty-mitchell-in-hot-seat-for-post-about-fire-island-parties/ [Accessed 13 March 2023]

Kagan, D., 2018. *Positive images: Gay men and HIV/AIDS in the culture of "post crisis"*. London: Bloomsbury.

Ledin, C. and Weil, B., 2021. 'Test Now, Stop HIV': COVID-19 and the idealisation of quarantine as the 'end of HIV'. *Culture, Health & Sexuality*, 23 (11), 1470–1484. 10.1080/13691058.2021.1906953

Lewis, S., 2020. What does the pandemic reveal about the private nuclear household? *Bullybloggers*, 1 April. Available from: https://bullybloggers.wordpress.com/2020/04/01/the-virus-vs-the-home-what-does-the-pandemic-reveal-about-the-private-nuclear-household-by-sophie-lewis-for-bunkerbloggers-originally-published-on-patreon-reblogged-by-permission-of-the-author/ [Accessed 13 March 2023]

Mbembe, A. and Roitman, J., 1995. Figures of the subject in times of crisis. *Public Culture*, 7 (2), 323–352.

Møller, K. and Ledin, C., 2020. Viral hauntology: Specters of AIDS in infrastructures of gay sexual sociability. In M. Stavning Thomsen, J. Kofoed, and J. Fritsch, eds. *Affects, interfaces, events*. Lancaster, PA; Vancouver, BC: Imbricate! Press, 147–162.

Moore, D., et al., 2017. Challenging the addiction/health binary with assemblage thinking: An analysis of consumer accounts. *International Journal of Drug Policy*, 44, 155–163. 10.1016/j.drugpo.2017.01.013

Murphy, D., et al., 2021. *Experiences after HIV diagnosis: Report on findings from a qualitative cohort study of people recently diagnosed with HIV*. Sydney: UNSW. 10.26190/bp16-2307

Murphy, D., et al., 2023. How to have sex in a pandemic: The development of strategies to prevent COVID-19 transmission in sexual encounters among gay and bisexual men in Australia. *Culture, Health & Sexuality*, 25 (3), 271–286. 10.1080/13691058.2022.2037717

Pienaar, K. and Dilkes-Frayne, E., 2017. Telling different stories, making new realities: The ontological politics of 'addiction' biographies. *International Journal of Drug Policy*, 44, 145–154. 10.1016/j.drugpo.2017.05.011

Pienaar, K., et al., 2017. Diffracting addicting binaries: An analysis of personal accounts of alcohol and other drug 'addiction'. *Health*, 21 (5), 519–537. 10.1177/1363459316674062

Pienaar, K., et al., 2021. Making publics in a pandemic: Posthuman relationalities, 'viral' intimacies and COVID-19. *Health Sociology Review*, 30 (3), 244–259. 10.1080/14461242.2021.1961600

Prestage, G., et al., 2022. COVID-19 vaccine uptake and its impacts in a cohort of gay and bisexual men in Australia. *AIDS and Behavior*, 26 (8), 2692–2702. 10.1007/s10461-022-03611-x

Race, K., 2022. An epidemic of rebuttal. *Homotectonic*, 16 August. Available from: https://homotectonic.com/2022/08/16/an-epidemic-of-rebuttal [Accessed 28 October 2022].

Razzhigaeva, N., 2022. HIV history can't repeat itself with monkeypox, UNSW social scientist warns. *UNSW Sydney* [online], 18 August. Available from: https://newsroom.unsw.edu.au/news/social-affairs/hiv-history-cant-repeat-itself-monkeypox-unsw-social-scientist-warns [Accessed 31 October 2022].

Roitman, J., 2014. *Anti-Crisis*. Durham, NC: Duke University Press.

Thorne Harbour Health, 2020. *Info sheet: Sex, intimacy and coronavirus*. Available from: https://thorneharbour.org/documents/420/CORONAVIRUS_SEX_INFO_SHEET.pdf [Accessed 20 March 2023].

Treichler, P., 1999. *How to have theory in an epidemic: Cultural chronicles of AIDS*. Durham, NC: Duke University Press.

United Nations News, 2022. Monkeypox declared a global health emergency by the World Health Organization, 23 July. Available from: https://news.un.org/en/story/2022/07/1123152 [Accessed 28 October 2022]

Watney, S., 1987. The spectacle of AIDS. *October*, 43, 71–86. 10.2307/3397565

WHO, 2023. 2022–23 Mpox (Monkeypox) outbreak. Global Trends. *World Health Organization* [online]. Available from: www.who.int/emergencies/situations/monkeypox-oubreak-2022 [Accessed 20 March 2023].

Zumla, A. et al., 2022. Monkeypox outbreaks outside endemic regions: scientific and social priorities. *Lancet Journal of Infectious Disease*, 22 (7), 929–931. 10.1016/S1473-3099(22)00354-1

9 People, politics and death

International, national and community responses to HIV and COVID-19

Richard Parker and Peter Aggleton

Introduction

Global epidemics (often now described as pandemics), such as HIV as well as COVID-19, provide important windows into the political dimensions of health. Perhaps because they are often linked to public health emergencies – and too often to what might be described as public health panics – global epidemics/pandemics highlight political issues, making them especially visible. They provide insight into the political dimensions not just of policymaking and formal political and legal processes, but also the politics of social and cultural reactions, as well as the interactions of political and economic systems and processes. By their very definition, they also offer insights into the relationship between the local and the global, shedding light on the ways in which transnational connections and flows both influence and are influenced by political forces and processes.

It is at the point of intersection between the social and political dimensions of epidemics that the analysis developed here is focused. Epidemics are complex events that involve not only viral transmission but a wide range of responses at local, community, national and international levels. These social responses arise in relation to changing epidemiological patterns and biomedical prospects, but they also take on a life (and a complexity) of their own – and may sometimes be even more important than biomedical factors in determining the impact that any epidemic will have. Analysing and interpreting these responses demand the use of social science theory and methods that are distinct from those employed by epidemiology and biomedicine. This social analysis requires its own distinct epistemological principles and conceptual frameworks and plays its own role in relation to confronting the challenges that any epidemic poses.

This chapter focuses on these social and political responses in comparative perspective, highlighting both important differences as well as unexpected similarities in relation to HIV and COVID-19. It draws heavily on our experience working with the global HIV epidemic (which was only rarely described as a pandemic at the time when it emerged) over roughly 40 years. It was during this time period, and in large part because of HIV and AIDS,

DOI: 10.4324/9781003322788-11

that the field of global health in its most recent incarnation has taken shape and consolidated itself, impacted by a series of political crosscurrents and processes that have been the focus for important analyses, but which are nonetheless worth continued consideration (Brown et al. 2006; Brandt 2013; Packard 2016). This is especially true today, following COVID-19, the first truly global pandemic to have emerged since the beginning of the HIV crisis – and which, by historical accident, came on the scene at roughly the same time that the field of global health was promising an imminent end of AIDS. In our view, it is the intersection between these two sets of events that offers key insights into, while at the same time raising major concerns about, some of the most serious social and political challenges confronting us in the early twenty-first century.

On the intersecting histories of the HIV and COVID-19 pandemics

Looking back at the social history of the HIV epidemic – both at the key events that shaped the epidemic and at the ways in which the global response to it changed over time, it is useful to think of change in terms of a series of waves (historical phases or periods) that washed over us as we have tried to understand the epidemic and responses to it (Parker 2011). The idea of waves provides a helpful metaphor in that it simultaneously captures the sense of being battered by powerful forces of nature, as well as by a series of events that can only be perceived as separate phenomena with some difficulty. Both the characteristics and the moment at which one wave becomes separate from the next are somewhat unclear, yet the changes from one wave to the next can have important consequences both for those who are personally affected by illness and disease and for society more generally.

Because of the later onslaught of COVID-19 since 2020, which has also been analysed as a series of 'waves' (this time, waves of ever-changing viral variants), it is important to stress that the waves we analyse in relation to HIV are *social* rather than epidemiological in character. Paralleling (and in some cases running ahead of) viral transmission are deep-seated social, cultural and political processes, which are often more powerful than the waves of viral infection themselves. It is in a *social* sense that we seek to understand what can be seen as distinct aspects of the response to HIV and AIDS – as well as more recent social and political responses to COVID-19 in recent times.

In developing this comparative analysis of HIV and AIDS, on the one hand, and COVID-19, on the other, it is important to recognise the very different historical periods we are working with. In the case of HIV and AIDS, we focus on a global epidemic that has been with us for more than 40 years now, whereas in the case of COVID-19, we are looking at a 3-year period at the time we are writing. These very different time frames impact knowledge and understanding of biomedical developments as well as of social and political responses – and our interpretations must keep these significant differences in mind. But precisely because of significant temporal differences, the longer record associated with HIV and AIDS makes it possible to pose questions in relation to both pandemics that we might not think about if we were not developing this analysis comparatively. In short, the contrasting time frames of these two global health crises create both limitations and possibilities for comparison, and it is important to keep both of these in mind throughout what follows.

With this comparative frame as a backdrop, it is possible to distinguish between at least four (and now possibly five) relatively distinct periods in the HIV epidemic as experienced over the course of its first four decades. The first wave, running from 1981 to roughly 1990 or 1991, may best be described as a time of crisis, characterised by intense forms of stigma and discrimination (Parker and Aggleton 2003), as the epidemic initially affected a range of highly marginalised and excluded communities and populations. But it was also a time of resistance, as affected communities began to mobilise politically, and societies (and, ultimately, the international governance system) struggled to understand and respond to the challenges posed by an epidemic with devastating human consequences.

A second wave, running from approximately 1990 or 1991 through to 2000 or 2001, was characterised by the development of new conceptual and institutional structures to provide the foundation for a more effective response to HIV, emphasising the role of power in driving the epidemic and the need to confront inequality in order to effectively respond to it (Parker and Aggleton 2003). During this second wave, an international social movement emerged advocating for treatment access based on human rights principles following the development of effective treatment options in the middle of the 1990s (Parker 2011). Key allies in international agencies such as the newly created Joint United Nations Programme on HIV and AIDS (UNAIDS) as well as in the diplomatic corps of a number of leading middle- and lower-income countries helped open up space in international relations processes through the United Nations (and the 2001 UNGASS Declaration of Commitment) and the World Trade Organization (WTO; and the Doha Declaration on TRIPS and Public Health). Together, these actions made it possible to imagine universal treatment access as a reasonable possibility (Piot 2015; Amorim 2017; Stuenkel 2019).

A third wave, roughly from 2001 to 2011, was associated with what has come to be described as the 'scale-up' of a reasonably coherent HIV response, incorporating comprehensive prevention and greater access to antiretroviral treatment as it became available in countries around the world (Kenworthy and Parker 2014), together with the growth of the global AIDS industry, or simply 'Global AIDS', as Hakan Seckinelgin (2017) has termed it. However, this third phase of the international response was also a time of fragmentation and regression, as the priorities and resources committed to the HIV epidemic gradually began to fail, and the earlier emphasis on human rights and the fight against stigma and discrimination gave way to a re-biomedicalisation of the epidemic, stressing biomedical approaches to prevention rather than broader social and political mobilisation as a response (Aggleton and Parker 2015). A so-called 'AIDS Backlash' (England 2007; Smith and Whiteside 2010), decrying unacceptably high investment in the AIDS response when compared to other 'higher impact' (in terms of the 'global burden of disease' [Hessel 2008]) global health challenges coincided with the 2007–2008 global financial crisis. This suggested that the 'boom era' in global health funding might be coming to an end (Fidler 2009; World Health Organization 2009) and led to demands for policymaking to be informed primarily by epidemiology and global health expenditure rather than other factors (Adams 2016; Tichenor and Sridhar 2019).

Beginning in about 2011 or 2012, we can identify a fourth wave, in which wildly optimistic claims began to be made about the imminent end of AIDS and the possibility of 'an AIDS-free generation', alongside more empirically grounded (but similarly grandiose) claims concerning the effectiveness of biomedical prevention in real-world situations (Kenworthy et al. 2018; Sandset 2020). By the time the United Nations was developing its Political Declaration on Ending AIDS and setting itself on a 'fast track to accelerate the fight against HIV and to Ending the AIDS epidemic by 2030' (United Nations General Assembly 2016), it was clear that the funding streams that had been so central to scale-up of the global HIV response were beginning to wane (Kates et al. 2017; see, also, Haakenstad et al. 2019) leading to yet further emphasis on targeted biomedical interventions as the primary means of confronting the global epidemic (Geng et al. 2019). By 2018, widespread doubt was beginning to be expressed not only about whether or not claims about the imminent End of AIDS bore any relationship to reality, but also whether they might in fact be a smokescreen cover-up for a global 'scale-down' rather than a 'scale-up' of international effort (Kenworthy and Parker 2014; Kenworthy et al. 2018). Within just a few years of the 2016 Political Declaration, international donors had already begun to withdraw from middle- and lower-income countries (Resch and Hecht 2018), and numerous HIV initiatives and agencies were showing signs of internal crisis (Fidler 2018; Marten and Hawkins 2018). Neoliberal policies and reforms (aided and abetted by a global financial crisis so persistent and extended that it had become 'the new normal') were growing in strength, rolling back conceptual and programmatic advances that had once seemed solid and sustainable (De Vogli 2011; Keshavjee 2014).

By the late-2010s, the official (both governmental and intergovernmental) response to the global HIV epidemic had increasingly lost both their veracity and legitimacy. Perhaps nowhere was this clearer than in repeated promises of the imminent 'End of AIDS', not so much as an aspirational goal (which might have been a reasonable policy strategy), but as a marketing slogan aimed at selling a vision of the global response to the epidemic as an exemplary success story of global health and development (Kenworthy et al. 2018). What such claims ignored was the fact that millions of people living with HIV in countries around the world still did not have access to antiretroviral treatment and that almost nowhere was access to HIV prevention guaranteed as a fundamental human right. They also ignored many of the other important lessons learned from community responses to the HIV epidemic (Aggleton and Parker 2015). Because of this, the world was increasingly at risk of what Boaventura de Sousa Santos has described, in a different context, as 'the waste of experience' (Santos 2015, p. 157). It seemed as if the HIV response was in danger of throwing away much of what had been learned over nearly 40 years, and of being forever condemned to reinventing the wheel time and again.

But this troublesome state of affairs was interrupted, and the status of the HIV epidemic as a focus of global attention was further displaced, in 2020 when the COVID-19 pandemic arrived (first reported in Wuhan in late 2019 and then declared a global pandemic in early 2020). Other epidemics had of course impacted the field of global health in the period in between – Ebola, SARS, MERS and Ebola again, to name but a few. But none of them had reached the scale of a global pandemic, and perhaps because of this, none had come close to eclipsing HIV as the world's biggest health and development concern, until 2020 at least. COVID-19, in contrast, arrived exactly at the point when the fourth wave of the AIDS epidemic was coming to a close, at least in part based on the realisation that claims to success in achieving the end of AIDS had begun to unravel. Just two years after the UN General Assembly passed the Political Declaration on HIV and AIDS (United Nations General Assembly 2016), UNAIDS itself had to admit that progress towards the end of AIDS was slowing (UNAIDS 2018; UNAIDS Press Release 2018). By the time Winnie Byanyima replaced Michel Sidibé as the Executive Director of UNAIDS in November of 2019, COVID-19 was just around the corner. And by mid-2020, shortly after COVID-19 had been granted the status of a truly global pandemic, it was already being identified as a key reason why the previously stated goal of ending AIDS by 2030 was unlikely to be met (UNAIDS Press Release 2020). In short, confidence in the imminent End of AIDS evaporated at the very moment COVID-19 arrived, and the serious disruptions caused by the COVID-19 pandemic provided an 'honourable' way out of the dead-end the administrators of the HIV epidemic had dug themselves into (Global Fund 2021; Global Fund Press Release 2021).

In the wake of COVID-19 and with growing failure in the international response to HIV, we find ourselves at the beginning of a fifth wave in the global response to HIV and AIDS. Although it is still too early to definitely characterise this wave, presently it might best be described as one of 'busy irrelevance' – characterised by a continued emphasis on technical fixes (inherited from the third and the fourth waves of the HIV response), wildly grandiose and unattainable target setting (such as the eradication of world poverty) (UNAIDS 2021, 2022) and lack of relevance in the face of anti-democratic populist conservatism/illiberalism (Stavrakakis 2018; Duppel 2020) and 're-traditionalisation', linked to gender and other culture wars

(Sajó et al. 2021). Within this context, AIDS does not end, but simply fades from view – in both public debate and global consciousness. Unable to compete with the immediacy and priority that COVID-19 had assumed (although it is also striking how quickly COVID-19 has already faded from public view in contexts where vaccines have led to a sense of biomedical triumphalism), HIV has become just another health issue for nations, both rich and poor, to contend with amidst other pressing items on the agenda including famine, climate change, mass migration, civil unrest and war.

Stigma, discrimination and denial / Knowledge, ignorance and power

Within this broad history of epidemic responses, it is worth pausing to consider the ways in which the biomedical sciences, public health and related disciplines have been convoked within them. In the case of HIV, both science and public health were relatively slow to act, taking several years to identify and isolate the virus and understand its complexity. Almost certainly because the first 'victims' of AIDS (many of them gay men or people in poverty) were considered socially marginal, undesirable, deviant and expendable, part of the problem lay in the stigma and discrimination directed towards those most affected (and even the scientists investigating it). In the case of COVID-19, in contrast, where the potential for widespread impact on the 'general' population was perceived as inevitable, biomedical science and public health were quicker to act, not initially with 'evidence-based' solutions such as proven means of prevention, treatment and cure, but with epidemiology as the leading science. As with HIV, the language of 'waves' was quickly appropriated to speak about the new pandemic – but conceived this time only as waves of COVID-19 viral variants rather than the more complex social and political processes described above. These epidemiological discourses (and, subsequently, media and popular representations of them) quickly eclipsed the language of a 'global epidemic' and the need for solidarity within and between nations that had been used to talk about AIDS in the 1980s. They replaced it instead by talk of a 'pandemic' in ways that are worth reflecting upon.

The denial and negation that had been a central part of the early history of HIV and AIDS, with leaders in countries as diverse as the USA, India, the former USSR and South Africa denying at different times that AIDS would be a problem for 'their' populations (Sabatier 1988; The Panos Institute 1990), and some scientists such as Peter Duesberg questioning whether HIV was the true or only cause of AIDS (Duesberg 1996; Specter 2007) was reproduced with perhaps even greater fervour in the early days of COVID-19. But there were significant differences in this dynamic that it is important to recognise. The stigma and discrimination associated with populations and communities affected by HIV – gay, bisexual and other men who have sex with men, transgender women and occasionally men, sex workers, injecting drug users, and supposedly promiscuous cisgender heterosexuals, for example – largely drove the dynamic of denial in relation to HIV.

In the case of COVID-19, in contrast, denial was more frequently linked to rejection of scientific information about the virus, its modes of transmission, or knowledge about prevention and effective treatment (Ortega and Orsini 2020; Falkenbach and Greer 2021; Parker and Ferraz 2021). This was linked to political manipulation of a type that had certainly existed in relation to HIV (with conservative politicians such as Ronald Reagan seeking political gain by stigmatising vulnerable minority populations, for example), but which this time took the form of extreme right-wing rage fuelled by conspiracy claims, often promulgated by social media, directed against anything that might hint of, or be construed as, state control. In the case of COVID-19, this led important actors (not just scientists, and much of the mainstream media) to engage in fervent defence of the truths of viral transmission in the face of rampant denialism and speculation concerning the viral origins of COVID-19. These events highlight the importance of paying attention not only to knowledge and its relation to power, but also to what might be described as the social and cultural 'construction of ignorance' (Proctor and Schiebinger 2008; Gross and McGoey 2015). In the case of both COVID-19 and HIV, social and political forces and economic interests actively constructed ignorance in complex ways, shaping the rapid development of the epidemics – and have their most serious impact on racial and ethnic minority populations, as well as on those who are poor (Fairchild et al. 2020; Timmermann 2020) in rich-, middle- and lower-income countries alike. This use of ignorance for strategic purposes has sought also to individualise responsibility for the everyday management of the epidemic, with the abdicating near-total responsibility on the part of the governments all over the world for anything other than mass vaccination, often ineffective public information campaigns, and on–off lockdowns (Ortega and Orsini 2020; Falkenbach and Greer 2021).

Much more in the case of COVID-19 than with HIV, this strategic deployment of ignorance raised questions about the apparent neutrality of epidemiological claims, with some high-profile politicians (such as Donald Trump in the USA and Jair Bolsonaro in Brazil) rejecting evidence-based science in its near entirety, while political leaders in countries such as the UK, Canada and much of continental Europe tended more easily to acknowledge the 'science' they were presented with – at least when it aligned with broader national and political priorities (Greer, Jarman et al. 2021; Greer, King et al. 2021).

The social and political determinants of death

In the case of HIV, limited success in developing vaccines together with a slower-moving epidemic created the opportunity for social research and advocacy to understand the structural forces driving the epidemic. This took time – nearly a decade to seed the beginnings of an insightful and critical social research agenda – and it was really only in the second decade of the global epidemic (during the 1990s) that insight into the social drivers of infection began to emerge. But the longer trajectory of HIV response was also a double-edged sword, and during the third major wave of the AIDS response in the mid to late-2000s, as the re-biomedicalisation of the epidemic took place, concern for the social diminished, with consequences we can now recognise as profoundly negative.

In the case of COVID-19 in contrast, a more massive scientific effort focusing on vaccine development moved matters forward (in marked contrast to the history of vaccine development in response to HIV), as did research on clinical approaches to reduce the initially high rates of morbidity and mortality associated with the pandemic. Social research was also quicker to mobilise, and insights that were only slowly achieved in the response to HIV – especially concerning the role of structural violence in driving viral transmission – were more quickly understood in relation to COVID-19. Activists, scholars and at least some policymakers (though more rarely) identified racism, gender oppression, colonialism, capitalism and neoliberalism as key drivers behind the new pandemic (Parker and Ferraz 2021).

Building on the analysis of structural factors and social inequalities identified as key drivers of HIV, much initial research on COVID-19 highlighted to role of health disparities and social vulnerability in shaping the impact of COVID-19 on different populations. In spite of the viruses' very different forms of transmission, gender, race/ethnicity and class/poverty were quickly found to be equally important in relation to COVID-19 as they had been in relation to HIV (Patel et al. 2020; Paremoer et al. 2021) – and while they received much less attention, inequities related to sexuality and sexual diversity have also been highlighted by social research (Döring 2020; García-Iglesias et al. 2021), as was the importance of stigma and discrimination in fuelling the new pandemic (Roelen et al. 2020). Research on COVID-19 also exposed the ways in which healthcare systems, capitalism's supply chains, work conditions, forced migration, migratory labour and a range of related issues affected access to personal protective equipment, medicines, vaccines and related health services and technologies (McClure et al. 2020; Sell 2020; Green 2021; De Genova 2022; Lee et al. 2022; Sparke and Levy 2022; Sparke and Williams 2022).

Yet what is perhaps most striking is that while these insights received significant scholarly and media attention, they have had remarkably little impact on the ways in which elected representatives, officials and the public health system responded to the new pandemic. Concern with the impact of social inequalities may have received the occasional polite 'lip-service', but rarely if ever has it influenced policy or programme development – contrasting markedly with the case of HIV during the second and third waves of the HIV response. Other key learning from the HIV response could also have been incorporated into the COVID-19 response. The importance of human rights, for example, was largely ignored, with notions of 'global health security' quickly trumping the defence of individual rights (Nunes 2020; Patterson and Clark 2020). Perhaps most strikingly, the considerations that led to the Doha Declaration on the TRIPS Agreement and Public Health and which resulted in increased access to medicine and medical technologies in relation to HIV were quickly outmanoeuvred by commercial and financial interests in debates and policies related to COVID-19 related vaccine equity and availability (Zaitchik 2021; Zarocostas 2022; Sparke and Levy 2023).

While a full account of the behind the scenes machinations cannot be provided here, one of the key things that COVID-19 has revealed however is the extent to which the pharmaceutical industry and its allies in intellectual property protection (including the Bill and Melinda Gates Foundation) had come to dominate not only the field of global health, but also key international institutions such as the World Health Organization (WHO) and the WTO (Torreele and Amon 2021). In the midst of a fast-moving global emergency, these groups succeeded in dominating the 'global governance' mechanisms aimed at promoting vaccine equity through COVAX, 'the vaccines pillar of the Access to COVID-19 Tools (ACT) Accelerator' (a public-private partnership between the Coalition for Epidemic Preparedness Innovations [CEPI], GAVI [the Vaccine Alliance], WHO and UNICEF) (Banco et al. 2022), which some saw as the world's primary vaccine charity initiative (Sparke and Levy 2022). At the same time, the same constellation of allies managed to slow deliberations in the WTO for a temporary patent waiver on COVID-19 vaccines as requested by a coalition of Southern nations led by South Africa and India, for nearly two years, and to gut the final agreement of its most important elements by excluding diagnostics and therapeutics (Torreele and Amon 2021; Zaitchik 2021; Zarocostas 2022).

What the debates and negotiations played out over the worst period of suffering and death caused by the COVID-19 pandemic between 2020 and 2022 demonstrated was not an advance in defence of health as a fundamental human right, but rather how the global health industry had learned how to roll back such advances. It essentially succeeded in undercutting any real emphasis on human rights with superficial marketing claims related to biomedical triumphalism (which guaranteed commercial access to rich countries and populations while simultaneously camouflaging short-term charity initiatives to poor countries and populations) combined with more or less draconian regulations employed to control population movement both across borders and within countries.

Looking back at health policies and politics internationally over the course of the past four decades, and at the HIV and the COVID-19 pandemics and the responses they generated, it is clear there remains an ongoing challenge to address the social as opposed to the biomedical dimensions of these concerns. One of the most important developments in the health-related social sciences over the course of the past 40 years has been growing awareness of what have been described (largely in parallel) as the 'fundamental causes of disease' (Link and Phelan 1995) and the 'social determinants of health' (Marmot and Wilkinson 2005). Such approaches, first developed in the later part of the twentieth century (Braveman et al. 2011), have had some influence over policy and programme design, being taken up by leading international organisations such as WHO as well as by a few national agencies in both the Global North and the Global South (Friel and Marmot 2011). While these developments have been important, it is shocking to see how limited the focus on fundamental social causes and determinants of health has been in the response to global health crises. Instead of addressing the social dimensions of infection and disease, both initial and ongoing responses to diseases such as HIV and COVID-19 have consistently prioritised biomedical perspectives, products and technologies. This has been paralleled by the development of the 'global health industry' (itself an outgrowth of the earlier 'AIDS industry') as an assemblage of commercial, philanthropic, academic, and civil society organisations, institutions and interests, that has developed over the past four decades to become the major apparatus for responding to newly emerging global health threats.

What our analysis of responses to HIV and COVID-19 suggests is that these responses were not shaped, at least in the first instance, by a focus on the fundamental causes of disease or even on the social determinants of health. On the contrary, in viral times, and in times of crisis and public health panic, a very different logic has come into play – one that might more accurately be described and understood as the social and political determinants of *death*. In keeping with a focus on 'structural violence' (Galtung 1969) or 'necropolitics' (Mbembé 2003), the social and political power that determines how some people may live – but others must die – comes to dominate the priorities that are set and the decisions that are made. As we close this chapter, it is on this dimension and its veritable appropriation by official and institutional responses on the part of established powers – that we wish to focus.

What both HIV and COVID-19 clearly demonstrated was that who would become ill and who would die in each of these global epidemics was never at random, and certainly never simply biologically determined. Instead, risk of infection, vulnerability to illness, resilience in response to care, and every other aspect of lived experience in both of these global epidemics depended as much on social and political factors as on biological or medical considerations. Racism, gender oppression, sexual stigma and discrimination and class oppression have undeniably been the key drivers of both epidemics, and these drivers, while undeniably social, are *also* political – they exist and continue to operate in the ways that they do because they are grounded in relations of power. Ultimately, they determined who would die, and who might live, and under what circumstances. To effectively confront both epidemics therefore requires engagement with the social and political determinants of *death*, and it is precisely because of this that collective practices of resistance have proved to be exceptionally important in responses to both HIV and COVID-19.

What we think has been less clearly recognised and addressed is the extent to which concern for the social and political determinants of *death* has also infiltrated the responses of governments, of intergovernmental systems, and the globalised neoliberal capitalist system more broadly. Quite clearly, in both pandemics, some people, some communities and some whole elements of society have been regarded as dispensable, both during the crisis and in its aftermath. Affected communities, activists, and at least some sectors of civil society may have resisted these forces, but with the passage of time and both in the case of HIV and COVID-19 they were silenced and side-lined by an established but complex political order. The result of this is that both HIV and COVID-19 remain with us today, affecting those who are poor, those who are marginalised, and those who are otherwise excluded, far more than others – with no end of either pandemic in sight but paralleled by the growth of a biomedical establishment more concerned with maintaining its own ascendancy and funding flows, than truly addressing the suffering and death it claims to be able to end.

References

Adams, V., 2016. *Metrics: What counts in global health.* Durham, NC: Duke University Press.

Aggleton, P. and Parker, R., 2015. Moving beyond biomedicalization in the HIV response: Implications for community involvement and community leadership among men who have sex with men and transgender people. *American Journal of Public Health*, 105 (8), 1552–1558. 10.2105/AJPH.2015.302614

Amorim, C., 2017. *Acting globally: Memoirs of Brazil's assertive foreign policy.* Lanham, MD: Rowman & Littlefield.

Banco, E., Furlong, A., and Pfahker, L., 2022. How Bill Gates and his partners used their clout to control the global Covid response – with little oversight. *Politico.* www.politico.com/news/2022/09/14/global-covid-pandemic-response-bill-gates-partners-00053969

Brandt, A.M., 2013. How AIDS invented global health. *New England Journal of Medicine*, 368 (23), 2149–2152. 10.1056/NEJMp1305297

Braveman, P., Egerter, S., and Williams, D.R., 2011. The social determinants of health: Coming of age. *Annual Review of Public Health*, 32, 381–398. 10.1146/annurev-publhealth-031210-101218

Brown, T.M., Cueto, M., and Fee, E., 2006. The World Health Organization and the transition from "international" to "global" public health. *American Journal of Public Health*, 96 (1), 62–72. 10.2105/AJPH.2004.050831

De Genova, N., 2022. Viral borders: Migration, deceleration, and the re-bordering of mobility during the COVID-19 pandemic. *Communication, Culture and Critique*, 15 (2), 139–156. 10.1093/ccc/tcac009

De Vogli, R., 2011. Neoliberal globalisation and health in a time of economic crisis. *Social Theory & Health*, 9 (4), 311–325. 10.1057/sth.2011.16

Döring, N., 2020. How is the COVID-19 pandemic affecting our sexualities? An overview of the current media narratives and research hypotheses. *Archives of Sexual Behavior*, 49 (8), 2765–2778. 10.1007/s10508-020-01790-z

Duppel, W., 2020. The paradox of (neo)liberal society: Collective consent for an anti-democratic project. *Confluence*, 2 (1), 132–151.

Duesberg, P., 1996. *Inventing the AIDS virus.* Washington, DC: Regnery Press.

England, R., 2007. Are we spending too much on HIV? *British Medical Journal*, 334 (7589), 334–344. 10.1136/bmj.39113.402361.94

Fairchild, A., Gostin, L., and Bayer, R., 2020. Vexing, veiled, and inequitable: Social distancing and the "rights" divide in the age of COVID-19. *The American Journal of Bioethics*, 20 (7), 55–61. 10.1080/15265161.2020.1764142

Falkenbach, M. and Greer, S.L., 2021. Denial and distraction: How the populist radical right responds to COVID-19; comment on "A scoping review of PRR parties' influence on welfare policy and its implication for population health in Europe". *International Journal of Health Policy and Management*, 10 (9), 578–580. 10.34172/ijhpm.2020.141

Fidler, D.P., 2009. After the revolution: Global health politics in a time of economic crisis and threatening future trends. *Global Health Governance*, 2 (2), 1–21.

Fidler, D., 2018. *PEPFAR's impact on global health is fading*. Council on Foreign Relations. www.cfr.org/expert-brief/pepfars-impact-global-health-fading

Friel, S. and Marmot, M.G., 2011. Action on the social determinants of health and health inequities goes global. *Annual Review of Public Health*, 32, 225–236. 10.1146/annurev-publhealth-031210-101220

Galtung J., 1969. Violence, peace, and peace research. *Journal of Peace Research*, 6 (3), 167–191.

García-Iglesias, J., Nagington, M., and Aggleton, P., 2021. Viral times, viral memories, viral questions. *Culture, Health & Sexuality*, 23 (11), 1465–1469. 10.1080/13691058.2021.1976564

Geng, E.H., et al., 2019. Personalized public health: An implementation research agenda for the HIV response and beyond. *PLoS Medicine*, 16 (12), e1003020. 10.1371/journal.pmed.1003020

Global Fund, 2021. *Results report 2021*. Geneva: The Global Fund to Fight AIDS, Tuberculosis and Malaria.

Global Fund Press Release, 2021. *Global fund results report reveals COVID-19 devastating impact on HIV, TB and Malaria programs* [press release], 8 September. www.theglobalfund.org/en/news/2021-09-08-global-fund-results-report-reveals-covid-19-devastating-impact-on-hiv-tb-and-malaria-programs/

Green, T., 2021. *The Covid consensus: The new politics of global inequality*. Oxford: Oxford University Press.

Greer, S.L., Jarman, H., et al., 2021. Social policy as an integral component of pandemic response: Learning from COVID-19 in Brazil, Germany, India and the United States. *Global Public Health*, 16 (8-9), 1209–1222. 10.1080/17441692.2021.1916831

Greer, S. L., King, E., et al., 2021. *Coronavirus politics: The comparative politics and policy of COVID-19*. Ann Arbor: University of Michigan Press. 10.3998/mpub.11927713

Gross, M. and McGoey, L., eds., 2015. *Routledge international handbook of ignorance studies*. Abingdon: Routledge.

Haakenstad, A., et al., 2019. Potential for additional government spending on HIV/AIDS in 137 low-income and middle-income countries: an economic modelling study. *The Lancet HIV*, 6 (6), e382–e395. 10.1016/S2352-3018(19)30038-4

Hessel, F., 2008. Global burden of disease. In W. Kirch, ed., *Encyclopedia of public health: Volume 1: A-H*. Cham: Springer Science & Business Media, 94–96.

Kates, J., Wexler, A., and Lief, E., 2017. *Donor government funding for HIV in low-and middle-income countries in 2016*. Menlo Park, CA: Kaiser Family Foundation and UNAIDS.

Kenworthy, N.J. and Parker, R., 2014. HIV scale-up and the politics of global health. *Global Public Health*, 9 (1-2), 1–6. 10.1080/17441692.2014.880727

Kenworthy, N., Thomann, M., and Parker, R., 2018. From a global crisis to the 'end of AIDS': New epidemics of signification. *Global Public Health*, 13 (8), 960–971. 10.1080/17441692.2017.1365373

Keshavjee, S., 2014. *Blind spot: How neoliberalism infiltrated global health.* California Series in Public Anthropology vol. 30. Oakland, CA: University of California Press.

Lee, R.S., Collins, K., and Perez-Brumer, A., 2022. COVID-19 violence and the structural determinants of death: Canada's seasonal agricultural worker programme. *Global Public Health*, 17 (5), 784–793. 10.1080/17441692.2022.2053735

Link, B.G. and Phelan, J., 1995. Social conditions as fundamental causes of disease. *Journal of Health and Social Behavior*, 35 (extra issue), 80–94.

Marmot, M. and Wilkinson, R., eds., 2005. *Social determinants of health.* Oxford: Oxford University Press.

Marten, R. and Hawkins, B., 2018. Partnering over the limit: The Global Fund's brewing crisis. *The Lancet*, 391 (10131), 1675. 10.1016/S0140-6736(18)30856-0

Mbembé, J.A., 2003. Necropolitics. *Public Culture*, 15 (1), 11–40.

McClure, E.S., et al., 2020. Racial capitalism within public health – How occupational settings drive COVID-19 disparities. *American Journal of Epidemiology*, 189 (11), 1244–1253. 10.1093/aje/kwaa126

Nunes, J., 2020. The COVID-19 pandemic: Securitization, neoliberal crisis, and global vulnerabilization. *Cadernos de Saúde Pública*, 36 (4), e00063120. 10.1590/0102-311X00063120

Ortega, F. and Orsini, M., 2020. Governing COVID-19 without government in Brazil: Ignorance, neoliberal authoritarianism, and the collapse of public health leadership. *Global Public Health*, 15 (9), 1257–1277. 10.1080/17441692.2020.1795223

Packard, R.M., 2016. *A history of global health: Interventions into the lives of other peoples.* Baltimore, MD: Johns Hopkins University Press.

Paremoer, L., et al., 2021. Covid-19 pandemic and the social determinants of health. *British Medical Journal*, 372. 10.1136/bmj.n129

Parker, R., 2011. Grassroots activism, civil society mobilization, and the politics of the global HIV/AIDS epidemic. *The Brown Journal of World Affairs*, 17 (2), 21–37.

Parker, R. and Aggleton, P., 2003. HIV and AIDS-related stigma and discrimination: A conceptual framework and implications for action. *Social Science & Medicine*, 57 (1), 13–24. 10.1016/S0277-9536(02)00304-0

Parker, R. and Ferraz, D., 2021. Politics and pandemics. *Global Public Health*, 16 (8-9), 1131–1140. 10.1080/17441692.2021.1947601

Patel, J.A., et al., 2020. Poverty, inequality and COVID-19: The forgotten vulnerable. *Public Health*, 183, 110. 10.1016/j.puhe.2020.05.006

Patterson, A. and Clark, M.A., 2020. COVID-19 and power in global health. *International Journal of Health Policy and Management*, 9 (10), 429–431. 10.34172/ijhpm.2020.72

Piot, P., 2015. *AIDS between science and politics.* New York: Columbia University Press.

Proctor, R.N. and Schiebinger, L., eds., 2008. *Agnotology: The making & unmaking of ignorance.* Stanford, CA: Stanford University Press. https://philarchive.org/archive/PROATM

Resch, S. and Hecht, R., 2018. Transitioning financial responsibility for health programs from external donors to developing countries: Key issues and recommendations for policy and research. *Journal of Global Health*, 8 (1), 010301.

Roelen, K., et al., 2020. COVID-19 in LMICs: The need to place stigma front and centre to its response. *The European Journal of Development Research*, 32 (5), 1592–1612. 10.1057/s41287-020-00316-6
Sabatier, R., 1988. *Blaming others: Prejudice, race and worldwide AIDS*. London: Panos Publications.
Sajó, A., Uitz, R., and Holmes, S., eds., 2021. *Routledge handbook of illiberalism*. Abingdon: Routledge.
Sandset, T., 2020. *'Ending AIDS' in the age of biopharmaceuticals: The individual, the state and the politics of prevention*. Abingdon: Routledge.
Santos, B.S., 2015. A critique of lazy reason: Against the waste of experience. In I. Wallerstein, ed. *Modern World-System in the Longue Durée*. Abingdon: Routledge, 157–197.
Seckinelgin, H., 2017. *The politics of global AIDS: Institutionalization of solidarity, exclusion of context*. Cham: Springer.
Sell, S.K., 2020. What COVID-19 reveals about twenty-first century capitalism: Adversity and opportunity. *Development*, 63 (2), 150–156. 10.1057/s41301-020-00263-z
Smith, J.H. and Whiteside, A., 2010. The history of AIDS exceptionalism. *Journal of the International AIDS Society*, 13 (1), 1–8. 10.1186/1758-2652-13-47
Sparke, M. and Levy, O., 2022. Competing responses to global inequalities in access to COVID vaccines: Vaccine diplomacy and vaccine charity versus vaccine liberty. *Clinical Infectious Diseases*, 75 (S1), S86–S92. 10.1093/cid/ciac361
Sparke, M., and Levy, O., 2023. Immunizing against access? Philanthro-capitalist COVID vaccines and the preservation of patent monopolies. In K. Mitchell and P. Pallister-Wilkins, eds. *The Routledge handbook of critical philanthropy and humanitarianism*. New York: Routledge, 71–93.
Sparke, M. and Williams, O.D., 2022. Neoliberal disease: COVID-19, co-pathogenesis and global health insecurities. *Environment and Planning A: Economy and Space*, 54 (1), 15–32. 10.1177/0308518X211048905
Specter, M., 2007. The denialists: The dangerous attacks on the consensus about HIV and AIDS. *The New Yorker*, 12 March, 32–38.
Stavrakakis, Y., 2018. Populism, anti-populism and democracy. *Political Insight*, 9 (3), 33–35. 10.1177/2041905818796577
Stuenkel, O., 2019. *India-Brazil-South Africa dialogue forum (IBSA): The rise of the global South*. Abingdon: Routledge.
The Panos Institute, 1990. *The 3rd Epidemic: Repercussions of the fear of AIDS*. London: Panos Publications.
Tichenor, M. and Sridhar, D., 2019. Metric partnerships: Global burden of disease estimates within the World Bank, the World Health Organisation and the Institute for Health Metrics and Evaluation. *Wellcome Open Research*, 4 (35). 10.12688/wellcomeopenres.15011.2
Timmermann, C., 2020. Epistemic ignorance, poverty and the COVID-19 pandemic. *Asian Bioethics Review*, 12 (4), 519–527. 10.1007/s41649-020-00140-4
Torreele, E. and Amon, J.J., 2021. Equitable COVID-19 vaccine access. *Health and Human Rights*, 23 (1), 273.
UNAIDS, 2018. *Miles to go: Closing gaps, breaking barriers, fighting injustice*. Geneva: Joint United Nations Programme on HIV/AIDS. www.unaids.org/en/resources/documents/2018/global-aids-update
UNAIDS, 2021. *Unequal, unprepared, under threat: Why bold action against inequalities is needed to end AIDS, stop COVID-19 and prepare for future*

pandemics. Geneva: Joint United Nations Programme on HIV/AIDS. www.unaids.org/en/resources/documents/2021/2021-World-AIDS-Day-report

UNAIDS, 2022. *Dangerous inequalities: World AIDS Day report 2022*. Geneva: Joint United Nations Programme on HIV/AIDS. www.unaids.org/sites/default/files/media_asset/dangerous-inequalities_en.pdf

UNAIDS Press Release, 2018. *UNAIDS warns that progress is slowing and time is running out to reach the 2020 HIV targets* [press release], 18 July. www.unaids.org/en/resources/presscentre/pressreleaseandstatementarchive/2018/july/miles-to-go

UNAIDS Press Release, 2020. *UNAIDS report on the global AIDS epidemic shows that 2020 targets will not be met because of deeply unequal success; COVID-19 risks blowing HIV progress way off course* [press release], 6 July. www.unaids.org/en/resources/presscentre/pressreleaseandstatementarchive/2020/july/20200706_global-aids-report

United Nations General Assembly, 2016. Political declaration on HIV and AIDS: On the fast-track to accelerate the fight against HIV and to end the AIDS epidemic by 2030. New York: United Nations. https://digitallibrary.un.org/record/831426?ln=en

World Health Organization, 2009. *The financial crisis and global health: Report of a high-level consultation, Geneva, Switzerland, 19 January 2009* (No. WHO/DGO/2009.1). Geneva: World Health Organization.

Zaitchik, A., 2021. How Bill Gates impeded global access to Covid vaccines. *The New Republic*, 12. https://newrepublic.com/article/162000/bill-gates-impeded-global-access-covid-vaccines [Accessed 19 September 2022]

Zarocostas, J., 2022. Mixed response to COVID-19 intellectual property waiver. *The Lancet*, 399 (10332), 1292–1293. 10.1016/S0140-6736(22)00610-9

10 Viral times and governance

The Philippines

Michael Lim Tan

When I was invited to contribute to this anthology, I immediately thought about a focus on governance and leadership in the Philippines in relation to HIV and AIDS and to COVID-19, and how differing modes of governance led to major differences in the way the pandemics unfolded and affected the country.

Shortly before the pandemic, I had read about the 2019 Global Health Security (GHS) Index (John Hopkins Center for Health Security and the Nuclear Threat Initiative 2019), a report that rated the USA number one in terms of preparedness for health security. I looked up the report on the Internet when COVID-19 broke out and found a PLOS journal article (Abbey et al. 2020) with the title: 'Global Health Security (GHS) Index is not predictive of coronavirus pandemic responses in the OECD (Organization for Economic Cooperation and Development)', noting that the top five countries ranked by the GHS Index countries were among those worst affected by COVID-19. The PLOS article concluded that the COVID-19 situation was 'directly influenced by the decisions made by a country's leadership in mobilizing critical resources and engaging proper stakeholders' (Abbey et al. 2020).

The report's inadequacy may as well have concerned not just the OECD but the world. Comparing the rankings in the report with how countries fared in the battle against COVID-19, it became clear that the GHS Index's main weakness lay in its inability to capture the importance of governance in relation to health security.

Against this background, this chapter focuses on the Philippines to reveal some of the dynamics behind governance and health security. The theme of the book in which it appears, 'Viral Times', could not have been more apt as I found myself using HIV and AIDS and COVID-19 as adjectives, thinking of the pandemics as HIV and AIDS and COVID-19 times. During the more recent COVID-19 pandemic, I had just finished a six-year stint as chancellor of the University of the Philippines Diliman. The university kindly allowed me to stay on in the campus, using the chancellor's official residence for a few more months after the end of my term. During this time, I was able to move around the sprawling campus and observe what was going on among the remaining

DOI: 10.4324/9781003322788-12

faculty, staff and some students, as well as in the large slum communities of informal settlers or 'squatters' occupying nearby land illegally.

As COVID-19 unfolded, I was invited to many online meetings with health professionals, consulted as a medical anthropologist and interacted with mass media practitioners because of a newspaper column I write weekly in the country's largest English language broadsheet. The exchanges, including those with readers of my column, provided many insights into the problems of the pandemic, as well as the reasons for the many lapses that occurred in the management of COVID-19.

HIV and AIDS, which seemed to be fading to a distant past, took on new significance as I recalled my work, during the early years of AIDS in the 1980s, with Health Action Information Network, a non-governmental organisation (NGO) that was among the first in the country to be supported by USAID for initial HIV prevention programmes and, later, by the Philippine government as it sought to develop community partnerships.

This chapter describes the impact of two Philippine presidents with radically different leadership and governance styles. First, I will describe the response to the early years of AIDS under Fidel Ramos, who was president of the Philippines from 1992 to 1998. I will then write about COVID-19 under President Rodrigo Duterte, one of several right-wing populist authoritarian presidents, notably Donald Trump in the USA and Jair Bolsonario in Brazil, who were heads of state in COVID-19 times. Duterte became president in 2016 on a law-and-order platform that included a war on drugs that led to the killings of, according to official figures, some 6,000 suspected drug users, with human rights groups estimating the actual figure may have been more than 30,000.

HIV and AIDS times

President Fidel Ramos was a key military official during the martial law regime and the Marcos dictatorship, but he turned against Marcos in 1986 in the 'People Power' uprising that led to Marcos' deposition. He was voted into office as a civilian and kept his distance from the military throughout his six-year presidency. Ramos was the first Protestant to be elected president in a predominantly Catholic Philippines and held his ground dealing with powerful and vocal Catholic bishops who were on the frontlines of culture wars around reproductive and sexual health. On HIV, the Catholic bishops opposed the promotion of condoms and sexuality education in general, insisting on abstinence and monogamy as the only effective measures against the epidemic.

Ramos' Health Secretary was Juan Flavier, also a Protestant known for his work with community-oriented health programmes and family planning before he entered government. Once appointed as Health Secretary, Flavier pushed hard for reproductive health. The message sent out by Ramos and Flavier was clear: uphold science in health care. The Ramos administration reached out to civil society, inviting them to become partners in health care, but without asking the NGOs to compromise on a history of critical health activism. Many of the organisations dated back to martial law and the Marcos dictatorship (1972–1986) with much organising work. HIV saw this health organising work extended to populations that had hitherto been discriminated against, even by progressives; in particular sex workers and gay men.

The Ramos administration created a Philippine National AIDS Council (PNAC), which helped to advance a progressive agenda that was later codified in an AIDS Act passed in 1999, putting an end to the calls for mandatory testing and isolation, or even the incarceration of people living with HIV. Most importantly, the new law assured civil society representation in the PNAC, notable in its inclusion of seats reserved for sex workers, gay men (later expanded to LGBT communities) and people living with HIV. Filipino HIV and AIDS activists actively participated in a wide spectrum of activities, from public education to caring for populations affected by HIV. Anti-retroviral drugs were made available for free and paid for by the government, helped by global efforts to make these drugs accessible.

The commitment to civil society participation has been maintained in HIV-related work, with strong links with women's organisations and reproductive health networks. The power of these groups was reflected in the successful lobbying and passage of a new AIDS Act in 2018. This newer version strengthens support for many HIV-related programmes. It allowed minors, aged 15 and up, to undergo an HIV test without parental or guardian's consent, a radical provision in a country where the minimum age for marriage is 18 and only with parental permission if the contracting parties are below the age of 21.

Certainly, 'HIV and AIDS times' in the Philippines were not always easy. Discrimination remained strong against groups like injecting drug users, and harm reduction programmes involving the distribution of syringes and needles to drug users were fiercely opposed in several cities. The fortunes of these harm reduction programmes depended on local government officials, who could easily open or close down the programmes. By and large though, the HIV pandemic allowed previously marginalised groups to become more visible and vocal, providing strong evidence that community mobilisation was vital in responding to public health emergencies. When COVID-19 emerged in the Philippines in 2020, there were many times when I thought of how our earlier experiences of handling HIV, particularly in getting communities involved, could have mitigated the adverse impacts of the new pandemic.

COVID-19 times

On 15 March 2020, Philippine President Rodrigo Duterte imposed a lockdown. The day before the lockdown began, I visited my children, who were about an hour and a half's drive away from where I lived, to assure them that, based on our experience with the SARS pandemic some 20 years earlier, the lockdown would probably be brief. Who would have known that it would be another three months before I would be reunited with my children, armed with all kinds of identification cards and permits to hurdle checkpoints in what was to be one of the world's longest and most restrictive lockdowns.

The government initially used the term 'lockdown' to describe the changes brought about but, realising how ominous it sounded, switched to 'community quarantine', with all kinds of acronyms to follow over the next two years. Enhanced community quarantine (ECQ) was the most well-known of these, an abbreviation that came to be a butt of jokes as the lockdown stretched, with frustrated Filipinos joking that 'e' meant 'eternal'. The presidential order was severe, closing down all business establishments except those providing essential services. Classes were suspended at primary, secondary and tertiary levels. Strict restrictions were imposed on the movement of people, requiring quarantine passes, limited to one member per household, to be able to leave home and then only to purchase groceries and medicines. Public transportation was banned. Minors (defined as those below the age of 18) and senior citizens (those over 60) were prohibited from leaving their homes without special permission.

Other measures reminded many older Filipinos, including myself, of martial law imposed in 1972 by then President Ferdinand Marcos. 'Mass gatherings' were prohibited, a night-time curfew was imposed and a 'heightened presence' of 'uniformed personnel' was ordered.

The lockdown also gave immense powers to local government executives, with governors, mayors and even *barangay* (village) officials allowed to declare their own quarantines and lockdowns. Towns and cities became mazeways of checkpoints and 'do not enter' signs.

As in many other countries, the COVID-19 pandemic revealed the many fault lines in society, or what we might call, to borrow medical terms, 'pre-existing or underlying conditions'. Medical pre-existing conditions such as diabetes and hypertension were constantly named in government press releases and information materials as increasing one's risk for COVID-19 but not the socioeconomic context or the social environments of risk that affect one's chances of being infected, and of surviving a serious infection. Some of these pre-existing social conditions are rooted in history. COVID-19 became payback time for the neglect of public housing amid urbanisation marked by massive migration and the growth of slums.

Many barangays in Metro Manila have populations of more than 30,000 people, even larger than the average rural municipality or town. The dense populations and crowded housing conditions were perfect for the spread of COVID-19. For the first few months of COVID-19, the National Health Department issued statistics on a daily basis, listing new infections by barangay, as well as by offices and institutions (e.g. jails). The grim statistics showed how COVID-19 raced through urban poor communities, a few initial cases quickly exploding to several hundred within a week or two. This was not surprising given that quarantine requirements kept people sequestered in their homes, which were often just shacks closely clustered together with poor ventilation.

The day the lockdown was implemented, I watched a television newscast showing pop-up shop vendors dismantling their tents and expressing their fear that eventually, it would be hunger and not the COVID-19 virus that would kill them. A Social Amelioration Package (SAP), targeting 18 million households, would have provided a monthly subsidy of P5000 to P8000 (about US$90–145) but only two actual payments were made during the pandemic and the subsidies were much too small to make a difference. Moreover, the funds were channelled through local government units and often tied to political connections.

COVID-19 also affected large numbers of undocumented populations, notably 'locally stranded individuals' or LSIs, usually rural migrants such as construction workers who were abandoned by their employers on construction sites, without salaries, food aid and documentation that would have made them eligible for assistance. Also put at risk were PDLs or 'persons deprived of liberty', the perversely politically correct term used to refer to jail inmates. Their numbers had swelled during the Duterte presidency and his war on drugs, with thousands of prisoners who languished in prison without formal charges ever being filed. Not surprisingly, COVID-19 outbreaks were recorded in these jails.

A failed health care system

COVID-19 exposed the consequences of the neglect of social safety nets. For example, the Philippines has no unemployment insurance, with many workers without formal work contracts and coverage by social security. Small-scale businesses comprise 99% of the country's commercial establishments (University of the Philippines Institute of Small-Scale Industries 2020); during the COVID-19 pandemic, many were closed down by the quarantine, never to reopen.

The Philippine health care system was totally unprepared for COVID-19. Besides the lack of equipment for such a communicable disease as COVID-19, health financing has always been problematic, with 48% of total health expenditures coming out of the individual or family pocket (World Bank 2023). A separate insurance system called PhilHealth only covers, for the most part, expenses incurred during hospitalisation. Worse still, massive corruption was exposed in 2020 with PhilHealth defaulting on many of its debts, as the result of covering reimbursements to private hospitals.

The corruption in PhilHealth was matched by exposés surrounding the purchase of COVID-19-related supplies. A probe by the Right to Know, Right Now! Coalition (2021) looked into P10.85 billion (US$197 million) worth of contracts for protective equipment, masks, testing kits and face shields. The face shields received much media attention because health professionals had long argued a face shield mandate was scientifically unsound. I wrote about the farce with face shields in my newspaper column, describing how I had searched through Chinese government directives on the Internet and could not find any administrative order requiring face shield use; yet, the shields being sold in the Philippines were all manufactured in China. A Senate probe noted the contracts went mainly to companies linked to China (Buan 2021). One such company, Pharmally, was registered in 2019 with paid-up capital of P625,000 (US$11,000) but won contracts worth P8.6 billion (US$156 million). The Senate probe ended on 2 June 2022, after more than a year of hearings, finding evidence of culpability on the part of several government officials. Only nine of the 24 senators signed the committee report, non-signers arguing that President Duterte was named in the committee despite the lack of evidence linking him to the contracts. The head of the committee, Richard Gordon, from the political opposition, said he was leaving the issue 'to the conscience of his colleagues'.

Nurses and health frontliners

The Philippines graduates many physicians, nurses, midwives and other health professionals each year, large numbers of whom migrate overseas. In December 2020, newspapers all over the country jubilantly featured the first COVID-19 vaccination being administered in the United Kingdom by a Filipina migrant and midwife, May Parsons. I shared in the national pride, but wished greater coverage had been given as well to the paradoxes surrounding Filipino health workers, many of whom ended up on the frontline during COVID-19. The export of Filipino health workers, particularly nurses, has been going on for decades (Ceniza Choy 2003). It has helped many Filipino families to improve their standard of living, sometimes producing second- and even third-generation caregivers and health workers who were themselves exported. But this export had its social costs, from the workers' families having absentee parents to the chronic lack of health workers to take care of Filipino patients.

COVID-19 put Filipino health workers in high-risk situations given the lack of preparedness in the health care system at home. During the first month of the lockdown, the Philippines' Health Department announced that 766 health workers had been infected. Only 2 weeks after that report, the number of infected health workers had risen to 1,694, including 33 deaths (Magsambol 2020b; Rey 2020). COVID-19 introduced still another dimension to the costs of nurse exports. High infection rates have been reported as well for the many Filipino health professionals who went overseas to work. In the first few months of the pandemic, deaths of overseas Filipino health workers in the line of duty exceeded those of similar frontline workers at home (Gulf News Report 2020; Soichet 2020). A *Guardian* newspaper article that appeared on 14 June 2020 described how a UK government report on the deaths of minority health workers had not been released because of fears of a backlash (Campbell 2020). The suppressed report's language was direct: 'Stakeholders pointed to racism and discrimination experienced by communities and more specifically BAME

(Black, Asian and Minority Ethnic) key workers as a root cause to exposure risk and disease progression'.

Despite the greater risks of working overseas compared to serving in the Philippines, Filipino nurses interviewed by local media still talk about applying for overseas work. I was also able to talk with health workers who had been evicted from their rented homes when the pandemic broke out and they pointed out how this discrimination had left them demoralised, but even more determined to migrate. One nurse put it this way: 'I know the risks are high as well overseas but here at home, I live with the risks of COVID-19 as well as the risk of my family not having enough to live on'. The Philippine government's response was to put a cap limiting nurses' overseas deployment to 7,500 a year. Despite this cap, the Health Department admitted in September 2022 that it still faced a shortage of 106,000 nurses (Magsambol 2022). This was not from a lack of nurses but from nurses choosing to remain unemployed or seeking work outside of nursing. Throughout the pandemic, nurses and other health workers were among the most militant, holding protest rallies to demand overdue hazard pay for working in COVID-19 wards.

Militarisation of COVID-19

Unlike his fellow populist presidents Trump (USA) and Bolsonaro (Brazil), the Philippines' Duterte did acknowledge the seriousness of COVID-19 but relied on an Interagency Task on Emerging Infectious Diseases (IATF-EID), composed of former military generals, to craft the government's response to COVID-19. This IATF-EID became the main policy-making and executive agency for dealing with COVID-19. Perhaps not surprisingly, a distinct military jargon emerged. It included reference to PUIs (Persons Under Investigation), referring to people who had symptoms but had not yet tested positive. The police and military were deployed en masse, with police uniforms changed to resemble the camouflage uniforms of the military. Uniformed personnel, armed with long-guns, were deployed at checkpoints and, later, in public transport throughout the country, assigned to check passengers' health certificates. The inter-agency committee came to be known, and criticised, for its calls for mandatory testing, hiring 'whistle-blowers' to report suspected cases and even conducting house-to-house searches, limited of course to urban poor communities.

A climate of fear, introduced at the very start of the Duterte presidency with his war on drugs, intensified during COVID-19. When, in April 2020, residents in Sitio San Roque, an urban poor community in Quezon City, launched a rally protesting the lack of government assistance for families displaced by the pandemic, President Duterte responded the same day with a speech, blaming the protest action on 'leftists' and threatening them with detention 'until the COVID-19 outbreak ends'. For quarantine violators, his warning was more ominous: 'I will not hesitate. My orders are to the police and the military, also the barangay, that if there is trouble or the situation arises that people fight and your lives are on the line, shoot them dead. Do you understand? Dead' (Magsambol 2020a; the quote has been translated from the original mix of English and Filipino).

As COVID-19 unfolded, the pandemic was used as an excuse to ban mass political action. Arrests were actually made at some of the rallies, citing the violation of public health laws. In July 2020, President Duterte Congress signed into law an Anti-Terrorism Act (Republic of the Philippines 2020) that allowed warrantless arrest and detention of up to 24 days and barred automatic compensation if wrongful detention occurred. A total of 37 petitions were filed with the Supreme Court by various groups questioning the constitutionality of this law, all of which were thrown out by the Supreme Court in December 2021.

Fears have been particularly strong about a powerful Anti-Terror Council set up to implement the law, with powers that include the naming of individuals and groups as 'terrorists'. This legitimised 'red-tagging' or accusing individuals and organisations of being communists, which had been going on since the 1950s but has intensified under President Duterte and which activists criticised as inviting the harassment and assassination of those who were tagged. One chilling example was the case of a 70-year-old physician, Natividad Castro, who had been working in remote communities, mainly with Indigenous people. Castro was first arrested in February 2022 and charged with kidnapping, based on her having brought several Indigenous people to Geneva to testify to government violations of Indigenous people's human rights. A court eventually ordered her release and the police had to comply, but in January 2023 she was again arrested, this time with no charges filed other than her having been designated as a terrorist by the Anti-Terrorism Council.

This red-tagging and harassment should be understood in the context of the Duterte government's attempt to monopolise anti-COVID-19 programmes. When Vice President Leni Robredo, who had been vocal in criticising President Duterte, began a shuttle system to assist essential workers with transport, a government prosecutor, the Presidential Anti-Corruption Commission ordered a probe for her 'competing with the national government' (Aguilar 2020). In 2021, a woman named Patreng Non put up a community pantry in her neighbourhood, offering free food supplies including vegetables, fruit and rice, as well as canned products. Volunteers came forward with their own donations, as well as offers to help with distribution. In a talk she gave to my college students, she described how touched she was by the first group of volunteers, tricycle drivers who helped to pack the food without asking for privileged access to the items. Government officials reacted quickly, describing Non as a 'communist'. Non kept on with her community pantry, with dozens of similar projects sprouting up throughout the country in open defiance, and inviting more red-tagging from the government.

It is not surprising government officials began to use the term 'pasaway' to refer to these many citizens' initiatives, 'pasaway' referring to stubborn disobedience. The term had first been used to describe people who were not using masks or conforming with quarantine, but was extended to people who initiated self-help projects such as the community pantries. Accompanying the label were calls for greater discipline, and for even stricter lockdown measures.

Biopower, biopolitics and bioregulation

There was more to the police model than outright threats and coercive force. What we saw during the COVID-19 lockdown were multiple strategies and multiple scripts used by government in the exercise of what Michel Foucault (2008) described as biopower. Government critics in the Philippines use the term 'weaponization' to refer to the way Duterte has gone beyond the usual judicial forms (the use of direct punitive force for example) to embrace biopower, further described as 'the subjugation of bodies and the control of populations government's campaigns' (Foucault 1978, p. 140).

In COVID-19 times, biopower came to include attempts to impose new norms such as the many rules around quarantine but also what the US journalist Derek Thompson (2020) calls 'hygiene theater', or the use of highly visible but largely ineffective measures in response to disease. In the Philippines, there was no lack of this hygiene theatre, with business people capitalising on these performances through sales of footbaths, gas masks and fogging machines. Hygiene theatre became political theatre in the Philippines, dramatically in some instances as in the deployment of tanks and drones as uniformed personnel swept into the slums to arrest people breaking lockdown rules. The most extreme and dramatic case involved political activist Reina Mae Nacino, who was arrested in 2019. She was pregnant at the time of her arrest and delivered in prison. She was initially allowed to keep her child with her in prison but was eventually separated from the child, in line with penitentiary regulations. The child died shortly after being taken away from her mother. Following the child's death, Nacino requested permission to attend the wake and funeral. A court allowed her two three-hour furloughs. At both the wake and the funeral, she was surrounded by guards – up to 40 at the funeral – several decked out in body armour and toting high calibre firearms. Nacino herself was made to use personal protective equipment (PPE) covering her entire body. The police and military refused to remove her handcuffs during the last few moments before the child was interred (ABS/CBN News 2020).

The editor of *The Lancet*, Richard Horton (2020), takes the position that greater state intrusion is acceptable when guided by principles such as transparency, equality, and indivisibility of rights. Both COVID-19 and HIV provided glimpses into what could be achieved if such principles were upheld. In the case of HIV, a National AIDS Council with government and civil society representation provided transparency. No such safeguards existed for COVID-19 so it was not surprising that so much corruption affected the very agencies that were supposed to mitigate the impact of COVID-19. 'Indivisibility of rights', meaning consistency in the application of the law, was particularly important during COVID-19, with the public quick to react whenever there were exposés of violations of COVID-19 rules by officials. When the press featured photos of a police general's birthday party showing him blowing out birthday candles and surrounded by unmasked birthday celebrations, the public reacted with anger, and some wishful thinking in social media that perhaps the celebrants might have caught COVID-19 through the reckless celebration. A few weeks later, a protest rally against the Anti-Terrorism Act was publicised as a *mañanitas*, the term normally used to refer to birthday celebrations.

Governance and social solidarity

HIV and AIDS and COVID-19 times in the Philippines were studies in contrast. The fight against HIV in the Philippines was marked by strong civil society participation and social solidarity that countered discrimination and taught people the value of empathy and responsibility. In contrast, COVID-19 times were marked by a militarisation that targeted civil society and community participation, pitting people against each other through red-tagging and the calls for whistle-blowing of people suspected to have COVID-19. The consequences of the two models of governance are also studies in contrast. With HIV, civil society participation encouraged social solidarity and trust. I saw how this translated into many self-help projects and volunteerism not just among people living with HIV, or with groups at risk, but with entire families and communities. Working with HIV programmes, I found myself taking up shifts to care for people with advanced AIDS, accepting invitations to become a godfather at the weddings of people with HIV, and grieving with and consoling bereaved families.

With COVID-19, one of the most adverse effects of the police or military model of public health was the erosion of social trust. In conversations and interviews with people – in the academe, in gatherings of friends and relatives, and in research settings – I often hear them say the pandemic is 'gawa-gawa lang ng gobyerno' (just fabricated by government) and when I asked what government had to gain from 'fabricating' COVID-19, the response always was that the 'fake' pandemic opened up more opportunities for corruption and the plunder of public funds. The erosion of social trust offers another angle with which to examine the exodus of nurses and other health professionals from the Philippines. COVID-19 made the choices – to stay or to migrate – more difficult. The continuing desire to migrate remains but those who stay on in the Philippines did not practise their professions, cognisant of the COVID-19 risks in local hospitals, compounded by frustration with government corruption that included overpriced purchases of protective equipment at a time when hazard pay was delayed or non-existent.

Viewed in retrospect, COVID-19 created new sites of conflict and resistance. To some extent, this was 'pasaway' or stubborn resistance, the term used by government against citizens. But it was pasaway that allowed people to look for ways to survive, even to thrive, amidst adversity and precarity. I referred earlier to the community pantries but there were many other examples of pasaway as social solidarity. One example of this took the form of the 'underground' tricycles that continued to run in the first few weeks of the lockdown when public transport was banned, with the tricycle drivers using routes that evaded the police. Food shortages also spurred collective action. In rural areas especially, people set up backyard vegetable gardens and created informal barter networks for groceries. As transport restrictions were lifted, people found ways to link farmers to urban consumers, with weekend deliveries of produce, all done without government assistance.

The sites of resistance were exemplary. When government began to offer relief goods during COVID-19, one mayor of a town in the northern Philippines, with a population comprised predominantly of Indigenous people, refused the relief goods, saying that they would survive by depending on their own traditions of mutual help. The mayor suggested that the relief goods be distributed instead to the more needy urban poor communities (Lapniten 2020).

The road ahead

National elections were held in May 2022. The new president is Ferdinand Marcos Jr, son of the dictator who was president from 1965 until his deposition in 1986. The vice president is Sarah Duterte, daughter of President Rodrigo Duterte. President Marcos declared the end of the health emergency on 19 July 2023, the declaration itself becoming part of continuing political theatre as government proclaimed victory over COVID-19 and a return to normalcy.

The new normal seems to be a return of the old abnormal, including the neglect of social and health services. The 'new normal' takes on perverse twists as well. One business article I read in 2022, as COVID-19 was described to be retreating to becoming 'endemic', talked about how real estate prices in the wealthier residential areas had soared during the pandemic, with expectations that this would speed up in the months ahead.

The Indian writer Arundhati Roy (2020) talks about the COVID-19 pandemic as 'a portal, a gateway between one world to the next', with optimism that people might 'break with the past and imagine their world anew'. I would like to be optimistic too but am sometimes overwhelmed by despair, having handled, since the pandemic began, a college set up for low-income students with generous endowments that included free laptops and modems for all, only to realise that a significant number of our students were living in areas that did not even have Wi-Fi. Halfway through the semester, we realised we had to bring the students to the national capital, Manila, where they could have assured access to Wi-Fi.

All of our students are now back in Manila attending face-to-face classes, but lecturers quickly noticed that the freshmen batch that entered college in August

2022, students whose last two years of high school had taken place exclusively online, came into college lagging far behind in reading and comprehension.

But education is more than a matter of reducing the learning losses in schools. Students and faculty find it important to talk about our viral times, sometimes almost as a form of therapy for the increasing incidence of mental health problems, but more often to identify COVID-19 narratives of social solidarity even as we set up new models. Early on, we moved into face-to-face classes, urging students to think of protecting each other through the early reporting of symptoms and self-quarantine, together with the use of home testing kits which the government had opposed for several months, insisting that people test in government-designated centres that were much more expensive.

In conclusion

I would like to end with some trans-pandemic reflections, taking off from a thought-provoking special issue of the journal *Culture, Health and Society* on the theme of 'viral times, viral memories, viral questions' (García-Iglesias et al. 2021).

Although HIV programmes were more productive and socially responsive than those of COVID-19, I keep finding reminders that they too did not respond to some of the more important structural needs, in the form of the 'pre-existing conditions' I referred to at the beginning of this chapter. About one month after the COVID-19 lockdown was declared, I found myself having to provide phone counselling to a fellow member of faculty at the University of the Philippines who was in a gay relationship. His partner had come down with respiratory symptoms and had to be rushed to a nearby government hospital. The faculty member explained to hospital personnel that his partner had cancer, but the hospital personnel insisted that new COVID-19 protocols required the confinement of 'suspects' in isolation tents until COVID-19 test results came back. The faculty member was also barred from being with his partner because the Philippines does not legally recognise any form of same-sex relationship. The faculty member's partner died three days after admission, still without any test results. His body was cremated a few hours after death, and COVID-19 protocols barred attendance even by relatives because of the fear of infection. The test results came back two days after the cremation, negative for COVID-19.

Many slogans have emerged as COVID-19 subsided, including references to a 'new normal' which, unfortunately, looks more like the old dispensation of health inequities. COVID-19 is showing how incredibly short people's memories are, almost as if they want to forget the trials and tribulations. Now more than ever, we need the narratives of HIV and COVID-19 times to give more substance to the term 'governance' as a dynamic process that must include social resistance, social solidarity and protection, given that scientists now refer to future pandemics not so much as 'if' than as 'when'.

References

Abbey, E.J. et al., 2020. The Global Health Security Index is not predictive of coronavirus pandemic responses among Organization for Economic Cooperation and Development countries. *PLOS One*, October 7, 2020. doi:10.1371/journal.pone.0239398

ABS/CBN News, 2020. Final goodbye: Reina Mae Nasino attends baby River funeral amid tight security. *ABS/CBN News* [online], 17 October. https://news.abs-cbn.com/news/multimedia/slideshow/10/17/20/baby-river-nasino-burial

Aguilar, K., 2020. PACC to NBI: Probe Robredo for competing with national government in fight against Covid-19. *Inquirer*, 2 April. https://newsinfo.inquirer.net/1252839/pacc-to-nbi-probe-robredo-for-competing-with-national-govt-in-fight-vs-covid-19

Buan, L., 2021. We swindled gov't': Pharmally changed expiry date of medical-grade face shields. *Rappler*, 24 September. https://www.rappler.com/nation/pharmally-admits-changed-expiry-date-medical-grade-face-shields/

Campbell, D., 2020. Racism contributed to disproportionate UK BAME coronavirus deaths, inquiry finds. *The Guardian*, 14 June. www.theguardian.com/world/2020/jun/14/racism-disproportionate-uk-bame-coronavirus-deaths-report

Ceniza Choy, C., 2003. *Empire of care*. Durham, NC: Duke University Press.

Foucault, M., 1978. *The history of sexuality*. Trans. R. Hurley. New York: Pantheon Books.

Foucault, M., 2008. *Birth of biopolitics: Lectures at the Collège de France 1978-79*. Basingstoke: Palgrave MacMillan.

García-Iglesias, J., Nagington, M., and Peter Aggleton, P., 2021. Viral times, viral memories, viral questions. *Culture, Health & Sexuality*, 23 (11), 1465–1469. doi:10.1080/13691058.2021.1976564

Gulf News Report, 2020. Coronavirus: Faces of Filipino nurses/porters who died in the UK. *Gulf News*, 13 April. https://gulfnews.com/world/asia/philippines/coronavirus-faces-of-filipino-nurses-porters-who-died-in-the-uk-1.1586762487253

Horton, R., 2020. *The Covid-19 catastrophe: What's gone wrong and how to stop it happening again*. Cambridge: Polity Press.

Johns Hopkins Bloomberg School of Public Health, Nuclear Threat Initiative (NTI), 2019. *Global Health Security Index 2019*. Washington, DC: Nuclear Threat Initiative (NTI).

Lapniten, K., 2020. Coping with crisis: The Cordillera way. *Inquirer*, 26 April. https://newsinfo.inquirer.net/1264788/coping-with-crisis-the-cordillera-way

Magsambol, B., 2020a. 'Shoot them dead': Duterte orders troops to kill quarantine violators. *Rappler*, 1 April.

Magsambol, B., 2020b. PH health workers infected with virus rise to 1694. *Rappler*, 1 May. www.rappler.com/nation/259637-health-workers-coronavirus-cases-philippines-may-1-2020/

Magsambol, B., 2022. Philippines lacks 106,000 nurses – DOH. *Rappler*, 30 September. www.rappler.com/nation/philippines-shortage-nurses-hospitals-doh/

Republic of the Philippines, 2020. *Anti-Terrorism Law (Republic Act 11479)*. Available from: www.officialgazette.gov.ph/2020/07/03/republic-act-no-11479/ [Accessed 31 July 2023].

Rey, A., 2020. 766 PH Health workers infected with coronavirus. *Rappler*, 27 April. https://www.rappler.com/nation/258270-health-workers-coronavirus-cases-philippines-april-17-2020/

Right to Know, Right Now! Coalition, 2021. Pharmally, 29 other firms bagged 42% of P65-B pandemic supply projects. *Philippine Center for Investigative Journalism* [online], 15 October. https://pcij.org/blog/2294/pharmally-other-firms-bagged-p65-billion-pandemic-supply-projects

Roy, A., 2020. The pandemic is a portal. *Financial Times*, 4 April. www.ft.com/content/10d8f5e8-74eb-11ea-95fe-fcd274e920ca

Soichet, C., 2020. Covid-19 is taking a devastating toll on Filipino-American nurses. *CNN Health*, 11 December. https://edition.cnn.com/2020/11/24/health/filipino-nurse-deaths/index.html

Thompson, D., 2020. Hygiene theater is a huge waste of time. *The Atlantic*, 27 July. www.theatlantic.com/ideas/archive/2020/07/scourge-hygiene-theater/614599/

University of the Philippines Institute of Small-Scale Industries, 2020. 2020 MSME Statistics. *University of the Philippines Institute of Small-Scale Industries* [online]. Available from: https://beta.entrepreneurship.org.ph/msme-statistics [Accessed 31 August 2023]

World Bank, 2023. Out-of-pocket expenditure (% of current health expenditure). *World Bank Health Expenditure Database* [online]. Available from: https://data.worldbank.org/indicator/SH.XPD.OOPC.CH.ZS [Accessed 7 April 2023]

Part III

Professional, practitioner, and community perspectives

11 When The Clapping stops

Mourning and the spectacle of public sacrifice during COVID-19

Bernard Kelly

Outside, police drones hover overhead, haunting the landscape, trying to catch someone out. When I used to walk to work, I rarely caught anyone's eye, but social distancing has led to a strange kind of intimacy. To avoid each other, you first must acknowledge that both of you are there to successfully navigate the little dance around death that meeting someone now involves. Inside my office, I have unpacked the day and I am ready to make my way home. Usually, I follow the main road running alongside the cemetery which stands testament to the site's former life as an old fever hospital. Tonight though, to inject some distraction into a narrowed existence, I take a route past the repurposed isolation blocks, stepping out of the hospital into darkened side streets. All is quiet, and I am the only one on the road. After a while, I hear something up ahead, and as I keep on walking it gets louder and louder. I don't know what it is at first, and then I see it, but it's too late to turn back now. People are on their doorsteps, standing by their gates, and they are all clapping. I stride on like the one-person parade I have become, eyes fixed straight ahead, trying to make myself invisible. It goes on and on, the sound filling my body, then someone calls out my name and everything stops. Even though this had never happened before, it seemed that everyone already knew that nobody was meant to be there. That was the first night of The Clapping.

The Clapping as a conjuring of spectacle

A person stands between you and the picture. They face away, and on the back of their shirt is written, 'BLACK DEATH SPECTACLE.' You cannot look at the picture without seeing these words. The artist and activist, Parker Bright, is holding a vigil in front of a painting called, 'Open Casket.' The painting proports to show the mutilated body of 14-year-old Emmett Till who was abducted, tortured and lynched by two white men in 1955. For his funeral, Emmett's mother, Mamie, demanded an open casket as, 'There was no way I could describe what was in that box. No Way. And I just wanted the world to see.' A photograph of Emmett's brutalised body was widely shared, an image, the reality of which, is virtually impossible to unsee. Parker Bright

DOI: 10.4324/9781003322788-14

and other activists view the painting, made by white artist Dana Schutz, as appropriating the reality of Emmett Till's suffering and remaking it along with other Black deaths into, 'a spectacle, something to be watched, recorded by bystanders and plastered into abstract forms' (Akolo 2020).

The morning after the first night of The Clapping, all the bodies of the Black healthcare workers have been disappeared, as the front pages of the newspapers, awash with whiteness, are 'totally ignoring any form of applause to the multiplicity of diversity in the National Health Service' (Adebayo 2020). In the spectacle, the realities of human suffering are framed and edited so as to render 'some lives meaningful while dismissing others as disposable.' The spectacle 'operates through a hidden structure of politics that colonises the imagination, denies critical engagement, and pre-emptively represses alternative narratives' (Evans and Giroux 2015, p. 32). The Clapping first appears as an act of solidarity with those willing to face death, yet thousands have already died, and there is no sense or sign of loss in the applause. This has been displaced such that 'everything that was directly lived has moved away into representation' and 'the common ground of the deceived gaze and of false consciousness, and the unification it achieves is nothing but the official language of generalised separation' (Debord 1977 p. 3). Separation was the overriding experience for many during COVID-19, and The Clapping, which presented itself as 'something enormously positive and indisputable' (Debord 1977, p. 22), was positioned as our 'we are all in it together' moment. A doctor is cycling away from the hospital when he is confronted by a man shouting, 'Get off your bike!' The man asks if he had read the signs and the doctor says he has and replies, 'you read the signs, look who can cycle in the park.' The man keeps saying 'get off your bike' and as it's a Thursday, the doctor asks, 'are you going to clap the NHS tonight?' The man says, 'Oh yes,' and the doctor just looks at him and replies, 'Don't,' and cycles off. Usually, this doctor wouldn't have stopped, but today he feels the anger of 'seeing so many people out when we're living in a day of deaths' (Haywood 2020, ep. 3). Across the hospital, I hear staff ask, 'How can I feel this angry and still be professional?'

In January 2020, in the locked-down city of Wuhan in China, anonymous cries of support for healthcare workers were heard. In Italy, people started banging on pots, playing accordions and singing arias, although the city of Florence soon stops the practice out of respect for the dead, and those in mourning. In Madrid, a man says the applause 'serves as an oasis for those of us who have been indoors for 13 days and counting … I was a ghost on my street until I started going to the balcony and establishing a relationship with my neighbours' (Booth and Adam 2020). One month after COVID-19 is declared a pandemic The Clapping begins in the UK. From 26 March, every Thursday at 7 pm, for ten weeks, millions take to the street to applaud 'frontline workers,' in an action that becomes the nation's defining public act during COVID-19 (see Figure 11.1). 'Oh my God they're clapping. What are they talking about? Do they even know what happens inside?' (Jesuthasan et al. 2021, p. 6).

30
"Why are we clapping every night?" asks John.
"Because our brave workers are at war with germs," says Mummy.
"And our neighbours can see us clapping."
new words
evening
virtue
signalling

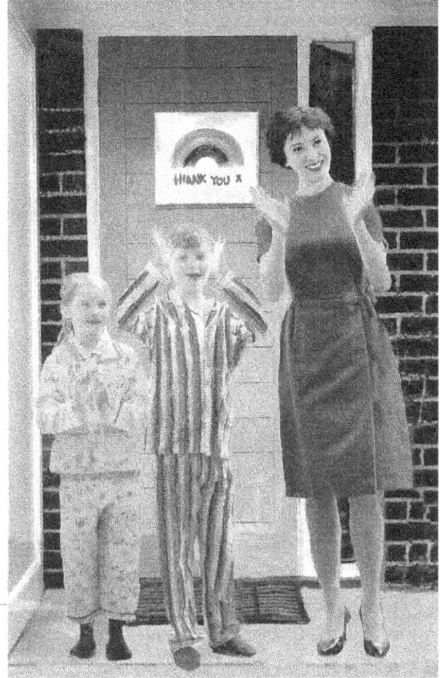

Figure 11.1 'Evening virtue signalling' from 'We do Lockdown' published by Dung Beetle Books ©Miriam Elia 2020. Reproduced with permission.

By the fifth week of The Clapping, although people from 'Black, Asian and Minority Ethnic' backgrounds make up 21% of NHS workers, they were accounting for 63% of the 106 NHS staff reported to have died from COVID-19. Fully 95% of all doctors and consultants who had lost their lives in the UK at that point in the pandemic were from a 'Black, Asian and Minority Ethnic' background (Cook et al. 2020). Over twice as many doctors from 'Black, Asian and Minority Ethnic' backgrounds said they had faced shortages of or were using sub-standard personal protective equipment (PPE) compared to 'White British' colleagues, leaving some feeling like 'sacrificial lambs.' 'There was one time when I was on-call, and I hadn't been mask fitted yet ... but ... my senior was like "it doesn't matter, can you just go and see the patient" ... I remember thinking this is really unsafe, I didn't feel like I could speak up because I was very junior' (Qureshi et al. 2022). While some lives during the pandemic were considered worthy of protection, others were stripped 'of any political, ethical and human value.' As the spectacle curates 'who and what is human even though the physical body might still be in existence' (Evans and Giroux 2015, p. 7), many had already been consigned to the realm of the 'still living dead' (Kear and Steinberg 1999, p. 172).

In the absence of those being ritually praised, the clappers were the audience to their own performance, which without the 'shared lived experience of real bodies in real spaces' (Fischer-Lichte 2005, p. 26) lacked the contact and catharsis of real drama. 'For the subject to take up a position as a subject, it must be able to be situated in the space occupied by its body' (Grosz 1994 p. 47) a 'body which implies mortality, vulnerability, agency: the skin and the flesh expose us to the gaze of others, but also to touch, and violence' (Butler 2020, p. 26). The bodies of those being clapped are not there, and the bodies of the already and soon-to-be dead are elsewhere, untouched and unseen. If theatre is like the plague, 'this is not because it is contagious, but because like the plague it is a revelation, urging forwards the exteriorization of a latent undercurrent of cruelty through which all the perversity of which the mind is capable, whether in person or a nation, becomes localized' (Artaud 2010, p. 20). 'They are out to be seen and will have been seen … If someone falls and breaks a leg, they will stare like the people of the Colosseum stared' (Cousins 2021, p. 262).

In The Clapping, 'the ethical imperative towards social transformation is replaced by a civic-minded but passive ideal of empathy. The political as a place of acts orientated towards publicness becomes replaced by a world of private thoughts, leanings, and gestures' (Berlant 1998, p. 641). As active citizenship is increasingly curtailed, 'sacrificial citizenship expands to include anything related to the requirements and imperatives of the economy' (Brown 2015, p. 211) and becomes a kind of folk horror. Like the islanders in the film *The Wicker Man*, we are clapping as the body burns.

Whilst 'murder inspires horror' (Girard 1977, p. 15) and 'violence is easily condemned when it appears exceptional' (Evans and Giroux 2015, p. 7), state-sanctioned killing 'is the final guarantee of civility' (Eagleton 2018, p. 17) and often 'inspires awe and respect.' Horror is all about looking; what can and can't be seen, what is and isn't there. 'The spectacle harvests and sells our attention, while denying us the ability for properly engaged political reflection' (Evans and Giroux 2015, p. 32). As The Clapping distances itself from the scene, it creates 'a sense of innocence and detachment yet provides a means to feel one has been authentically close to an event' (Sturken 2007, p. 12). Everyone is looking at each other, as there is nothing else to see. In The Clapping, 'The world was fully present, fully visible, but somehow not there; it had become possible to look fixedly at it without seeing it' (Bersani 2018, p. 107). This event of unseeing, of looking through the other, can be seen as constituting 'the veritable death of the witness' (Evans and Giroux 2015, p. 241).

The Clapping as a sacrifice of others

The night before The Clapping started in the UK, Sansari Ojha, a priest of the Goddess Brahmani temple in the eastern Indian state of Odisha, had a dream. In his dream, the Goddess appears and promises to rid the world of the Coronavirus, as she has with many plagues before, if he makes a sacrifice to her. When the 72-year-old priest enters the temple, a villager, Saroj Kumar Pradhan, is bowing before an effigy of the Goddess. Unseen, the priest emerges out of the shadows, and wielding a scythe, he severs the head of Saroj Kumar Pradhan from his body. Narasinghpur police station sits just above the Brahmani temple, and detective Ashish Kumar Singh is soon on the scene within the shrine. The priest recounts the dream, but under further interrogation it emerges that the two men shared a room together and shortly before the killing they had an alcohol and drugs fuelled argument regarding a longstanding dispute over a mango orchard in the village. Sometimes what looks like a sacrifice is something else, and sometimes what looks like something else is a sacrifice.

When institutions have lost 'their vitality' and 'the whole cultural structure seems on the verge of collapse' (Girard 1977, p. 49) there is often a turning towards the sacred. During COVID-19, a God embodying the 'spirit of community,' who is there 'at some of the most profound moments in our lives' (Welby and Stevens 2020) became the presiding deity, when all churches, synagogues, temples and other places of worship were closed. The National Health Service (NHS) itself a child of sacrifice, brought into being after and its existence forever bound to the countless losses of the Second World War, had risen again. The government declared that the NHS was to be preserved at all costs, but it was the sacrificial system that had really to be saved, and anyone sacrificed to that end.

The function of sacrifice is to restore harmony to a community under threat, through the performance of an ambiguity which 'plays out the paradox of the affirmation of life through its destruction' (Flood 2013, p. 129). Whilst 'the modern state's hunger for human sacrifice is insatiable' (Halbertal 2012, p. 105), this is 'hidden from sight by the awesome machinery of ritual' (Girard 1977, p. 19) which relies 'on its ability to conceal' and 'a certain degree of misunderstanding' as the celebrants 'must not comprehend the true role of the sacrificial act' (Girard 1977, p. 7). 'The more critical the situation, the more "precious" the sacrificial victim must be' (Girard 1977, p. 18), and who is seen as more precious than a doctor or nurse during a pandemic?

Ellis, Telford, Lloyd and Briggs (2021) in their paper, *For the Greater Good: Sacrificial Violence and the Coronavirus Pandemic*, follow Girard and Halbertal in suggesting that sacrifice always takes place within a hierarchical structure and have conceptualised this for the COVID-19 pandemic in the UK (see Figure 11.2).

They cast NHS and care home staff as 'sacred sacrificers' and care home residents, the elderly and the vulnerable as being 'primary sacrificers.' At the bottom of the pyramid sits wider society, with its sacrifices of mental health, personal freedoms, education, and the other harms and threats that COVID-19 posed. This sacrificial structure echoes existing power imbalances. Within the NHS, one healthcare worker observed, 'The distribution of PPE

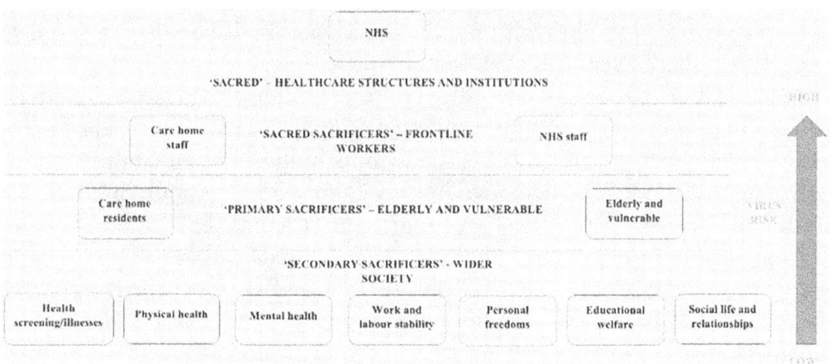

Figure 11.2 'Conceptualising the relationship between the "sacred" and "sacrificed"' taken from Ellis et al. (2021). Reproduced with permission of the authors.

seems to have followed a hierarchical structure. So, medics are walking around with 3M rubber fit-sealed masks, although they do not spend that much time in COVID areas, while some Filipino nurses are struggling to find a 3M mask that fits them. And then when it comes to risk assessing the domestic staff, they're an afterthought' (Jesuthasan et al. 2021).

Sacrifice always requires an intermediary so that 'the two worlds that are present can interpenetrate and yet remain distinct' (Hubert and Mauss 1964, p. 99). Those doing The Clapping cannot involve themselves in the rite to the very end, as there they would find 'death, not life' (Hubert and Mauss 1964, p. 98). In ancient Athens, the city kept a group of people at public expense, the Pharmakos, who were on hand to face sacrifice when plague, famine or foreign invasion threatened. In classical Greek, Pharmakon, means, 'both poison and the antidote for poison, both sickness and cure' (Girard 1977, p. 95). 'This homeopathic creature cleanses by being contaminated' (Eagleton 2018, p. 143) and had to be kept separate from the populous in ways similar to health workers during COVID-19. Whilst colleagues were stripping off on doorsteps to protect others, it still proved impossible for some to escape being praised as pure through The Clapping and treated like poison at home. One doctor was confronted by her husband,

> 'You still walked through that filthy place until you got out of it. You're putting our lives at risk. A thirteen-year-old died! Didn't you know that?' And despite yourself, you start to argue and justify yourself, even though you're the doctor and you know that your actions are safe and don't need defending.
>
> (Farooki 2022, p. 69)

Willing victims assuage collective guilt, and it became imperative during COVID-19 to portray healthcare as an act of self-sacrifice with the health worker as hero; 'a destroyer of monsters' whose 'own death - or triumph-transforms into a guarantee of order and tranquillity' (Girard 1977, p. 87). A hero can both carry out the sacrifice and be its victim. Like 'frontline workers,' they are essential because they are expendable. As one nurse said, 'I disagree with the "hero worship" idea that went along with the clap – we're not heroes, we are professionals doing a job – calling us heroes just makes other people feel better when we die' (Manthorpe et al. 2021). Like the chorus in Greek tragedy, The Clapping bestows a flaw to the hero that rightly 'belongs exclusively to the crowd' (Girard 1977, p. 203), and with this 'the ceremony of sacrifice is drowned, not in blood but in pity' (Williams 1966, p. 157).

Wrapped in the rhetoric of war, 'frontline workers' became easier to kill, as 'the language of war legitimizes emergency and authoritarian measures' and 'makes our crumbling healthcare systems appear to be the result of an enemy virus rather than the outcome of public policy' (Neocleous 2022, p. 39). War talk aligns the healthcare worker with the figure of 'the soldier' whose 'arena of war is first and foremost his own body; a body poised to penetrate other bodies and mangle them in its embrace' (Kemp 2013, p. 42), taking us out of care and cure, and into combat. Most of those working with people living with HIV in the 1980s and 1990s actively chose to do so, but during COVID-19, many staff simply felt compelled, or were compelled to do their job, as others, still classed as civilians, were suddenly working remotely. As ever, the higher up the command structure you were, the more likely you were to be saved. The first members of staff to die in the hospital from COVID-19 were three cleaners, their sacrifice outsourced to a private company which trades on consigning people 'to zones of abandonment, containment, surveillance, and incarceration' (Evans and Giroux 2015, p. 50) as the operator of the UKs largest migrant detention and removal service.

'Kinship connections between the living and the sacrificed dead carry significant cultural capital during times of national crisis' (Bennett 2009, p. 40), and The Clapping gave 'a protective sanctity' (Hubert and Mauss 1964, p. 102) to those made divine with flattery. Queered in the image of a rainbow and clapped even unto death, these 'hero victims' carried the communities fears away to a place beyond, as the clappers were 'transported into the world of life' (Hubert and Mauss 1964, p. 62), through a ritual enactment of a triumph over death. By wearing the mask of celebration, The Clapping concealed itself as a primary site of sacrifice during COVID-19, where so many found their death upon the 'altar of the nation.'

The Clapping as a summoning of ghosts

At the centre of the room stood a bright pink fluffy dressing gown, looking as if Stuart had just stepped out of it. In life, Stuart was always stepping out of it. If you had visited our gay communal house in the 1980s, the door was likely to be opened by Stuart either in his pink dressing gown or in nothing at all. Stuart was diagnosed with HIV aged 18 and now at 26 he was dead. After

Stuart's funeral in a sex club in San Francisco, some of us set off for the crematorium, him in a cardboard box, a fluorescent pink feather boa on top. We stood around the box singing, each trying on the pink boa in turn. Once he had disappeared into the flames, every time the man opened the furnace's iron door and raked over his remains, we looked inside and shared all that we saw.

On the HIV wards back then, it was commonplace to see a frail body, curled up on a hospital bed, in the warm embrace of a lover or friend. As one nurse remembered,

> Everybody knew our patients were dying and every moment was charged with bravado and bravery. Something very honest was going on. It was so different to every other nursing experience. Young men were planning their funerals and deciding how they should be done. It was inspiring to see those patients take control of their own life and death.
>
> (Mendel 2022)

Closeness through authentic repetition, 'the renewal and redetermination of legacy, rather than merely its pious reproduction' (Pogue Harrison 2003, p. 95), enabled a reconfiguring of the relationship between the living, the dying and the dead. As challenges of isolation and separateness were articulated, communities were consciously reimagined as sites of contact and care. It was a time when we insisted, 'on the importance of clinging to ruined identities and to histories of injury. Resisting the call of gay normalization means refusing to write off the most vulnerable, the least presentable, and all the dead' (Love 2009, p. 30). When AIDS bodies were deemed disposable and not worthy of sacrifice, death was reclaimed as a queer rite, and through the burying of our dead within us, they took up their rightful place with all 'the charisma of the ancestor' (Pogue Harrison 2003, p. 94).

During COVID-19, clinicians were often separated from the dying by the fear of being overwhelmed or infected.

> We thought that we should probably minimise unnecessary contact, that sounds so sort of clinical and brutal of us, but basically if we didn't need to do something that involved going and getting right face to face with someone, because we were getting a lot of staff sickness, we thought we should probably avoid it.
>
> (Haywood 2020, ep. 2)

Shortages of PPE, 'was one of the things that stopped us popping our head in and having a chat. So, you'd look through the window and you'd see someone just lying there, staring blankly at a wall, looking as bored as anything and you'd feel rubbish' (Haywood 2020, ep. 2). 'Communications got a bit better with iPads and FaceTime … but it is just a violent, horrible, horrible time' (Haywood 2020, ep. 3). These voices were amongst many captured in the hospital during the pandemic's first wave by doctor and playwright Serena Haywood and screenwriter Joseph Lidster, in their podcast *Unmasked.*

Despite the hospital where I work having the largest mortuary in London, it could still not cope with the bodies now overflowing, and temporary freezers had to be set up in the Chapel of Rest, which prevented families from viewing the dead. Our bereavement assistants were faced with the distress that this caused. 'She said, "I want to come and visit my husband," and I told her "No" and she was a Black woman and that makes it even worse, we like to touch and look. I felt like it was my mother I'm telling you can't come and see my father' (Haywood 2020, ep. 3). In the absence of the families, our medical examiners did their best to prepare the dead. 'I say, "pardon me" and "sorry" to the dead as I turn them gently from side to side, looking for metal hip screws, pacemakers, anything that could damage a crematorium. I take a breath in the quiet and whisper a "goodbye"' (Haywood 2020, ep. 3).

Whilst within the hospital attempts were made to include the dead, outside, The Clapping, continued to distance and deny them. In the weekly ritual, there was no sense of loss, sign of grieving or markers of mourning. In the era of thousands of HIV-related deaths in the UK, there was a sense that we had 'to answer for this death of the other' and that 'the other becomes my neighbour precisely through the way the face summons me, calls for me, begs for me and in so doing recalls my responsibility' (Levinas 1989, p. 83). As the corpses piled up, the clappers kept on clapping, the joggers kept on jogging, and the sun worshipers kept on looking up at the sky. The spectacle had robbed death of its reality.

In 1955, the English anthropologist, Geoffrey Gorer, wrote about the distancing of the dead, 'If we dislike the modern pornography of death, then we must give back to death – natural death – its parade and publicity, re-admit grief and mourning' (Gorer 1955, p. 52). In more recent years, we have witnessed, 'not only a commodified popular culture that trades in extreme violence, greed and narcissism as a source of entertainment but also the emergence of a predatory society in which the suffering and death of others becomes a reason to rejoice rather than mourn' (Evans and Giroux 2015, p. 11).

As a particularly virulent strain of nationalism infected the system, unmasked men were stalking down hospital corridors, accusing doctors of being 'ventilator killers,' and attempting to persuade very sick patients to leave their beds to be treated at home with zinc and vitamin C. 'HIV deniers' were no different, with over 300,000 lives sacrificed in South Africa alone, to those beliefs (Nattrass 2008). In the UK, this retreat from the real into the viral, where fantasy is, 'internalized, digested and manifested as new spectacle' (Peak 2014, p. 42), was partly a symptom of 'a nation sickened by nostalgia' (Judah 2016) for an empire which 'was never mourned or buried' (Hirsch 2018, p. 270). For the virulent nationalist, sacrifice only happens in the past, made by unknown soldiers whose tombs, void as they are of identifiable mortal remains, 'are nonetheless saturated with ghostly national imaginings' (Anderson 1983, p. 9). A haunting 'can be construed as a failed mourning. It is about refusing to give up the ghost or – and this can sometimes amount to the same thing - the refusal of the ghost to give up on us' (Fisher 2014, p. 22). Whilst those clapping did not mourn because there was no body there, the viral vigilante, for whom 'the ultimate sacrifice comes only with an idea of purity, through fatality' (Anderson 1983, p. 144) avoids mourning by sacrificing the body that is there. The burden of the past 'demands loyalty, since betraying it means retroactively stripping the sacrifice of meaning' (Halbertal 2012, p. 90), and so 'melancholia appears in place of mourning' (Freud 2005, p. 203).

I am wandering through an abandoned Jewish school, the coat pegs no higher than my waist, a child's picture of the Star of David still stuck to a wall. One day this building will bear the inscription, 'REBUILT BY MANY HANDS, FOR LONDON LIGHTHOUSE, A CENTRE FOR PEOPLE FACING THE CHALLENGE OF AIDS.' But today, in the winter of 1986, the words 'AIDS DEATH HOUSE' have been scrawled on the front door of the founder's house across the road. He is receiving phone calls, 'It's not that I object to what you h-o-m-o-sexuals get up to in private, I just don't want my children caught in the crossfire when you get beaten up in the street.' A public meeting is called in a local church and as one side shouts down the other, an elderly woman slowly makes her way to the front and there with the altar behind her says, 'I arrived in this country as a refugee in the Second World War, escaping with my sister on the last children's train out of Czechoslovakia where the rest of my family perished. I find it very hard to understand how it is that you, the people of this country who reached out the hand of welcome to me, a foreigner, then, won't now look after your own.' In the silence as she made her way back to her seat, a man stood up, gave the Nazi salute, and shouted, 'Heil Hitler!' (Spence 1996, pp. 17, 19).

Six years later, thousands are marching, some carrying urns, boxes or plastic bags filled with ashes. The AIDS Coalition To Unleash Power (ACT UP) is holding a demonstration in Washington, DC to make the reality of AIDS visible and to create a space to grieve. There is nothing fake about the protest, these are the real remains of real people. 'They have turned the people we love, into ashes, into bone chips, into corpses.' As mounted police charged at them, they scattered the ashes across the President's lawn. It's been said that 'for all its grave stillness there is nothing more dynamic than a corpse' (Pogue Harrison 2003, p. 93), and six months later, the friends of Tim Bailey were attempting to lay his body on the steps of the White House. 'It was very much about, literally bringing the bodies of our dead to where we thought the blame (lay) and making that quantifiable … Here's a dead body – this was someone who we loved, who we valued' (Shulman 2021, pp. 606, 622). Like the burial vaults of the first Black churches where those escaping slavery were hidden, ACT UP's political funerals were acts of 'imaginative resistance' (Evans and Giroux 2015, p. 10) where the dead were deployed to make a spectacle of themselves for the living.

In Tarkovsky's final film, *The Sacrifice*, a man is given a fifteenth-century map of the world which he assumes must be a reproduction. When he is assured that it is authentic and not a copy, he is reluctant to accept as although 'it's no sacrifice ... it's far too dear a gift.' The giver responds, 'Of course it's a sacrifice. Every gift involves a sacrifice, if not what kind of gift would it be?' One of our doctors said, 'When you enter intensive care, you come with a certain amount of courage, and you leave a piece of your soul behind which you don't get back.' In exchange, you receive 'the privilege and honour' of working 'with everyone you were surrounded with' and of being able 'to enter into lives at their most critical moment.' Death reopens ritual space, offers an opportunity of return, possibilities of transformation and the realisation that 'If you feel the pain of thresholds, you are not a tourist: the transition can occur' (Handke 1983, p. 13).

> It's peculiar because at the start of it we were in darkness, as the clocks hadn't gone back. The Thursday clapping for key workers was in pitch black darkness ... but it's now an incredible burst of bright sunshine, and green and colours and blossom and butterflies ... My son gave me £7.50 in an envelope and wrote, he can just about write, he's written: 'Dear Doctors, please care for everyone and survive.'
>
> (Haywood 2020, ep. 1)

Nine months after The Clapping stopped, a single red heart appears on a hospital wall opposite the UK Houses of Parliament. Ten days later, 150,000 hearts are painted there. The COVID-19 bereaved had come for, and were naming and counting, their dead. Across one heart is written: 'You died without the soft touch of a loved one's hand, without the feathered kiss upon your forehead, without the muted murmur of familiar voices gathered around your bed. Our sister is not a statistic of Covid.' Another says: 'To all the patients I could not save - I'm so sorry. I promise I tried so hard.' Unlike The Clapping, this memorial is both a site of mourning and an avowedly political act.

The day before The Clapping started, the residents of Pristina, the Kosovan capital, took to their balconies with their pots and pans and brought down their government for mishandling the Coronavirus outbreak. Seven months after The Clapping stopped, an attempt to resurrect it was thwarted by nurses who dismissed it as a 'hollow gesture.' 'I have seen too much Covid denial, general abuse and harshness towards the medical profession since then to fully believe the sentiment is real' (Mitchell 2021). Two years after The Clapping stopped, with all health workers facing mandatory COVID-19 vaccination or dismissal, a paramedic remarked, 'Back in 2020 we were all being clapped and come 2022 they're saying we are sacking you' (Meierhans 2022). Three years after The Clapping stopped, nurses and doctors, no longer considered 'bodies of sacrifice,' were striking in the streets against their disposability, chanting the words on their placards, 'CLAPS DON'T PAY THE BILLS.'

Where The Clapping was complicit with spectacles of violence that thrive on the 'accelerated death of the unwanted' (Evans and Giroux 2015, p. 44), disappearing them into 'phantasmagoric scenes' (Biehl 2005, p. 4), the wall brings them back and makes them visible again. With their dead behind them, the living face those in power with the reality of loss. Our then prime minister, Boris Johnson visited the wall under cover of darkness the day after he denied ever saying, 'let the 'bodies pile high in their thousands.' The bereaved, who he had avoided meeting responded: 'These "bodies" were our loved ones.'

The Clapping happens at the threshold, on a doorstep, over a balcony, the ways between interior and exterior worlds. As in every place of passage, 'death is always inscribed in the threshold' as beyond it 'a completely different state of being begins' (Han 2018, p. 34). The clapper's failure to cross over this boundary and identify with the death of the other, rendered them 'consumers of violence as spectacle, adepts of proximity without risk,' who 'will do anything to keep themselves from being moved' (Sontag 2019, p. 97). During COVID-19 there was 'a loss of difference between the living and the dead,' and when homes became tombs, the people emerged through The Clapping into the collective living room of the street, where they tried 'to recapture through ritual the element of complete spontaneity' (Girard 1977, pp. 254, 131). It made the living feel more alive, and the dead (seem) less dead. Those being clapped were 'simultaneously present, yet absent, dead yet living, corporal yet intangible' (Coverley 2020, p. 205). They had already become ghosts.

References

Adebayo, D., 2020. Why were black NHS staff whitewashed out of Clap for Our Carers? *The Voice* [online], 31 March. www.voice-online.co.uk/news/coronavirus/2020/03/31/why-were-black-nhs-staff-left-out-of-clap-for-our-carers/

Akolo, D., 2020. Abstract pain: George Floyd and the viral spectacle of Black death. *bitch media [online]*, 17 June. www.bitchmedia.org/article/black-death-george-floyd-viral-spectacle

Anderson, B., 1983. *Imagined communities*. London: Verso.

Artaud, A., 2010. *The theatre and its double*. V. Corti, trans. London: Alma Books.

Bennett, J.A., 2009. *Banning queer blood: Rhetorics of citizenship, contagion, and resistance*. Tuscaloosa: University of Alabama Press.

Berlant, L., 1998. Poor Eliza. *American Literature*, 70 (3), 635–668.

Bersani, L., 2018. *Receptive bodies*. Chicago: University of Chicago Press.

Biehl, J., 2005. *Vita: Life in a zone of social abandonment*. Berkeley: University of California Press.

Booth, W. and Adam, K., 2020. In fight against coronavirus, the world gives medical heroes a standing ovation. *The Washington Post*, 26 March.

Brown, W., 2015. *Undoing the demos: Neoliberalism's stealth revolution*. New York: Zone Books.

Butler, J., 2020. *Precarious life: The powers of mourning and justice*. London: Verso.

Cook, T., Kursumovic, E., and Lennane, S., 2020. Deaths of NHS staff from covid-19 analysed. *Health Services Journal*, 22 April.

Cousins, M., 2021. *The story of looking*. Edinburgh: Canongate.
Coverley, M., 2020. *Hauntology: Ghosts of futures past*. Harpenden: Oldcastle Books.
Debord, G., 1977. *Society of the spectacle*. Detroit: Black and Red.
Eagleton, T., 2018. *Radical sacrifice*. New Haven: Yale University Press.
Ellis, A., et al., 2021. For the greater good: Sacrificial violence and the coronavirus pandemic. *Journal of Contemporary Crime, Harm, and Ethics*, 1 (1), 1–22. 10.19164/jcche.v1i1.1155
Evans, B. and Giroux, H.A., 2015. *Disposable futures: The seduction of violence in the age of spectacle*. San Francisco: City Lights.
Farooki, R., 2022. *Everything is true*. London: Bloomsbury.
Flood, G., 2013. Sacrifice as refusal. In J. Meszaros and J. Zachhuber, eds. *Sacrifice and modern thought*. Oxford: Oxford University Press, 115–131.
Fischer-Lichte, E., 2005 *Theatre, sacrifice, ritual: Exploring forms of political theatre*. Abingdon: Routledge.
Fisher, M., 2014. *Ghosts of my life*. Winchester: Zero Books.
Freud, S., 2005. *On murder, mourning and melancholia*. London: Penguin.
Girard, R., 1977. *Violence and the sacred*. Baltimore: John Hopkins University Press.
Gorer, G., 1955. The pornography of death. In G. Gorer, ed. *Death, grief and mourning*. New York: Doubleday, 192–199.
Grosz, E., 1994. *Volatile bodies: Toward a corporeal feminism*. Bloomington: Indiana University Press.
Halbertal, M., 2012. *On sacrifice*. Princeton: Princeton University Press.
Han, B-C., 2018. *The expulsion of the other*. Cambridge: Polity Press.
Handke, P., 1983. *Phantasien der Repetition*. Frankfurt: Suhrkamp.
Haywood, S., 2020. *Unmasked*. [Podcast]. https://shows.acast.com/unmasked
Hirsch, A., 2018. *Brit(ish): On race, identity and belonging*. London: Vintage.
Hubert, H. and Mauss, M., 1964. *Sacrifice: Its nature and function*. Chicago: University of Chicago Press.
Jesuthasan, J., et al., 2021. 'We weren't checked in on, nobody spoke to us': An exploratory qualitative analysis of two focus groups on the concerns of ethnic minority NHS staff during COVID-19. *BMJ Open*, 11, e053396. 10.1136/bmjopen-2021-053396
Judah, B., 2016. England's last gasp of empire. *The New York Times*, 12 July.
Kear, A. and Steinberg, D.L., 1999. *Mourning Diana: Nation, culture and the performance of grief*. Abingdon: Routledge.
Kemp, J., 2013. *The penetrated male*. Santa Barbara: Punctum Books.
Levinas, E., 1989. *The Levinas reader*. S. Hand, ed. Oxford: Blackwell.
Love, H., 2009. *Feeling backward: Loss and the politics of queer history*. Cambridge, MA: Harvard University Press.
Manthorpe, J., et al. 2021. Clapping for carers in the Covid-19 crisis: Carers' reflections in a UK survey. *Health & Social Care in the Community*, 30 (4), 1442–1449. 10.1111/hsc.13474
Meierhans, J., 2022. Covid vaccines: The unvaccinated NHS workers facing the sack. *BBC*, 27 January.
Mendel, G., 2022. *The ward*. London: Trolley.
Mitchell, G., 2021. Clap for heroes: Nurses say that they do not want return of applause. *Nursing Times*, 7 January.
Nattrass, N., 2008. AIDS and the scientific governance of medicine in post-apartheid South Africa. *African Affairs*, 107 (427), 157–176. 10.1093/afraf/adm087

Neocleous, M., 2022. *The politics of immunity: Security and the policing of bodies.* New York: Verso.
Peak, D., 2014. *The spectacle of the void.* USA: Schism Press.
Pogue Harrison, R., 2003. *The dominion of the dead.* Chicago: University of Chicago Press.
Qureshi, I., et al., 2022. Health workers from diverse ethnicities and their perceptions of risk management during the COVID-19 pandemic: Qualitative insights from the United Kingdom – REACH Study. *Frontiers in Medicine*, 9. 10.3389/fmed.2022.930904
Shulman, S., 2021. *Let the record show: A political history of ACTUP New York, 1987–1993.* New York: Farrar, Straus and Giroux.
Sontag, S., 2019. *Regarding the pain of others.* London: Penguin.
Spence, C., 1996. *On watch: Views from the Lighthouse.* London: Cassell.
Sturken, M., 2007. *Tourists of history.* Durham, NC: Duke University Press.
Welby, J. and Stevens, J., 2020. Community Spirit: Let's build a bright future by coming together to celebrate the 72nd birthday of the NHS. *The Sun*, 9 June.
Williams, R., 1966. *Modern tragedy.* London: Chatto and Windus.

12 Memorialisation within an ongoing crisis

Learning from COVID-19, HIV and AIDS, and the Overdose Response Activists

Theodore (ted) Kerr

In May 2020, a 13-year-old girl in California started encouraging people to send her fabric representing loved ones who had died due to COVID-19. From there, she began the COVID Memorial Quilt project, inspired by her mother's stories of earlier working on the AIDS memorial quilt. On 28 May 2023, a group of New Yorkers physically pulled the Global Pandemics Touchstone, a two-ton memorial artwork honouring people who died of HIV and COVID-19, from the former Mount Sinai Coronavirus Field Hospital to St John the Divine, where it remained until it was laid at the potter's field at Hart Island. These are but two of many powerful examples of people and communities who have turned to and built upon the legacy of HIV and AIDS as a model for how to memorialise the COVID-19 pandemic.

Several writers have done the same. Two months into quarantine, scholar Micki McElya wrote about the lack of collective pandemic mourning in the Washington Post. The reason, she suggested, 'is as simple as it is terrible: We share no understanding of these staggering losses as *ours*' (McElya 2020). At such inflection points, she wrote, shared experiences of reckoning are needed. She provided two AIDS-related examples: the AIDS memorial quilt, and the Ashes Action, during which members of the activist group ACT UP invited people to bring the ashes of loved ones who died with AIDS and scatter them on the White House Lawn.

In a 2022 feature for the New York Times, writer Mark Harris considered the impact of a variety of memorials, ending with an expression of gratitude for AIDS memorials. He wrestled with how to even conceive of how to memorialise COVID-19:

> … it is harder to imagine what such a memorial will, or should, look like — perhaps because memorials, while they are locations for collective remembrance and mourning, also carry within them a kind of reassurance: *That happened. We lived through it.*
>
> (Harris 2022, emphasis in original)

DOI: 10.4324/9781003322788-15

As Harris pointed out, with COVID-19, like AIDS, there is an additional reality to consider: the urge to memorialise is happening while the crisis is still ongoing. Other memorialisation projects often take place after the fact, be it after violence has occurred, or when a historical figure has died. In her early work on AIDS memorials, respected scholar Marita Sturken wrestles with this order of things when she writes, 'the desire to memorialize the AIDS epidemic while it is still occurring reveals the need to find healing amid death' (Sturken 1997, p.16). The same can be said for COVID-19.

There is something else to consider when it comes to COVID-19 and HIV: the two pandemics are not being pitched against each other when it comes to memorialisation. This is unlike other situations when there is debate about what can and should be remembered (as happened when the construction of a new museum or monument gets proposed on the National Mall in Washington DC). The pitching of memories against each other that happens within memorialisation is a phenomenon historians call competing memories, and as memory scholar Michael Rothberg points out, it suggests that the public sphere is made up of '... limited space in which already established groups engage' (Rothberg 2009, p. 5). Rothberg sees competing discourse as antithetical to how memory – specifically violent memory – is shared and understood in public. He proposes multidirectional memory to illuminate how different histories can co-inform one another. We don't have to choose between atrocities; instead, looking at COVID-19 and HIV together, as an example, helps to articulate the differences and the similarities between the pandemics, including how ill people are treated while they are alive, and how the dead are remembered after they are gone.

Rothberg and Sturken's scholarship is part of a larger network of memory studies scholarship that interrogates and expands how we look at the past. Central to this work is theorist Pierre Nora's thinking around memory and history. As he stated in 1989, 'there are *lieux de memoire*, sites of memory, because there are no longer *milieux de memoire*, real environments of memory' (Nora 1989, p. 7). Nora argued that with the demise of close-knit societies 'that had long assured the transmission and conservation of collectively remembered values, whether through churches or schools, the family or the state' (Nora 1989) we have had to create new ways of collectively remembering. Where we once had memory, we now have history. Where we once had kinship and familial bonds tying us to the present, which he thinks of as memory, we have history, 'a representation of the past' (Nora 1989).

Below, I write about a one-day overdose prevention site (OPS), created by a group of activists that took place near the Toronto's AIDS memorial on World AIDS Day 2018 as a call to action regarding the opioid overdose crisis. An OPS is a place where people can consume the drugs they bring in with them, among volunteers or staff who can support them as they use, and step in if anything goes wrong. OPSs are harm reduction settings, in which people can do drugs, build community and learn about housing opportunities, local safety information and health services.

Initially, I saw the pop-up OPS primarily as an example of multidirectional memory in action, as it related both to HIV and the overdose crisis. But it is also useful as an example to think further about the multidirectional engagement of HIV and COVID-19 memorialisation projects. In a memory circle I conducted with four of the organisers, additional dimensions of their action emerged, most powerfully around what counts as a memorial and the uses of a memorial in an ongoing crisis such as COVID-19, HIV and overdose deaths. With their permission, I share quotes from the memory circle in this chapter. In doing so, it becomes clear that in terms of memorialisation, a realm where, to reflect back on Nora, memory and history loom large, the distinction between memory and history matters. The inflection point to understanding this centres on the group's ambivalence towards the Toronto AIDS memorial itself.

Among the three prongs Rothberg offers that constitute multidirectional memory, the second concerns how 'collective memories of seemingly distinct histories are not easily separable from each other, but emerge dialogically' (Rothberg 2014). To put it differently, one of the ways in which we first started to know COVID-19 was through other crises, such as HIV. Additionally, we can continue to learn how to memorialise COVID-19 and HIV as the crises continue, by learning from the opioid overdose crisis, specifically the one day OPS action.

Memorial ambivalence in the Village

On World AIDS Day 2018, in Toronto, Canada, a community of friends, drug users, activists, AIDS service organisation employees, harm reduction workers and others put up a one-day OPS. The primary audience for the action was the city's legacy AIDS service and queer community care organisations centred in the historic LGBTQ+ neighbourhood known locally as the Village. The message: stop ignoring the overdose crisis. In Toronto alone, according to a 2018 City status report (de Villa 2018), there were more than 300 deaths from opioid toxicity in 2017, an increase from the prior year, and from January to October 2017 in Ontario, there were over 1,000 opioid-related deaths (compared with under 900 in 2016). During this time, zero harm reduction services were offered by local AIDS service and LGBTQ+ organisations.

On a warm spring afternoon five years after the temporary Village OPS, some of the people involved got together for a memory circle to talk about the action. Many had not seen each other since that day in 2018. While much had changed since then – most notably, the arrival of COVID-19 – other things had not: the overdose crisis was still raging, and the response from LGBTQ+ and AIDS service organisations was disappointing. In 2020 and 2021, there were 545 and 593 overdose deaths in Toronto, respectively, and nearly 500 in 2022 (CBC News 2023). While this was down from previous years, largely due to the efforts of activists, the amount of death was still cause for alarm, most notably because no Toronto AIDS or LGBTQ+

organisations had yet to open an OPS and, according to activists, the harm reduction services they did offer were limited.

I facilitated the memory circle as someone who has worked within the HIV response for the last 20 years and is attuned to the ways in which activism, memorialisation and intersectional approaches to AIDS shape how we understand the past, present and future of epidemics. Of specific interest to me was the location selected for the Village OPS, the back corner of Barbara Hall Park, a stone's throw from the city's AIDS memorial and The 519 (a community service centre in the heart of the Village).

At one point in the memory circle, I asked why the AIDS memorial had been chosen as a site, to which the group responded that The 519 was more of the focus, the fact that the AIDS memorial was nearby was incidental. This surprised me. Part of what drew me to the one-day Village OPS story was the assumption the organisers saw an AIDS memorial as a place for mourning *and* present-day action, connecting the dots between the legacy of AIDS activism and the urgency of the ongoing opioid crisis. I was hoping they were working to blur the line between memorialisation and activism. This seemed all the more prescient given the attention AIDS memorials had received since the arrival of COVID-19. But as the memory circle continued, those participating shared something important: when it comes to memorialisation, process matters. This is especially true when the crisis being memorialised is ongoing.

In working through these ideas, I want to share some more information about the OPS and continue thinking about HIV and COVID-19 memorialisation in tandem. I am interested in how, for the OPS organisers, the past was not a site for engagement that they were interested in, rather the activation of memory is more than what can be recalled, it is what can be used to save and value life in the present.

AIDS and COVID-19 memorialisation projects

In the decades since the medical world first recognised HIV, there have been many advances: the rollout of life-saving medication from 1996 onwards, the understanding that if someone living with HIV is on treatment the virus is untransmittable, the functional cure of handful of people, and the introduction of pre- and post-exposure prophylaxis. Yet, the crisis of HIV remains with us. According to UNAIDS, worldwide almost 700,000 people died with HIV in 2021. Of the 38.4 million people currently living with the virus, 40% still do not have access to medication. Worldwide, people are regularly sentenced to jail for having HIV. The burden of the virus is intensified for women, people of colour, Black people, people living with disabilities, people detained in prison and people living in poverty. HIV is one more obstacle to survival. Amidst all this, there has emerged a robust culture of memorialisation.

The earliest recognised AIDS memorial project dates back to 1986, around five years into the AIDS response. A man named Michael Lee and a partner cultivated an abandoned plot of land in Houston, left by a railroad company, to create the Texas AIDS Memorial Garden. A year later, the NAMES Project's AIDS Memorial Quilt, imagined by the activist Cleve Jones, was first presented to the public; 1,920 handmade quilt panels that covered a space larger than a football field were positioned on the National Mall in Washington DC. Each panel was a tribute to a friend, lover, parent or stranger who had died with HIV.

Looking at the Quilt and the Garden together, both can be seen as counter-monuments and sites of communal happenings, in which participation is encouraged not merely through reverence, but through stitching, tending and witnessing. Unlike a statue to a US President, or even a gravestone, the Quilt and the Garden are memorialisation projects amidst an ongoing crisis and are constituted and reconstituted as the epidemic continues. Existing panels of the Quilt are stored and brought out again. New panels are made. Shrubs in the garden are pruned and flowers are planted. Conceived of at a time of mass death, intense activism, government neglect and public apathy, the Quilt and the Garden are assemblages responding to a variety of purposes: to honour the dead, provide shape to the crisis, educate the public, increase AIDS awareness and provide a platform for activism.

These early AIDS memorial projects informed both later AIDS memorials and some of those dedicated to COVID-19. But when it comes to the latter, there is an important difference. The first generation of COVID-19 memorials was created during quarantine within a digital native context. Among them was a website www.covidmemorial.online, created by Duncan Meisel and a friend, that collected and shared online tributes to loved ones who had died due to the Coronavirus. At the time the project began, there had been an estimated 13,000 COVID-19-related deaths in the USA. Two weeks into the project, Meisel and team hosted an offline public event. After sundown, content from the online memorial was projected onto two walls of a building in Washington DC. On one wall was a slideshow of memorials collected from the site, and on the other was a rotation of messages such as 'We Will Remember,' 'You Are Not Alone' and 'We Will Support Each Other.' By this time, over 30,000 people had died of COVID-19 in the USA.

Around the same time as Meisel was using the Internet and public space to share the names and stories of the dead, the folklorist and performer Kay Turner and NYC Council Member Alexa Avilés were working with a small group of people to create #NamingTheLost: A 24 Hour Covid Vigil. Using their personal connections and social media, the group, now known formally as Naming the Lost, collected the names of people from around the USA and beyond who had died of COVID-19 to have their names read out over the span of 24 hours by a rotating crew of volunteers broadcasting from their homes. It was recorded live on Zoom and broadcast on Facebook over the last weekend of May 2020.

More recent memorial projects

A silence permeated around HIV in western culture after effective treatment became available in 1996. AIDS memorials made at this time and into the early twenty-first century are intimate, hyperlocal and often tucked away or hiding in plain sight. They are the work of small yet mighty communities using modest means to remember dead friends, and the Herculean efforts that were mounted against their premature death. Examples include a walkway approaching White Street Pier in Key West, Florida, and a series of glass discs depicting the faces of local people living with HIV in New Orleans, Louisiana, and the AIDS Memorial sculpture in Brighton, UK.

What many of the earliest AIDS memorials and some of the ones that appeared during this period of silence have in common is a place to list the names of the dead, to be added to over time, and to be seen and read aloud at annual World AIDS Day vigils. The importance of naming is an example of what African American literature and art scholar Dagmawi Woubshet (2015), in his 2015 book, *The Calendar of Loss*, has lovingly called the 'trope of inventory taking' that permeated the earlier periods of AIDS cultural production, marked by compounded loss and trauma, and resulting in compulsions to say and re-say, share and share again, the names of the dead.

Of the few opioid overdose-related memorials that exist, most are similar in form and scope to these early AIDS memorials. A majority of the projects are online pages where the names and images of people who have died due to the war on drugs are shared. Exceptions include a 2022 pop-up overdose memorial park in Philadelphia, and a flame-shaped statue in Toronto, less than five miles from the AIDS memorial, where community members have engraved the names of lost loved ones and friends together with messages of encouragement.

More recent AIDS memorialisation projects are different. Not only are they in central, visible locations, but they have also moved away from the inventory trope. Central to the Provincetown AIDS Memorial, in Massachusetts, unveiled in 2018 near the City Hall, are engraved poems and the word 'remembering.' Similarly, in the latest New York City AIDS Memorial, opened in 2016 in the heart of Greenwich Village, which features a Jenny Holzer installation of a Walt Whitman poem. Beyond the East Coast, a different yet related tactic is becoming apparent. The AIDS Memorial Pathway in Seattle, which opened in 2021, and STORIES: The AIDS Monument in Los Angeles, set to open in 2024, are also in highly visible locations and both focus on incorporating stories from the community.

Similar to AIDS, as the COVID-19 crisis intensified, the names became less of a focus. Instead, as people began to emerge from quarantine, location became increasingly important to this second wave of COVID-19 memorials. During autumn 2020, there were two pop-up memorials on the National Mall in Washington DC. The community group, COVID Survivors for Change, used the Mall as a site upon which to put out 20,000 empty chairs with each one representing 10 lives lost. Less than a year later, the Mall was the site of another memorial installation. Entitled, *In America: Remember*, artist Suzanne Brennan Firstenberg presented over 620,000 white flags honouring the ever-increasing number of COVID-19-related deaths in the country. She had done an earlier version outside the nearby RFK stadium in 2020, which included over 200,000 white flags. That version was entitled *In America: How Could This Happen*. In both cases, people were invited to personalise the blank white flags with the names of people who died of COVID-19, along with a short message. A number of these flags were subsequently acquired by the Smithsonian Museum.

When a memorial is not a place

James Young, drawing from his own Holocaust research and his committee work connected to the 9/11 memorial in Lower Manhattan, asserts that the success of a memorial is not just measured by what gets made and how it is received:

> The monument succeeds only insofar as it allows itself full expression of the debates, arguments, and tensions generated in the noisy give and take among competing constituencies driving its creation. In this view, memory as represented in the monument might also be regarded as a never to be completed process, animated (not disabled) by the focus of history bringing it into being.
>
> (Young 2018, p. 16)

With this line of thinking, the 9/11 memorial is not just the twin reflecting pools around which the names of the dead are engraved, or the nearby museum, it is also the process that led up to the creation of those spaces.

Before his 9/11 work, one of Young's focus had been on counter-monuments, which he describes as, 'brazen, painfully self-conscious memorial spaces conceived to challenge the very premises of their being' (Young 1992, p. 271). These works were created at a cultural moment in Europe saturated by monuments and memorials emerging from the horrors of the Second World War, and a sense among a then-emerging generation of architects that such sites were actually places where the past was forgotten. People could walk past statues and plinths in parks and other public spaces, unmoved by and unaware of what was being represented.

In an attempt to refuse the act of storing history, these young architects created public spaces that used but then subverted the language of public memorial and instead put the work of remembering back onto the viewers. Among the most powerful examples of these counter-monuments is the Monument against Fascism in Harburg, Germany. The monument began as a 12-metre high column, surfaced in lead. The public was invited to mark the surface however they wished. From the day of dedication in late 1986 until late 1993, the monument was lowered into the ground until it was gone. In place of the column, there is now a plaque that reads: 'In the end it is only we ourselves who can rise up against injustice.'

This expansion of what we can understand as memorialisation is also present in the work of Marita Sturken. In her latest work, rooted in the post-9/11 era, she writes: 'Architecture and design have been particularly burdened with the role of shaping and guiding the emotional weight of traumatic events, designing both for loss and grief and for renewal and resilience' (Sturken 2022, p. 5). Memorialisation can take many forms, such as poetry, dance, oral tradition, film, activism and performance.

In a class I teach on AIDS memorials, informed by the work of Young and Sturken, my students and I came up with an argument: a memorial – regardless of form – should take place in ways that reflect aspects of the crisis itself. In relation to AIDS, this means it should be collaborative; involve risk and shared vulnerability; be replicable, while also being disruptive, educational and able to change (accumulating meaning, stories and history over time). Examples of this kind of work include Food For Thought in Forestville, California (a vegetable garden honouring those who have died with HIV, which is part of a food bank that serves chronically ill people) and The Wall Las Memorias Project in Los Angeles, which is a physical monument (with a wall of names and murals) but also a nearby health clinic for people impacted by HIV and other chronic illnesses.

As part of this expanded memorial-related thinking, others still remove the notion of a memorial from a stable site all together. In his 2015 text, *AIDS Memorialization: A Biomedical Performance from Viral Dramaturgies*, academic Marc Arthur (2015) wonders if PrEP isn't a memorial of sorts, a daily ritual undertaken by HIV-negative people to consider (and remember) the history that led them to be able to distance themselves from the stigma and the virus. And in a 2013 essay in which he provides a people's history of Clean Needles Now – a needle exchange programme that grew out of overlapping activist and artistic communities in LA in the 1990s – AIDS activist and artist Dont Rhine (2013) makes the case that needle exchange is as foundational to the stories we need to tell about AIDS as Freddie Mercury, red ribbons and ACT UP. As life-giving institutions, birthed in the earliest days of the HIV epidemic, Rhine positions needle exchange programmes and supervised injection sites as places of urgency and memory. All of these examples can be understood as AIDS counter-monuments, works pairing activism and action with the act of remembering.

As memorial forms expand, so too can their focus. Memorials do not have to be just about one thing. The examples above illustrate how AIDS memorial projects can be both about people who died with HIV, and also food insecurity, pharmaceutical intervention, and the war on drugs. This capaciousness is happening with COVID-19 too. In Brooklyn, a series of cloth masks affixed to a chain link fence started to appear in the late summer of 2020. On each mask, someone had stitched the name of a Black person who died due to police violence. That same year the Asian/Pacific/American Institute at NYU started documenting the effects of the COVID-19 pandemic on Asian/Pacific Americans through oral history, including the impacts of the Trump presidency on anti-Asian rhetoric and increased Chinatown gentrification. Three years after the project started, the general public had a chance to engage with what had been collected through an exhibition entitled *Archive as Memorial*. The exhibition (as memorial) was both the archive of audio documenting COVID-19 as well as related issues, and the ways in which the curators exhibited the audio and the public engaged.

In this emerging era of memory, AIDS and COVID-19 memorialisation projects are no longer limited by being only about the virus. In fact, illustrative of Rothberg's theory of multidirectional memory, the numerous crises being looked at in tandem are seen as connected. It is thereby possible to consider not only how crises intersect, but also acts of memorialisation.

More memory, less history

The Toronto AIDS Memorial was initially a pop-up site. Spearheaded by academic and activist Michael Lynch, it was an annual place during Pride for people to collectively mourn loved ones who had died that year with HIV. Looking at pictures from 1988 available online, one can see primarily young and youngish industrious men and a few women erecting temporary walls upon which they will affix slats that will hold the names of the dead. In one of the photos, a group of people pose in front of the memorial. Like so many photos from that time, there is something stunning and heart breaking seeing young people navigating death.

Fast forward 30 years and a similar memorial photo will be taken. Except instead of being in front of names, the Village OPS crew will pose in front of the pop-up site they made. Behind them, in their photo, is a tent and a trailer, providing a safe space for people to inject. There is a handmade unfinished banner that reads VILLAGE OPS. In other photos from this day, you can see the trailer had a disco ball, a purple boa hanging on the door and a handwritten land acknowledgement in the window.

OPSs are part of the long legacy of modern drug-related harm reduction starting in the 1970s by groups such as the Junkie Union in Rotterdam. They established an understanding that people who use drugs can be seen as something other than criminals or in need of help, they can be seen as people with agency. As early as 1980, the Union started to provide a variety of services, including needle exchange, a programme where people get unused needles by bringing in their used needles and syringes. The programme has been replicated globally and was key in reducing HIV transmission within communities of injection drug users in the first decade of the crisis and beyond.

OPSs became part of harm reduction in the mid-1980s when Switzerland opened up a supervised injection facility, in part to curb Hepatitis C and HIV transmission among people who use drugs. Such sites had been around in the late 1910s in the USA, after the passing of the Harrison Narcotic Act of 1914, but were shut down soon after (Trickey 2018). They did not legally exist again in North America until 2002 when the Dr. Peter Centre, a medical facility for people living with HIV in Vancouver, began providing supervised injection services.

The path to open more sites has been hard with a few wins, which is why, when overdose deaths were on the rise in 2016 and 2017, a group of experienced activists within the world of drugs and social services started the Toronto Overdose Prevent Services (TOPS). They opened up an unsanctioned, volunteer-run OPS in Moss Park, an area impacted by drug-related death. Within days, the site was preventing and reversing numerous overdoses (using tools like Naloxone). The City of Toronto started to sanction OPSs.

Amidst all this, TOPS noticed the AIDS organisations and related service providers' overdose silence. TOPS reached out to Queers Crash the Beat (QCB), a collective organising against cruising park raids perpetrated by the police. Together, the two collectives organised the Village OPS in less than a month over dumplings and beer, bringing together years of their own grassroots organising, along with the activist tactics from the drug user and AIDS response communities that came before them.

Contestation as memorial

The one-day Village OPS is what I and the AIDS class students would consider a good memorial. It builds on the activist goals of the movement; creates culture about the past, present and future of AIDS; uses tactics that earlier AIDS activists used to love, fight, die, etc.; and by targeting the AIDS service organisations, communicates the uniqueness of HIV, specifically as a site for social change. But something else is also at play; the Village OPS was confrontational, something Sturken explores. Providing different ways to categorise public memory projects, she writes:

> Memorialization can operate as a form of social cohesion that is needed more during times when other modes of cohesion are failing … Memorialization can also be a site for contestation, disruption and intervention.
>
> (Sturken 2022, p. 4)

In the first case, Sturken is referring to the numerous 9/11 memorials that emerged in the years after the 2001 terrorist attack, and with the second case, she is focusing on The Legacy Museum and National Memorial for Peace and Justice in Montgomery, Alabama, that works to memorialise those who have been lynched across the USA but also to educate the public on how slavery is not over. Instead, in the USA, it mutates and can be seen in the legacy of Jim Crow and racial segregation and, more recently, in mass incarceration.

With Sturken's vision in mind, the pop-up Village OPS can be seen as fitting the description of the second case, crafted as a literal site for contestation, disruption and intervention, with the goal of applying pressure and accountability regarding the overdose crisis. And much like the aims of the National Memorial for Peace and Justice, the Village OPS was a site that drew upon the past, while being rooted in the urgency of the present. Talking with some of the organisers about their experiences helped to unpack the swirling impacts of the past and present, alongside goals and intimate community desires for the project.

About an hour into the memory circle that I facilitated in Toronto in 2023, almost five years after the pop-up Village OPS took place, I asked, 'What are some either big impacts or personal impacts of that day, of December 1st, 2018?' Jonathan Valelly, from QCB, said he was proud of what they did. Michael Holmes, also from QCB, echoed him. TOPS organiser Amanda Leo agreed, and then provided some context about what motivated her involvement:

> Thinking back to that time, I had so much grief about where things were at in the HIV/AIDS movement because it is the single most effective, transformative social movement led by people and communities. And working in those spaces at the time I was like, 'What the fuck is going on? Why aren't you sharing this? … You guys have all this experience and all this knowledge and all of this history of resistance and getting things done. Why won't you help?' … And so what I loved about this project was that it was a way to, I don't know, address those feelings that I think a lot of us were maybe feeling. I definitely was. And it felt nice to be like, 'Oh yeah, no, this is a thing. We can do stuff. Fuck you guys.' There's a way to channel that spirit of activism, which I learned from people who are doing AIDS activism.

Later, Zoë Dodd, from TOPS, shared similar thoughts:

> And it was hard for a while. I've let it go, but there was a few years where I was like, 'It would be nice if some of the older people who were around could talk to us about this weird survivor's guilt we have. And how we keep going and the face of all this death could just show up.'

When listening to the organisers, what becomes clear is that when it comes to AIDS, they are not motivated by what Nora calls *lieux de memoire* (sites of memory), which he categorised as being 'fundamentally remains, the ultimate embodiment of a memorial consciousness that has barely survived in a historical age that calls out for memory because it has abandoned it.'

This is why the Toronto AIDS memorial was of no interest to them. Even the site's caretakers understand it as a relic. In 1993, two years after Lynch's AIDS-related death, it became a permanent place for people impacted by AIDS to remember and mourn. The 519, which manages the memorial now, states on their website, 'The AIDS Memorial reflects a particular place and time. It is a physical monument in a park in a neighborhood that was devastated by AIDS in the early years of the epidemic' (The 519 2023).

What also becomes clear is what the OPS organisers *were* interested in: AIDS as it relates to *memory*, which Nora defines as, 'a gigantic and breathtaking storehouse of a material stock of what it would be impossible for us to remember, an unlimited repertoire of what might need to be recalled' (Nora 1989, p. 13). In her remarks, Leo says she was moved by the AIDS activism she grew up with so much that she got involved. Now, in the middle of the opioid overdose crisis resulting in premature death, she wants to work alongside, learn with and share the work of care with the people whose footsteps she followed. So does Dodd, who wants to learn from others and is open to being a source of information as well.

Leo, Dodd and fellow organisers want to be drawing upon and adding to what Nora calls the breathtaking storehouse. They do not want mentorship or a history class, they want community. AIDS activism history is not a site for them, it is a way for life. The 1 December 2018 action was an intervention to capture the attention of Toronto LGBTQ+ and AIDS organisations, and an invitation to participate in collaborative life-saving AIDS memory work in the face of the opioid crisis and already experienced loss. It was memorialisation through activism, intended to save lives, instead of having to mourn them. Put another way, the Village OPS was a counter-monument amid a nexus of connected crises such as HIV and overdose deaths. The act of caretaking – and remembering what that includes – was dragged forward by the OPS organisers, embodying tactics of activism from previous generations, all done in the shadow of the Toronto AIDS memorial.

Conclusion

As I was finishing this chapter, a Toronto city councillor suggested that a homeless encampment be cleared, and in its place, as reported in a newspaper, 'she would like to see a peaceful memorial garden for people who have died on Toronto's streets, decorated with works by homeless artists.' What is suggested takes Nora's critique of memorialisation to a new level. Beyond just being a place for the past to be forgotten, one can read the call to replace temporary housing with a homeless memorial as an attempt to violently obliterate the present through displacement and obfuscation. It is also, one could argue, a kind of cruel inversion of a counter-memorial. Instead of creating something that empowers the public to remember, the councillor's call for a memorial can be seen as an attempt to help the general public further ignore the homeless crisis.

In response, the Village OPS's own Zoe Dodd tweeted, 'We don't need more memorials, we need to fight for lives, for people to LIVE. I'm so disgusted.' To be generous, what the councillor does capture is, as Sturken put it, an attempt to make meaning out of tragedy. What they fail to offer, though, is a humane way to address a crisis beyond mourning those the system has already failed. But of course, one need not have to choose between making meaning and taking action, especially within an ongoing crisis. What I hope this chapter has made clear is that among the many things that scholars invested in exploring COVID-19 and HIV together might be interested in is the way both pandemics have helped usher in a cultural understanding that memorialisation is no longer a public signifier that something is over. Even more than 40 years into the AIDS crisis, with no effective vaccine or cure in sight (but with life-saving treatment available) there continues to be premature death and memorialisation. Similarly, now almost a half decade into the COVID-19 pandemic, people continue to get sick and communities mourn the millions who have died and will die. At the heart of both crises are impacted people fighting for the dead and for the living; one of the sites where these forces meet is within the realm of memorialisation.

While the differences and similarities between COVID-19 and HIV are numerous, exploring their relationship to each other and connected to other issues is of value. When it comes to memorialisation, looking at pandemics together better enables us to see that memorial projects can be gardens, websites and art installations, and they can also be spaces for safe drug use and a place where someone's name is sewn into a quilt. AIDS and COVID-19 memorials provide examples of places where people can name loss and work with others to provide a way forward for, as Dodd puts it, people to LIVE.

References

Arthur, M., 2015. *AIDS memorialization: A biomedical performance from viral dramaturgies*. Cham: Palgrave Macmillan.

CBC News, 2023. Opioid-related deaths dropped in Toronto in 2022, expert says more robust response to crisis needed. *CBC News* [online], 15 May. www.cbc.ca/news/canada/toronto/opioid-related-deaths-1.6843960

de Villa, E., 2018. *Toronto overdose action plan: Status report 2018*. Toronto: Toronto City Council Board of Health. Available from: www.toronto.ca/legdocs/mmis/2018/hl/bgrd/backgroundfile-116008.pdf [Accessed 7 July 2023]

Harris, M., 2022. Imagining a memorial to an unimaginable number of Covid deaths. *The New York Times*, 9 November. www.nytimes.com/2022/11/09/t-magazine/public-memorials-monuments-covid.html

McElya, M., 2020. Almost 90,000 dead and no hint of national mourning. Are these deaths not 'ours'? *Washington Post*, 15 May. www.washingtonpost.com/outlook/national-mourning-coronavirus/2020/05/15/b47fc670-9577-11ea-82b4-c8db161ff6e5_story.html

Nora, P., 1989. Between memory and history: Les lieux de mémoire. *Representations*, 26, 7–24. doi:10.2307/2928520.

Rhine, D., 2013. Below the skin: AIDS activism and the art of clean needles now. *X-TRA Contemporary Art Journal*. www.x-traonline.org/article/below-the-skin-aids-activism-and-the-art-of-clean-needles-now

Rothberg, M., 2009. *Multidirectional memory: Remembering the Holocaust in the age of decolonization.* Stanford: Stanford University Press.
Rothberg, M., 2014. Multidirectional memory. *Témoigner. Entre histoire et mémoire* [online], 119. doi:10.4000/temoigner.1494
Sturken, M., 1997. *Tangled memories: The Vietnam War, the AIDS epidemic, and the politics of remembering.* Oakland: University of California Press.
Sturken, M., 2022. *Terrorism in American memory: Memorials, museums, and architecture in the post-9/11 era.* New York: NYU Press.
The 519, 2023. AIDS Memorial and Vigil. *The 519* [online]. Available from: www.the519.org/programs/aids-memorial-and-vigil/ [Accessed 7 July 2023]
Trickey, E., 2018. Inside the story of America's 19th-century opiate addiction. *Smithsonian Magazine.* www.smithsonianmag.com/history/inside-story-americas-19th-century-opiate-addiction-180967673/
Woubshet, D., 2015. *The calendar of loss.* Baltimore: Johns Hopkins University Press.
Young, J.E., 1992. The counter-monument: Memory against itself in Germany today. *Critical Inquiry*, 18 (2), 267–296.
Young, J.E., 2018. *The stages of memory: Reflections on memorial art, loss, and the spaces between.* Amherst: University of Massachusetts Press.

13 Critical hope and responses to pandemics

From HIV to COVID-19

Carmen H. Logie and Frannie MacKenzie

This chapter utilises the concept of 'critical hope' to analyse and compare responses in the HIV and COVID-19 epidemics to date. It signals the importance of hope in responses to HIV and the need to build hopeful, strengths-focused and creative approaches in relation to COVID-19. But hope by itself is not enough. There needs also to be recognition of suffering and pain as a shared human experience. Engaging people with acceptance, kindness and patience when experiencing life challenges encourages an awareness of our shared humanity. Combining this with recognition that the effects of any epidemic are socially patterned such that those who are economically and socially excluded suffer most leads to the need to position hope in broader struggles for social justice and equality. This is what 'critical hope' is all about. To what extent has hope of this kind been present in responses to COVID-19 to date? What – if anything – has been learned from earlier experiences of HIV? And how might critical hope be engendered for the future so as to move beyond the suffering and exclusion that constitutes the 'new normal'?

What is critical hope?

Believing in, striving for and nurturing hope in our struggles for social justice and equality are the essence of critical hope. In his recent foreword 'Paulo Freire's Pedagogy of Hope in Dark Times' to Freire's book, *Pedagogy of Hope*, Henry A. Giroux explains:

> For Freire, pessimism is the underside of apocalyptic thinking and functions largely to depoliticize people. Freire's Pedagogy of Hope encourages us not to look away in the face of such crisis or to surrender to such events as inescapable acts of fate, but to seize upon them as offering up new challenges and opportunities to make politics, hope, and education central to the challenge of rethinking politics and the possibilities of collective agency and resistance. Freire is not trying to locate redemption in the ruins that plague humankind as much as he

DOI: 10.4324/9781003322788-16

> believes that the impulses of hope can prevent us from becoming accomplices to the terror imposed by the [COVID-19] pandemic and its mounting catastrophes.
>
> (Giroux 2021, p. 2)

In this description, a few key principles underpinning critical hope are identified. First, lack of hope – pessimism – can produce barriers to political action for social change. It can reduce motivation and in turn political engagement – even towards fundamental political actions such as voting. As social and structural drivers embedded in laws and policies continue to re/produce health inequities, creating structural level change through political engagement of all forms – including protest and voting – is required. For instance, stigma embedded in laws has led to the criminalisation of health issues such as HIV. Even in the face of significant evidence that laws that criminalise HIV harm health and human rights, it is challenging to overturn these legal systems. Persistent advocacy for health and rights is thus required to dismantle harmful laws regarding HIV and other social justice issues.

Second, hope holds the potential to spark collective agency and the spirit of resistance. This collectivisation and resistance can emerge through awareness of – and response to – a lack of gender, racial, economic and social justice. For instance, critical hope and belief in the power of collective anti-racist action was evidenced in the ways in which Black Lives Matter sparked collective action and consciousness raising against racist social, legal, educational and economic systems. Organising for radical change – whether abortion rights, sexual rights or against sexual and gender-based violence – requires collective action to redefine space, networks and institutions. Transitional moments in history – such as the arrival of a pandemic – can produce new opportunities for connection and critical dialogue based on intersectional collective action. For Freire, critical pedagogy was rooted in the ways in which critical thinking and critical dialogue can expose power relations, promote problem solving, hold persons in power accountable and ultimately increase individual and collective agency in active struggles for social justice. To be effective, this organising also necessitates an intersectional lens that addresses interlocking oppression beyond one identity or experience, including gender, race, sexual orientation, class, im/migration status and dis/ability, among others.

Finally, without hope we can become, as described in the above quotation, 'accomplices' to not only the terror in a pandemic but also to the everyday terrors of injustice and inequity in mundane and ordinary life. Freire constructs hope as a warning and call to action rather than as a remedy for injustice (Freire 2014). Without hope, one can become disconnected and passive, not understanding or actualising personal or social responsibility, and not able to imagine and work towards a more just and equitable future. In this way, hope is courageous and 'an ontological category that was crucial to prevent individuals from falling into despair, cynicism, and passivity'

(Freire 2014, p. 11). Freire's work underscores hope as an essential ingredient that strengthens and stabilises our struggles for social justice:

> Hopelessness paralyzes us, immobilizes us. We succumb to fatalism, and then it becomes impossible to muster the strength we absolutely need for a fierce struggle that will re-create the world. I am hopeful, not out of mere stubbornness, but out of an existential, concrete imperative. I do not mean that, because I am hopeful, I attribute to this hope of mine the power to transform reality all by itself, so that I set out for the fray without taking account of concrete, material data, declaring, 'my hope is enough!' No, my hope is necessary, but it is not enough. Alone, it does not win. But, without it, my struggle will be weak and wobbly. We need critical hope the way a fish needs unpolluted water.
>
> (Freire 2014, p. 2)

In the description above, both hopelessness and hope are experienced from within the body. Freire framed hope as part of the human experience and a force that could be leveraged individually or collectively to struggle against inequity, dehumanisation and social division (Webb 2010) and 're-create the world'. This concept of re-creating the world reflects transformative hope – whereby collective and personal actions hold the possibility of dismantling and rebuilding social structures (Freire 2007). Such transformative hope has fuelled social change movements, including Civil Rights and anti-war movements (Van Hooft 2014). Critical hope is thus always in tension with social and structural forces of oppression and the status quo. At times, Freire described critical hope as grounded in patience during struggles for justice, while at other times he notes the need for passion, anger and 'just rage' (Freire 1972, 2007; Webb 2010). Importantly, critical hope is rooted in virtues such as patience and love, humility, courage and generosity (Freire 2016), yet it must be distinguished from false, simplistic or naïve ideas of hope. As the above quotation reminds us, hope on its own is not enough to create change but can help us move beyond only critiquing current problems to also envisioning solutions. In this way, the utopian hope described by Freire (2004) both rejects current societal inequities while offering new possibilities.

bell hooks has also discussed the importance of building solutions and ways forward while challenging social inequities in order to avoid the danger of cynicism.

> There have been many quiet moments of incredible shifts in thought and action that are radical and revolutionary. To honor and value these moments rightly we must name them even as we continue rigorous critique. Both exercises in recognition, naming the problem but also fully and deeply articulating what we do that works to address and resolve issues, are needed to generate anew and inspire a spirit of ongoing resistance. When we only name the problem, when we state complaint without a

> constructive focus on resolution, we take away hope. In this way critique can become merely an expression of profound cynicism, which then works to sustain dominator culture.
>
> (hooks 2003, p. 14)

In this way, hooks conceptualised hope as political, rooted in possibility and spanning time. hooks also situated hope as central to community building and empowering to educators, students, researchers and others in ways that nurture connections and a 'liberating mutuality' (hooks 2003, p. 15). In contrast to the isolation and despair that results from living in contexts of social inequity, social justice work rooted in hope can foster solidarity, trust, joy and care that leads to the awareness of individual and collective *interbeing* (hooks 2003). In part, this derives from an understanding of our shared humanity, whereby 'we are connected in our suffering. That connection is part of our understanding of compassion: that it is expansive, that it moves in a continuum' (hooks 2003, p. 159). The pain from being marginalised and disempowered can in fact provide the space to connect with others engaging in social change. hooks discusses how this space of marginality is 'much more than a site of deprivation, that it is also the site of radical possibility, a space of resistance' (hooks 1989, p. 20). This vision of hope and possibility detailed by hooks requires an openness to change, including being changed oneself, and imagination that opens up new ways to build communities rooted in social justice (hooks 2003). This perspective on critical hope shines a light on the strengths gained from being at the margins: 'it nourishes one's capacity to resist. It offers to one the possibility of radical perspective from which to see and create, to imagine alternatives, new worlds' (hooks 1989, p. 20). These marginal spaces of possibility offer a pathway to understand how to respond to pandemics in ways that nurture critical hope and social justice.

Critical hope and the HIV pandemic

Community responses to HIV have centred hope for more than four decades. For instance, there were dreams and hopes for a cure for HIV early in the HIV pandemic. As Herbert de Souza explained in the book 'The Cure of AIDS' with regards to dreams of a cure, 'suddenly, I realized that all had changed because there was a cure. That the idea of inevitable death paralyzes. That the idea of life mobilizes … To wake up knowing that you are going to live makes everything in life meaningful' (de Souza and Parker 1994, p. 48). This same hope also centred liberation and challenged stigma and social inequities towards HIV and towards sexually and gender-diverse communities. For instance, the San Francisco gay and lesbian theatre company Theatre Rhinoceros (1977–2001) explored empowering perspectives on HIV alongside challenges with coming out experiences among sexually diverse persons, illness from HIV and homophobic violence. They produced a show on the early days of the pandemic from 1980 to 1984 called the 'Artists Involved with Death and Survival: The A.I.D.S. Show' that portrayed hopeful perspectives on gay and lesbian life, including people living with HIV receiving care and social acceptance and engaging in HIV prevention. The show spotlighted both suffering and inequities alongside love and liberation, reflecting a critically hopeful perspective (MacDonald 1989). Other writers, such as Simon Watney, in his book *Imagine Hope: AIDS and Gay Identity*, conceptualised hope as central to healing among people living with HIV while also remaining precarious: 'if you hoped for too much you were bound to be disappointed. If you expected very little, you might even possibly be admirably surprised' (Watney 2000, p. 263).

More recent writings in the field of HIV have shown the ways that hope is relational and temporally sensitive among people living with HIV, and points to the need to provide opportunities to discuss both hope and hopelessness to move beyond a social script that prioritises *only* hope and positivity (Bernays et al. 2014). Others note how hope has been key to HIV responses and is contextually shaped by factors such as access to material resources, agency nurtured through social support and optimistic attitudes (Barnett et al. 2015). Among marginalised communities such as transgender women of colour, critical hope can be fostered through participatory research that provides space to discuss journeys of self-acceptance through experiences of pain, social exclusion and personal loss; through these spaces persons can find solidarity, community connections and personal and collective optimism (Logie et al. 2022).

Critical hope and the COVID-19 pandemic

The COVID-19 pandemic was shaped by fear of many unknowns – including the uncertain trajectory and future waves of the pandemic; unknown transmission routes; unknown long-term social, health and economic impacts; and the unknown future of the world as we know it. In the last few years, we have experienced collectively radical changes in how we work, socialise and access basic resources and services. Xenophobia and anti-Asian racism were amplified in the early days and have persisted throughout the pandemic, as have global inequities in access to vaccines and treatment. COVID-19 exacerbates pre-existing social and health disparities – and it can feel overwhelming to address the intersecting stressors of climate change, racism and health inequity.

At the same time, together within these feelings of overwhelm and despair, there is a sense of opportunity to redefine our collective futures. In fact, COVID-19 has been described as a portal (Roy 2020) for redefining and reimagining the future – including how and where we work, how we understand our global interconnectedness and responsibility to one another, and how we relate to persons in our close and distal proximity. Since the beginning of the pandemic, COVID-19 has had a devastating impact on people's livelihoods, health and well-being, and connections with one another. Indeed, the pandemic has reversed progress in addressing HIV, tuberculosis and malaria (Kuehn 2021). It has exacerbated gender inequities (World Economic Forum 2021) and contributed to mental health challenges (Phiri et al. 2021). Yet it has also offered possibilities of rethinking how societies and life in general are structured and imagining new possibilities. In Arundhati Roy's (2020) essay 'The Pandemic is a Portal', she described:

> Whatever it is, COVID-19 has made the mighty kneel and brought the world to a halt like nothing else could. Our minds are still racing back and forth, longing for a return to 'normality', trying to stitch our future to our past and refusing to acknowledge the rupture. But the rupture exists. And in the midst of this terrible despair, it offers us a chance to rethink the doomsday machine we have built for ourselves. Nothing could be worse than a return to normality. Historically, pandemics have forced humans to break with the past and imagine their world anew. This one is no different, it is a portal, a gateway between one world and the next. We can choose to walk through it, dragging the carcasses of our prejudice and hatred, our avarice, our data banks and dead ideas, our dead rivers and smoky skies behind us. Or we can walk through it lightly, with little luggage, ready to imagine another world. And ready to fight for it.
>
> (Roy 2020, p. 214)

Roy's piece reflects core elements of critical hope: the ability to hold in one's view injustice and broken social systems alongside dreams of new worlds and possibilities. Building community and social support, engaging in activism, and organising and solidarity are ways through which such critical hope can be nurtured. Indeed, in the COVID-19 pandemic, social movements aimed to effect structural and systemic change for a more equitable future, and concepts of solidarity, community and hope were seeds for growing and sustaining these initiatives. COVID-19 saw the adaptation of existing social movements, as well as the creation of new movements that provide the opportunity to consider how to foster critical hope in a new pandemic.

In the context of the COVID-19 pandemic, political action was needed to argue for social assistance for persons who lost their employment, to fight against global vaccine inequities that continue to be experienced by low-income countries, and to advocate for access to needed health resources such as masks, COVID-19 testing, sick and disability leave and treatment and care for long COVID-19 (Hargreaves and Logie 2020). Many social movements existing pre-COVID-19 had to adapt when the pandemic emerged and addressed the above calls for political action. Wood (2022) has examined how social movements in Toronto, Canada continued organising to provide essential services during the lockdowns early in the COVID-19 pandemic. For example, activists were successful in ensuring undocumented people could seek medical attention in the event of a health emergency and advocated for the release of immigrant detainees and persons incarcerated for non-violent offences. These successes offer insight into possibilities of the kinds of structural changes that can be made to benefit the most marginalised communities (Wood 2022).

Calvo (2020) explored how the 15 M movement was adapted by other social movements to respond to COVID-19. In 2011, activists and residents in Spain took over public squares to call for social reform and political transformation in what was referred to as the 'Indignados' or 15 May movement (15 M movement). This movement shifted from large demonstrations and occupations to address neighbourhood-level issues, largely concerning housing and social solidarity (Dufour et al. 2016). During COVID-19, a racial justice group in Spain used the 15 M method to bring to light the unequal effects and consequences of the pandemic. It shifted thinking from COVID-19 as a *pandemic* to COVID-19 as a *social movement* bringing awareness to social inequalities, collective solidarity, shared solutions and defence of public services. By tying the pandemic to social movements, people came together to develop shared solutions to build a better future (Calvo 2020).

Elsewhere, Mendes (2020) has explored how urban social movements, fighting for equality in access to housing in Lisbon, responded to the COVID-19 pandemic. Although always present, housing scarcity in Lisbon emerged as a prominent issue during the pandemic, and social movements were successful in the government taking tangible action, including suspending evictions and deferring housing loan payments. In this way, the exposure of extreme housing inequities during COVID-19 mobilised communities to expand their mutual support networks, and ultimately advanced policy changes aligned with their pre-pandemic social movement goal of ensuring all people have the right to adequate housing (Mendes 2020).

Under the impact of COVID-19, some social movements shifted from in-person to online and digital activism in the pandemic. Pinckney and Rivers (2020) surveyed activists in 27 countries to explore how social movements themselves adapted to the COVID-19 pandemic. There was an observed decrease in street protests and public activism at the beginning of the pandemic. However, there was no decline in interest of social movements, but rather a shift to digital and online activism. A key takeaway here is the fact that activists were optimistic for the future, as they saw COVID-19 as an opportunity for systemic change (Pinckney and Rivers 2020).

Tabbush and Friedman (2020) also observed a shift to online and digital activism when examining feminist social movements on a global scale during the pandemic. They discussed how COVID-19 magnified rooted systematic inequalities for women and gender non-conforming people. Despite reduced visible activism, online and digital networks of women and LGBTQI+ activists continued to advance social justice. Tabbush and Friedman describe how,

> although pandemic policies have halted the most visible crest of the fourth feminist 'wave' and facilitated crackdowns on women and LGBTQI

> activists, deeply rooted, digitally enhanced networks are driving an unprecedented response to the COVID-19 outbreak, ranging from multilateral policy interventions to solidaristic actions in low-income urban neighborhoods.
>
> (Tabbush and Friedman 2020, p. 631)

The Feminist Alliance for Rights, which aims to develop a global policy agenda focused on women's human rights, published 'A Call for a Feminist COVID-19 Policy' in March 2020 which was endorsed by 1,600 people and organisations spanning 100 countries. The Call applied a rights based and intersectional lens to advocate for pandemic responses regarding food security, health care, education, social inequality, water and sanitation, economic inequality, gender-based violence, information, and power abuse. The Association for Women in Development developed the online '#FeministBailout Campaign' to advocate for support to sex workers, care workers, migrant workers and seasonal agricultural workers. In addition to digital activism, grassroots feminist activists' groups throughout Latin America came together in solidarity to provide basic needs that the government failed to, including food, masks, hygiene products, gender-based violence support and prevention information. A feminist activist and teacher in Argentina, Laura Marquez, explained 'the *olla* [soup kitchen] is much more than an act of solidarity – [it] is a space for political transformation' (Tabbush and Friedman 2020, p. 635). These feminist movements provided a sense of hope and solidarity and addressed not only COVID-19 but also struggled for economic, reproductive and gender justice (Tabbush and Friedman 2020).

Pleyers (2020) has discussed the actions taken by social movements in early pandemic lockdowns across diverse global contexts between March and May 2020. These included defending workers' rights; mutual aid and solidarity; monitoring policymakers; and the delivery of popular education. His analysis advanced calls attention to the less-visible dynamics of social movements, how activism can be practised in day-to-day life, and how solidarity can extend to building community beyond other activists. It also describes the importance of exploring what meanings, knowledge and narratives are produced by social movements. It also highlights the ways in which activists and protests continued to be repressed during the pandemic by state forces, and how grassroots mutual aid groups arose in low-, middle- and high-income countries and helped to rebuild 'the social fabric based on concrete solidarity' (Pleyers 2020).

Focusing on the role of social movements between March and August 2020, Della Porta (2021) observed that social movements globally used COVID-19 as an opportunity for conversation about social injustice, the inequalities experienced by marginalised groups, and governments' role in ensuring human rights. As a result of these conversations, a collective identity came to be fostered through shared feelings of hope and change for the future. Unlike pre-COVID-19 movements which sought immediate short-term relief for social inequities, COVID-19 social movements pursued radical social change (Della Porta 2021).

New care collectives and mutual aid also emerged in the pandemic. Littman et al. (2022) explored the values underpinning mutual aid practices in the USA early in the pandemic by interviewing mutual aid organisers and participants. They identified shared values including reciprocity and beyond, shared humanity and community-driven care, and the redistribution of resources. The concept of *reciprocity and beyond* encompasses ideas of mutuality that expand beyond a binary of 'giver' or 'receiver' and are guided by solidarity and liberation and the underlying notion that mutual aid is for everyone. This concept of mutuality considers everyone as having something to offer as well as everyone having needs at some point in their life, both material and emotional. The idea challenges typical ideas of material transactions in mutual aid to also include social connection and friendships. Solidarity and liberation were values underlying mutual aid: 'mutual aid meant fighting to shift systems to take care of everyone and free everyone from oppression' (Littman et al. 2022, p. 102). The notion of compassion grounded in shared humanity also influenced mutual aid, as did notions of interdependence and collectivism. Participants also discussed mutual aid as a community-level practice grounded in trust, neighbourhood connection and recognising different needs within a community. To be able to practise, mutual aid requires community collaboration, creativity, cooperation, authentic connection building, and a dynamic process that remains responsive to changing needs (Littman et al. 2022).

In sum, existing social movements saw the COVID-19 pandemic as an opportunity for growth and systematic change (Calvo 2020; Mendes 2020; Pleyers 2020; Tabbush and Friedman 2020; Della Porta 2021; Mackenzie 2022). COVID-19 social movements harnessed support leveraging collective identities (Grant and Smith 2021), mutual aid (Pleyers 2020; Bielski 2022; Littman et al. 2022) and shared emotions such as grief and loss (Grant and Smith 2021; Mackenzie 2022) to engage in collective action. Much of the mobilisation of collective action has focused on government policy changes such as suspension of evictions (Mendes 2020) and rent stabilisation (Wood 2022), or financial support programmes such as the Canadian Emergency Response Benefit (Wood 2022). However, as action plans were developed in relation to COVID-19, once restrictions and the perceived severity of the pandemic declined, the movements saw a loss of motivation and resources (Mendes 2020; Della Porta 2021; Wood 2022). While temporary social change may have been brought about, much of the literature on COVID-19 social movements highlights the need for post-pandemic awareness and systemic change rather than temporary solutions to immediate problems (Calvo 2020; Mendes 2020; Pinckney and Rivers 2020; Pleyers 2020; Della Porta 2021; Mackenzie 2022; Wood 2022).

Critical hope and pandemic responses: From HIV to COVID-19 and beyond

COVID-19 challenged social structures, economic security and health globally (Littman et al. 2022). It increased pre-pandemic inequalities rooted in poverty, racism, sexuality and gender inequities, among others (Calvo 2020; Mendes 2020; Pleyers 2020; Tabbush and Friedman, 2020; Della Porta 2021; Bielski 2022; Littman et al. 2022; Mackenzie 2022; Wood 2022). Yet, as detailed above, there are fine examples spanning global contexts of social movements and resistance in the context of pandemic-related suffering. These movements can nurture critical hope. As Roy's (2020, p. 214) writing on the pandemic as a portal put it, 'Historically, pandemics have forced humans to break with the past and imagine their world anew'. This was also the case with HIV, where social movements and care collectives played a role in generating critical hope.

There are important parallels between the critical hope, care and social movements that arose in the context of HIV and those that arose in response to the COVID-19 pandemic. For instance, literature has examined similarities in community responses to COVID-19 in Canada and those that earlier arose in relation to HIV, finding that in both pandemics the most marginalised people did not have access to resources and support they needed, resulting in reliance on community networks of support (Bielski 2022). These community networks came together to share experiences, enhance credibility and bring more attention to the wide-scale effects of the pandemics. Other work has explored the role that emotion plays in social movement organising and found other similarities between COVID-19 and HIV responses. In both cases, social movements leveraged emotion, such as grief and loss, to motivate action for structural change (Mackenzie 2022). By centring emotion, individual trauma can be shared to develop a collective identity to address inequalities – this mobilisation can spark hope for change.

Pandemic-related care communities and mutual support can thus address structural inequities while also fuelling critical hope. The Care Collective's *The Care Manifesto: The Politics of Interdependence* frames the pandemic as a space 'in which carelessness reigns' (The Care Collective 2020, p. 1) and situates the care (and carelessness) that emerged in the COVID-19 pandemic within the larger histories of gay and lesbian liberation struggles. The family and social exclusion experienced by sexually and gender-diverse persons resulted in the formation of gay neighbourhoods and alternative kinship structures with chosen families. They describe, 'this was often out of necessity, but it was also advocated as part of the radical politics of gay liberation that sought to expand affective relations of care and intimacy beyond those sanctioned by and through heteronormativity' (The Care Collective 2020, p. 35).

State failure to effectively respond to HIV and provide care for people living with HIV later led to communities and community-based organisations addressing these care needs, including ACT UP, Gay Men Fighting AIDS, Buddies and the Terrence Higgins Trust. The Care Collective described how these new models of care by and for sexually and gender-diverse persons and people living with HIV created a new model of care network for 'strangers like me', whereby persons with shared social identities helped look after others (The Care Collective 2020). An advisory committee of people living with HIV in the USA developed the Denver Principles in 1983 that described the rights of people living with HIV, including 'to die – and to LIVE – in dignity', and made recommendations for all people to: 'Support us in our struggle against those who would fire us from our jobs, evict us from our homes, refuse to touch us or separate us from our loved ones, our community or our peers …' (People with AIDS Advisory Committee 1983). This frames social, emotional and material support needs directly within larger contexts of oppression while stressing the hope to LIVE – the only capitalised word in the Denver Principles – in dignity.

In its work, the Care Collective proposes an 'ethics of promiscuous care' that:

> proliferates outwards to redefine caring relations from the most intimate to the most distant. It means caring more and in ways that remain experimental and extensive by current standards. We have relied on the 'market' and 'the family' to provide too many of our caring needs for too long. We need to create a more capacious notion of care.
>
> (The Care Collective 2020, p. 41)

Importantly, promiscuous care does not discriminate, can be applied to distal and proximal connections, and expands our caring imaginaries. This framing of an ethics of promiscuous care builds on Crimp's (1987) writing, *How to have Promiscuity in an Epidemic* to reframe gay men's sexual cultures as experimental intimacies and alternative models of care. This care included developing safer sex practices, spanning from the early HIV pandemic to today. In its writing, The Care Collective (2020) characterises caring as inclusive of capacities, practices and imaginaries. It calls attention to the limits of caring, including the need to tackle structural inequalities (e.g. poverty, limited resources) and discusses how COVID-19 has sparked new forms of care, including mutual aid. A new and expansive vision of caring is proposed.

> What, we now ask, would happen if we were to begin instead to put care at the very centre of life? In this manifesto, we argue that we are in urgent need of a politics that puts care front and centre. By care, however, we not only mean 'hands-on' care, or the work people do when directly looking after the physical and emotional needs of others – critical and urgent as this dimension of caring remains. 'Care' is also a social capacity

> and activity involving the nurturing of all that is necessary for the welfare and flourishing of life. Above all, to put care centre stage means recognizing and embracing our interdependencies.
>
> (The Care Collective 2020)

This manifesto frames care as an activity and as a social dimension of life that is needed in order to flourish – and live a good life, whatever that may mean individually and collectively. It also highlights the concept of interdependency – our interconnectedness and shared humanity. In a similar vein, Freire's *Pedagogy of Hope* – 'written in rage and love, without which there is no hope' (Freire 2014, p. 18) – and his other writings conceptualise love for the self and others as a fundamental component of shared humanity and a necessary fuel for collective resistance and social justice work (Darder 2017).

Revisiting the core concepts on critical hope discussed at the beginning of this chapter, we recall that critical hope can help to overcome barriers to political action to effect social change; critical hope can spark collective agency and fuel resistance; and finally, critical hope can help to stop us from falling into passiveness and disconnection. When societal leaders failed to act during the HIV pandemic, critical hope fuelled communities and community organisations to engage in collective action, to challenge stigma and to provide care for one another in the face of stigma and social exclusion. In a similar vein, social movements during the COVID-19 pandemic engaged with critical hope to fuel collective action and advocate for systemic change.

Taken together and as explored in these examples from COVID-19 and HIV, critical hope is needed to catalyse engagement in social justice, care and mutual aid initiatives but can itself be an outcome from this engagement. Alternative models of care are necessary in social contexts characterised by global pandemics as they interface with serious resource inequalities, institutionalised discrimination and socioeconomic exclusion. Centring critical hope, capacious concepts of care and shared humanity in the work we do – as researchers, service providers and advocates – can inform how to advance justice and well-being not only in present and future pandemics but throughout day-to-day life.

References

Barnett, T., et al., 2015. Hope: A new approach to understanding structural factors in HIV acquisition. *Global Public Health*, 10 (4), 417–437. doi:10.1080/17441692.2015.1007154

Bernays, S., Rhodes, T., and Jankovic Terzic, K., 2014. Embodied accounts of HIV and hope: Using audio diaries with interviews. *Qualitative Health Research*, 24 (5), 629–640. doi:10.1177/1049732314528812

Bielski, Z., 2022. What does 'living with' COVID-19 mean? HIV/AIDS activists offer lessons from pandemics past. *The Globe and Mail*, 17 March. www.theglobeandmail.com/canada/article-what-does-living-with-covid-19-mean-hivaids-activists-offer-lessons/

Calvo, D., 2020. Social movements in a time of pandemic. *CCCB LAB*, 6 October. https://lab.cccb.org/en/social-movements-in-a-time-of-pandemic/
Crimp, D., 1987. How to have promiscuity in an epidemic. *October*, 43, 237–271. doi:10.2307/3397576
Darder, A., 2017. *Reinventing Paulo Freire: A pedagogy of love*. New York: Routledge.
de Souza, H. and Parker, R.G., 1994. *A cura da AIDS [The cure of AIDS]*. Rio de Janeiro: Relume-Dumará.
Della Porta, D., 2021. Progressive social movements, democracy and the pandemic. In *Progressive social movements, democracy and the pandemic*. De Gruyter, 209–226. doi:10.1515/9783110713350-014
Dufour, P., Nez, H., and Ancelovici, M., 2016. Introduction: From the Indignados to Occupy: Prospects for comparison. In P. Dufour, H. Nez, and M. Ancelovici, eds. *Street politics in the age of austerity*. Amsterdam University Press, 11–40. www.jstor.org/stable/j.ctt1d8hb8t.4
Freire, P., 1972. *Pedagogy of the oppressed*. London: Penguin.
Freire, P., 2004. *Pedagogy of indignation*. New York: Paradigm. doi:10.4324/9781315632902
Freire, P., 2007. *Daring to dream: Toward a pedagogy of the unfinished*. New York: Paradigm.
Freire, P., 2014. *Pedagogy of hope: Reliving pedagogy of the oppressed*. London: Bloomsbury.
Freire, P., 2016. *Pedagogy of the heart (Bloomsbury Revelations)*. London: Bloomsbury Academic.
Giroux, H., 2021. Paulo Freire's pedagogy of hope in dark times. In P. Freire, *Pedagogy of hope: Reliving pedagogy of the oppressed*. Trans. R. Barr. London: Bloomsbury Academic, 1–14. doi:10.5040/9781350190238.0004.
Grant, P.R. and Smith, H.J., 2021. Activism in the time of COVID-19. *Group Processes & Intergroup Relations*, 24 (2), 297–305. doi:10.1177/1368430220985208
Hargreaves, J. and Logie, C.H., 2020. Lifting lockdown policies: A critical moment for COVID-19 stigma. *Global Public Health*, 15 (12), 1917–1923. doi:10.1080/17441692.2020.1825771
hooks, b., 1989. Choosing the margin as a space of radical openness. *Framework*, 36 (36), 15–23.
hooks, b., 2003. *Teaching community: A pedagogy of hope*. New York: Routledge.
Kuehn, B.M., 2021. COVID-19 rolls back progress against HIV, TB, and malaria. *JAMA*, 326 (15), 1471. doi:10.1001/jama.2021.18252
Littman, D.M., et al., 2022. Values and beliefs underlying mutual aid: An exploration of collective care during the COVID-19 pandemic. *Journal of the Society for Social Work and Research*, 13 (1), 89–115. doi:10.1086/716884
Logie, C.H., et al., 2022. Eliciting critical hope in community-based HIV research with transgender women in Toronto, Canada: Methodological insights. *Health Promotion International*, 37 (Sup 2), ii37–ii47. doi:10.1093/heapro/daac017
MacDonald, E.L., 1989. Theatre Rhinoceros: A gay company. *TDR*, 33 (1), 79–93. doi:10.2307/1145946
Mackenzie, S., 2022. Social movement organizing and the politics of emotion from HIV to Covid-19. *Sociology Compass*, 16 (5), e12979. doi:10.1111/soc4.12979
Mendes, L., 2020. How can we quarantine without a home? Responses of activism and urban social movements in times of COVID-19 pandemic crisis in Lisbon. *Tijdschrift Voor Economische En Sociale Geografie*, 111 (3), 318–332. doi:10.1111/tesg.12450

People with AIDS Advisory Committee, 1983. *The Denver Principles.*

Phiri, P., et al., 2021. An evaluation of the mental health impact of SARS-CoV-2 on patients, general public and healthcare professionals: A systematic review and meta-analysis. *EClinicalMedicine*, 34. doi:10.1016/j.eclinm.2021.100806

Pinckney, J. and Rivers, M., 2020. Sickness or silence: Social movement adaptation to Covid-19. *Journal of International Affairs*, 73 (2), 23–42.

Pleyers, G., 2020. The pandemic is a battlefield. Social movements in the COVID-19 lockdown. *Journal of Civil Society*, 16 (4), 295–312. doi:10.1080/17448689.2020.1794398

Roy, A., 2020. The pandemic is a portal. *Financial Times*. Available from: www.ft.com/content/10d8f5e8-74eb-11ea-95fe-fcd274e920ca

Tabbush, C. and Friedman, E.J., 2020. Feminist activism confronts COVID-19. *Feminist Studies*, 46 (3), 629–638. doi:10.1353/fem.2020.0047

The Care Collective, 2020. *The Care Manifesto: The Politics of Interdependence*. A. Chatzidakis, et al., eds. London and New York: Verso Books.

Van Hooft, S., 2014. *Hope*. New York: Routledge.

Watney, S., 2000. *Imagine hope: AIDS and gay identity*. London: Routledge.

Webb, D., 2010. Paulo Freire and 'the need for a kind of education in hope'. *Cambridge Journal of Education*, 40 (4), 327–339.

Wood, L., 2022. Social movements as essential services in Toronto. In B. Bringel and G. Pleyers, eds. *Social movements and politics during COVID-19*. 1st ed. Bristol: Bristol University Press, 141–146. doi:10.2307/j.ctv2qnx5gh.22

World Economic Forum, 2021. *Global gender gap report*. World Economic Forum. Available from: www.weforum.org/reports/global-gender-gap-report-2021 [Accessed 15 March 2023]

14 HIV outreach for men who have sex with men during the COVID-19 pandemic in Indonesia, 2020–2021

Benjamin Hegarty, Amalia Puri Handayani, Sandeep Nanwani, and Ignatius Praptoraharjo

The COVID-19 pandemic generated a renewed focus on the impact of inequality on health and the role of research in critiquing the social and political decisions that drive such forms of inequality. Ethically grounded research conducted in collaboration with the communities most affected by health inequities has demonstrated how pandemics can amplify discrimination and stigmatisation (see for example Garcia-Iglesias et al. 2021; Manderson et al. 2022; Banerjea et al. 2022). In this chapter, we draw on findings from an ethnographic study of HIV peer outreach to men who have sex with men at one community organisation in Indonesia during the COVID-19 pandemic in 2020. During this time, the conditions of the COVID-19 pandemic placed great strain on 'Indonesia's brittle, patchy and under-resourced health system' (Bennett and Dewi 2022, p. 223). Under such conditions, ethnography is much more than a method that can offer context for public health interventions. Instead, it provides a critical interpretive framework for interrogating how normative models of data collection and evidence-making conceal the origins and even the violence of inequality.

The very different yet overlapping conditions of the HIV and COVID-19 pandemics lay bare the need for analyses grounded in the lives of those subject to the most significant impacts of inequality. Ultimately, this means that the questions asked and theoretical frameworks used must emerge from the methods that are only possible through long-term commitments to individuals recruited as participants in a study. Scholars have recently drawn on decolonising frameworks to grapple with the thorny ethical problem of whose and what interests global health research serves (Kelly-Hanku et al. 2021; Bhakuni and Abimbola 2021). One component of successful approaches – those that are embedded within and respond to the concerns of affected communities – is the proximity forged through close, long-term interactions. During the early AIDS pandemic, anthropologists drew on long-term research based on participant observation to develop ethnographic theories of 'the social body' (Scheper-Hughes 1994), highlighting the structural forms of inequality that give rise to disease and death.[1] Ethnographic research continues to provide an important basis for critiquing the assumptions of individual

DOI: 10.4324/9781003322788-17

agency and biomedical supremacy that characterise responses to both the HIV and COVID-19 pandemics.

Peer outreach workers, who are paid a nominal salary by community-based organisations, typically provide HIV-prevention packages and safe-sex information, and refer individuals to HIV testing, counselling and treatment through existing community networks. They are usually members of communities who are at greater risk of HIV and therefore have considerable expertise about the kinds of approaches needed to improve access to testing, treatment and care (Nugroho et al. 2019). Based on ethnographic research undertaken since 2017, we have documented the expansive roles played by peer outreach workers in the provision of HIV programmes to men who have sex with men in Indonesia (Hegarty et al. 2020, 2021). The term men who have sex with men is translated into Indonesian as *lelaki berhubungan seks dengan lelaki* (LSL) and is widely used in HIV programmes and everyday contexts among outreach workers.

In Indonesia, following the rollout of widely available HIV testing and anti-retroviral treatment, outreach workers now provide a vital link to affordable state-run healthcare services. Anti-retroviral treatment has been made widely available in Indonesia since 2013, with national government guidelines requiring that all state-run clinics be equipped and staffed to provide HIV testing and treatment (Lazuardi 2019). This includes supporting hard-to-reach people who receive a positive test result but do not continue to receive treatment, referred to as 'lost to follow up' (Hegarty 2021; Samuels 2020). The role of peer outreach workers has become particularly crucial for men who have sex with men and transgender women in Indonesia, who face complex structural barriers to accessing HIV testing and treatment as they navigate the Indonesian healthcare system.[2]

Following the declaration of the COVID-19 pandemic as a public health emergency of international concern by the World Health Organization on 30 January 2020, we developed a study to track how a group of HIV outreach workers contended with the impact of the COVID-19 pandemic, related public health restrictions, and shifting guidelines from international funding agencies. We developed the research questions, designed our methods and recruited participants in collaboration with Yayasan Pesona Jakarta (YPJ), a community organisation that delivers internationally funded programmes for men who have sex with men and transgender women, and with which we had an existing relationship. Our experiences conducting research during this period yielded new insights into how ethnographic methods could mobilise new forms of connection and action between researchers and participants.

Our research comprised participant observation, interviews and focus groups all conducted virtually, with participants who were HIV outreach workers in Indonesia between July and September 2020 (see Hegarty et al. 2021). Between July and September 2020, we conducted online interviews, and focus groups, and collected video diaries to understand the experiences of outreach workers at YPJ. We also invited participants to participate in focus groups designed to elicit their interpretation and analysis of the data collected (see e.g. Redman-MacLaren et al. 2014; Syvertsen 2020). This chapter contributes to renewed interest in alternative models for building knowledge in viral times by drawing on our experience of ethnographic research about HIV outreach workers in Indonesia during the COVID-19 pandemic. Ethnographic research creates room to alter the epistemological frame of what constitutes evidence, authority and meaning in international health programmes. This is only possible, however, if ethnographers remain open to the ethical and moral imperatives voiced by participants – and continue to develop research based on long-term relationships – in the context of ongoing epidemics.

Researching HIV during the COVID-19 pandemic

The COVID-19 pandemic had a significant impact on HIV programmes internationally, particularly in the underfunded healthcare systems of low- and middle-income countries (Pinto and Park 2020; Ponticiello et al. 2020). In Indonesia, people living with and at risk of HIV experienced disruptions in both access to anti-retroviral therapy and routine sexual and reproductive health services (Bennett and Dewi 2022; Gedela et al. 2022). On the other hand, some communities most heavily affected by the HIV epidemic drew on their experiences to mobilise an active response to the COVID-19 pandemic. The transgender activist Rully Mallay (Mallay et al. 2021) has reported on the central role that Indonesian *waria* (transgender women) played during the COVID-19 pandemic in 2020 and 2021, detailing how they maintained access to HIV services and economic support through community networks. In the Philippines, Quilantang et al. (2020) documented the role of HIV-focused community organisations in mapping the most vulnerable in their communities, to ensure the continued delivery of anti-retroviral therapy medication via courier services.

This chapter draws on ethnographic research which documented community-based HIV outreach work during the COVID-19 pandemic to theorise alternative models for transforming knowledge into theory, policy and programmes in international health. We found that Indonesian peer outreach workers found themselves at a specific juncture of the imperative to work towards the targets set by international donors and assembling limited resources to facilitate care in local settings. In recent years, the meaning of 'outreach' (*penjangkauan*) had been transformed by an international policy shift towards biomedical interventions for HIV treatment and prevention (Nguyen et al. 2011; Leclerc-Madlala et al. 2018). For outreach workers, the 'biomedical turn' (Kippax and Stephenson 2016) has reoriented their role in part towards the collection of evidence: counting and reporting the number of people tested, treated and with an undetectable viral load to the agencies that fund and provide technical assistance to programmes.

In 2020, when the majority of the data for this study were conducted, COVID-19 vaccines were not yet available, and there was considerable anxiety both about how long the pandemic would last and what its ongoing impact would be. Early in our research, together with participants, we were concerned about the vulnerability of outreach workers in light of a slow vaccination rollout, inconsistent responses at different levels of government, and a lack of community involvement. The fragility of outreach workers' position was revealed in July 2021, when the Delta variant of SARS-CoV-2 spread rapidly throughout Indonesia. The severity of the disease that the variant caused resulted in the collapse of the healthcare system. Our social media feeds were flooded with images of people overwhelming hospital services, long queues for oxygen tanks and neighbourhoods imposing their own forms of impromptu local lockdown. Soon after, we began to receive worried calls from our research participants, who found themselves without access to adequate testing, personal protective equipment (PPE) and healthcare.

In response, we quickly arranged community meetings, in which participants shared their concerns and asked questions to medical doctor volunteers we mobilised. Outreach workers also shared their significant anxieties with us. Some outreach workers spoke of the fear they would potentially transmit the virus to their families, and many wished to access separate accommodation so that they could continue to work safely. At this stage, however, test kits and PPE were difficult to obtain. Financial support for those isolating, in the form of food and physically distanced house visits, was not provided. Knowledge of how to treat COVID-19 at home was limited. Between July and September 2021, almost all of the outreach workers that we interviewed tested positive for COVID-19, and two of them tragically passed away. We experienced a moment of deep concern, urgency and sense of injustice. How was it that, almost two years into the COVID-19 pandemic, outreach workers supported by a well-resourced international programme could be left in such a vulnerable position?

In part, we understood this situation to have emerged due to the distance between those designing programmes and the lives of the outreach workers tasked with delivering them. Normative models of evidence-making generally did not account for the care work that outreach workers saw as comprising a significant component of what they did. Since 2020, HIV programmes had been adjusted to accommodate the shifting conditions of the COVID-19 pandemic. For example, in response to the strain on public clinics, international agencies funded private clinics in Jakarta to offer free testing and treatment to clients as an exceptional measure. However, these responses were based on evidence that was oriented towards a biomedical response. Outreach workers reported that their work continued to be concerned with 'meeting targets', overshadowing much of the care work that they otherwise performed. A lack of consideration of the care work that was a critical but largely unrecognised component of outreach work also meant that their vulnerability to the COVID-19 pandemic went largely unseen and unacknowledged.

The outreach workers who participated in our study were aged between 24 and 42 years old, and most had worked for more than 3 years at YPJ. All worked for more than 40 hours a week on tasks such as virtual outreach through social media and dating applications, in-person outreach, attending the clinic to accompany clients for an HIV test, and report writing. Almost all the outreach workers in the study reported spending more time undertaking virtual outreach early in the COVID-19 pandemic, while more of their time had been based in primary healthcare facilities prior to it. In general, the profile of research participants was similar to the community they served. Broadly speaking, they were men who have sex with men, migrants to Jakarta, vulnerable to economic precarity due to the nature of their employment, and whose safety net consisted largely of support from one another.

The COVID-19 pandemic placed additional economic stress on many outreach workers, meaning that they needed to secure additional sources of income. Outreach workers showed an easy-going attitude towards us and had a strong relationship with one another. When we created a WhatsApp group to share information about the research project with them and conducted focus group discussions, we found that conversations focused not only on the research, but also on other issues. Just as a great deal of their work hinged on maintaining relationships with the people they sought to provide information to, or accompany to an HIV test, so too did they maintain an ongoing relationship with us.

Meeting targets in a pandemic

Despite significant changes to the delivery of HIV programmes during the COVID-19 pandemic, our research found that outreach workers largely described the steps undertaken as part of outreach as unchanged from those employed prior to the pandemic. Even as funders introduced notable changes to programme requirements in response to the pandemic (including adjustments to targets), the role of community-based outreach workers remained positioned in relation to the goal of maintaining rates of HIV testing, treatment and retention in care.

At the onset of the pandemic, international agencies did make adjustments to the type and number of targets to align with the shift to virtual modes of outreach delivery. For example, rather than having to successfully 'make contact' with five people in person and provide them with information about HIV per month, each outreach worker was instead required to contact at least 60 people online every month. The enormous increase in the number of people contacted via online platforms demanded a great deal of time and effort, but it also rested on the incorrect assumption that all forms of in-person work had ceased.

Contrary to this assumption, our research found that, although outreach workers did adopt virtual methods for undertaking outreach during the pandemic, they often combined this with in-person activities as well. This was described as necessary for the delicate work of helping clients navigate access to testing and treatment. Although in-person work was in theory limited to 'urgent cases', on the ground this was defined as work with clients with any symptoms of sexually transmitted infections (associated with increased risk of HIV).

Moreover, outreach workers' concern for hands-on care made this difficult to achieve through virtual methods alone. Outreach workers therefore creatively combined virtual and in-person methods throughout the COVID-19 pandemic, accompanying clients for HIV testing and to access treatment, despite the risks to their own health that they faced.

Despite these on the ground changes, funders' expectations of outreach work did not shift, with the ultimate objective being to increase the number of people tested. In the case of a positive HIV test result, some programmes extended this objective to include the successful enrolment of a client in anti-retroviral therapy. We organised the narrative accounts gathered from interviews conducted during the COVID-19 pandemic into five steps of HIV outreach work, namely: 1. gain visibility; 2. build and maintain relationships; 3. provide HIV and safer-sex information; 4. follow up with clients; 5. refer to healthcare providers for testing/treatment. The organisation of narratives in this way ultimately reflected outreach workers' integration into a system in which HIV testing, treatment and adherence were organised around a biomedical model of intervention. A key finding from the analysis was that the mode of delivery of the outreach, be it virtual or in-person, was not understood as fundamentally important to the outcome. An ethnographic perspective revealed that it was the labour of outreach work – one primarily oriented and grounded in care – that was central to the successful delivery of HIV prevention.

Participants used three main platform types to gain visibility: dating applications, social media applications (e.g. Instagram, Facebook) and messenger services such as WhatsApp. Participants described how gaining visibility required a great deal of time spent online. In addition to posing significant ethical challenges, the anonymity of online communications and specific platform profiles meant that outreach workers found it difficult to verify that those whom they were speaking to formed part of their target population. Participants described employing a wide range of strategies to take the crucial step of obtaining a mobile phone number, which was needed in order to demonstrate that they had 'made contact' for the purpose of reporting targets. This included specific strategies to alter their appearance to make themselves appear more attractive:

> We edit our photos for use on dating applications, but not too much. Afterwards if we actually meet in person, it won't be good. What I mean is, the photo that we think is the best on social media, that is the kind of photo we should use on dating applications.
>
> (OW01, focus group, 21 August 2020)

Most dating applications make use of the geographical location data provided by mobile phones. During the pandemic, participants described a significant challenge in reaching areas which were the focus of outreach efforts when they were working from home. Participants tended to live in many different parts of Jakarta, a large and sprawling city, whereas the focus of outreach work shifted from time to time in line with the numbers of men who have sex with men testing positive for HIV at clinics in a particular district. To address this challenge, participants described making use of technologies, including virtual private networks and fake global positioning system applications, through which they could target or appear to be in a specific location.

The next step in successful outreach involved building and maintaining a relationship with clients. Obtaining a phone number was no guarantee of staying in contact. Participants shared narratives of being blocked by users or ignored when they asked for the personal information needed to facilitate access to HIV programmes. Participants described the importance of keeping in regular contact via mobile phone applications as particularly important during the COVID-19 pandemic. This, they described, demanded that they communicate in a similar manner as with friends, or similar to a salesperson. During the COVID-19 pandemic, outreach workers also adjusted from directly asking clients whether they wanted to take a test, to whether they had symptoms of STIs. This was because, at the height of restrictions, only those clients with symptoms, and who were therefore classed as 'urgent cases', were able to access HIV testing:

> After we met, he told me that he had suspicions that he had HIV … Because on his skin he had symptoms like an STI. That evening, that client underwent counselling, and the next day took a test. This kind of experience made me happy this week.
>
> (OW03, video diary, 20 July 2020)

Even as outreach workers were at times not permitted to attend clinics due to public health regulations, completing their work was more effective if they accompanied them to the clinic directly. The continued need to face demands to meet targets despite limitations on attending clinics in person was described as a challenge by one outreach worker, who continued to field requests from clients:

> We are still chasing the targets … but during the pandemic in April, a policy was introduced that we were not allowed to present at healthcare service. But in fact, there were many urgent cases that needed to present at clinics.
>
> (OW10, interview, 14 July 2020)

The final step in conducting outreach involved referring clients to healthcare services for testing and for some programmes, in the case of a positive test, linking them to treatment. During the COVID-19 pandemic, easy access to HIV testing became difficult to achieve due to the imposition of restrictions, including limitations in the opening hours of clinics and density requirements. Directives, issued by both funders and clinics, requested that outreach workers limit themselves to accompanying 'urgent' cases for regular testing. Nevertheless, and despite these limitations, outreach workers witnessed an increase in new HIV cases during the pandemic. As one of them explained:

> During the pandemic, we are afraid of going to health facilities. We only take clients who have STI or other symptoms. And, during the pandemic, there are a lot of [HIV] positive cases. Is it because there are fewer condoms being distributed?
>
> (OW10, focus group, 14 August 2020)

This outreach worker was concerned that newly diagnosed cases of HIV were not being adequately attended to because programmes had shifted their focus to adherence and maintaining access to anti-retroviral therapy for existing cases. This perspective, which may have originated from the view that lockdowns would result in fewer people being sexually active during the pandemic, contrasted with outreach workers' own experiences. Yet, within existing frameworks for recording and sharing evidence, they had little ability to convey this fact.

Regardless of the shift in focus to anti-retroviral adherence among existing HIV cases, outreach workers described working both in person and virtually throughout the pandemic in ways that exceeded the support made available to them. Several participants described regularly accompanying clients in person to obtain access to testing and treatment, helping them to navigate intermittent clinic closures. Public health regulations issued by provincial and national governments to address COVID-19 were in constant flux, further complicated by an inconsistent application of regulations by individual clinics:

> The health facilities applied the policy differently. I asked one health facility … to conduct a mobile health centre with limited patients and follow health protocol. But, it couldn't be done yet. Another facility … did that. It is confusing. We just hope that the clients have free time and really do need to have the test, and then we can refer one or two to that particular health facility [which was willing to do so].
>
> (OW03, interview, 9 July 2020)

Other outreach workers described how, despite their reduced capacity to enter clinics, they continued to coordinate closely with healthcare workers. This was especially important given shifting processes and the need to ascertain which cases would be classed as 'urgent'. One outreach worker described the level of coordination required in order to facilitate access to HIV testing:

> We are suggested to coordinate with the doctor when there is a client who wants to take the test. For example, how many clients can we take on that day? What are the health protocols? We need to make sure that clients can receive the service needed before taking them to the local health clinic … I sent

> a text to the doctor, 'How is the situation at the clinic? Can I take clients there? What is the protocol?' Because I haven't seen it myself [the situation at the health clinic].
>
> (OW03, interview, 9 July 2020)

Overall, the step of referring clients to healthcare providers appeared to be that which was most transformed by the pandemic. Outreach workers were largely expected to adjust their activities (whether to online, or modified forms of in-person work at clinics) with little additional support. Moreover, the focus on virtual outreach confounded some outreach workers, who continued to see at least part of their role as providing free condoms and lubricant. Outreach workers fretted about the fact that these efforts ceased at the onset of the COVID-19 pandemic.[3] Several outreach workers speculated that this was perhaps one reason why rates of HIV and sexually transmitted infections had anecdotally increased during the COVID-19 pandemic.

Ethnography and inequality

Our ethnographic account highlights how the role of HIV outreach workers during the COVID-19 pandemic was embedded within specific social contexts framed by forms of work associated with care. Even as the practice of outreach work was expected to align with the frameworks provided by donor-driven HIV programmes, the accounts that participants shared with us revealed the careful work and interpretive insights that outreach workers conducted as an everyday part of their role.

The impact of the COVID-19 pandemic on HIV outreach workers was most acutely felt in the form of an ongoing emphasis on targets, which made the needs of outreach workers subservient to externally determined programme imperatives. The assumption of there being a relatively linear 'cascade of care' through which people should be linked to HIV testing and treatment remained a common preoccupation in the narratives of outreach workers. One outreach worker explained the contradictory pull between the work that they undertook 'from the heart', or the work of care, and the need to meet monthly targets as follows:

> In NGOs, we do our work based on targets. It causes a conflict. Our work is a calling from our heart, but we also need to think about meeting targets. It means that we lessen our focus on clients.
>
> (OW04, interview, 9 July 2020)

In addition to fuelling such dilemmas, the emphasis given to meeting targets during the COVID-19 pandemic heightened a sense of stress for outreach workers at a challenging time. For example, in a video diary, one outreach worker explained the effects of alterations to targets:

> I have been thinking a lot within this week, 'Can I reach the target at the end of this programme? Does my organisation achieve the target? Will our

> programme be extended?' There was a rumour saying that if our targets are not achieved, this programme won't be extended. I am thinking a lot about this. If it is not extended, I need to start over from zero, and look for another job. I am confused, and meanwhile I am getting old. I also have personal problems, so I am overthinking things more and more.
>
> (OW09, video diary, 10 August 2020)

Beyond this pressure, a focus on targets based on programme outcomes had the effect of concealing other important information gathered by outreach workers, including evidence of the impact of a lack of condoms and lubricant. An ethnographic analysis that records the insights of outreach workers and values their interpretation as a source of theory can help to elevate these more socially focused insights, which remained concealed in the hegemonic focus on meeting targets modelled on biomedical intervention and individual behaviour change.

Outreach workers also had to contend with fast-changing public health guidance from local and national authorities, which at times was contradictory. This impacted how outreach work could take place but also revealed the gap between programme requirements during the pandemic versus reality on the ground. For example, as a result of the shift to virtual outreach, outreach workers no longer received payment for travel to clinics. Because of their sense of responsibility or care, some outreach workers accompanied people to clinics by using funds from their own pocket. This placed them at risk of contracting COVID-19, given that programmes did not provide adequate resources for testing, contact tracing and PPE.

Our participant's concern that he was 'chasing targets in a pandemic' offers a critique of the limitations of hegemonic paradigms of collecting and analysing evidence in international HIV programmes. Ethnographic analyses and interpretation, conducted together with participants, can help to unsettle taken-for-granted knowledge. As Jennifer L. Syvertsen writes, 'those of us working in global health settings know that power relations remain asymmetrical and research is too often an extractive process without genuine, sustained collaboration' (2020, p. 85). Such genuine forms of collaboration, as we have shown based on our experiences conducting research during the COVID-19 pandemic, are possible, even at a distance. Yet collaboration, like ethnography, is not a simple procedure which can be straightforwardly built into a project.

The narratives and experiences that we shared with HIV outreach workers during the COVID-19 pandemic reveal that one value of ethnographic research during pandemics lies in its capacity to unsettle assumptions of what counts as evidence. What was happening on the ground in Jakarta among men who have sex with men rarely aligned with the theories and models produced elsewhere during the COVID-19 pandemic. More than this, dominant methods of gathering evidence failed to listen to outreach workers' insights into the experience of HIV prevention, testing and treatment during the COVID-19 pandemic. To be sure, outreach workers juggled their responsibilities and improvised to connect people to care beyond what was visible or knowable in biomedical and individual paradigms. However, too often, this unrecognised work placed participants at significant risk. This gap between models and experiences meant that outreach workers were not supplied with adequate PPE the ongoing reality of accompanying clients to clinics, even at the height of lockdowns. It meant that their concerns about the fact that men who have sex with men were continuing to have sex but that condoms were not widely available, went unheeded.

Researchers have argued for maintaining many of the technical and biomedical HIV innovations pioneered during the COVID-19 pandemic (see e.g. Wilkinson and Grimsrud 2020). Ethnographic evidence highlights that another key lesson from HIV prevention during the COVID-19 pandemic is the need to provide adequate resources for the critical forms of care work that are unaccounted for within the hegemonic biomedical and individual paradigms of international health. Our ethnography of HIV outreach work in Indonesia during the COVID-19 pandemic in 2020 and 2021 offers one example of how the production and assumptions of expert knowledge can be held to account. Ethnographic research embedded in long-term relationships can challenge the dominant political and economic arrangements that perpetuate the inequality that pandemics so starkly make visible.

Acknowledgements

We are especially grateful to the participants who agreed to share their stories with us for this study, the outreach workers, and particularly Mas Eric at Yayasan Pesona Jakarta for his support. All of this took place during an exceptionally challenging time, and we are grateful for their time and insights. The research was conducted while Benjamin Hegarty was a McKenzie Fellow at the University of Melbourne. The University of Melbourne and Atma Jaya Catholic University ethics committees reviewed and granted permission for data collection. We also thank the Faculty of Arts Indonesia Initiative at the University of Melbourne and the Indonesia Democracy and Human Rights Hallmark Initiative for funding to conduct this research. Helen Pausacker of the Asian Law Centre at the Melbourne Law School provided support in her expert administration of the scheme. Finally, we thank Taylor and Francis the publishers of *Global Public Health* for allowing us to reproduce parts of Hegarty et al. (2021).

Notes

1 The AIDS pandemic provided a crucial but often forgotten backdrop and ethnographic subject for debates about the role of ethically engaged anthropology in the 1990s (see e.g. Scheper-Hughes 1995). The critical perspectives on the social mounted by Scheper-Hughes and other medical anthropologists, while

coming from different methodological and theoretical perspectives, resonate with some of the bolder experiments in queer theory from the same period (Halperin 1995).

2 As is the case in several other parts of the world, men who have sex with men and transgender women in particular regions in Indonesia are at greater risk of HIV. For example, data from the 2015 Indonesian Integrated Biobehavioural Survey found that HIV prevalence among men who have sex with men in the Greater Jakarta Capital Region was 32%, compared to an overall HIV prevalence of 0.3% in the country (UNAIDS 2022).

3 Outreach workers reported that condoms became unavailable in mid-2020, initially due to reported supply chain issues related to the COVID-19 pandemic. However, this situation persisted until at least May 2022, suggesting that other factors were at play. In a forum organised by the Center for HIV/AIDS Research at Atma Jaya Catholic University on 22 June 2022, speakers from community organisations and public health researchers speculated that not only supply chain issues but also a shifting politics of morality had led to shortages.

References

Banerjea, N., Boyce, P., and Dasgupta, R.K., 2022. *COVID-19 assemblages: Queer and feminist ethnographies from South Asia*. London: Routledge.

Bennett, L.R. and Dewi, S.M., 2022. The amplification effect: Impacts of COVID-19 on sexual and reproductive health and rights in Indonesia. In L. Manderson, N.J. Burke, and A. Wahlberg, eds. *Viral loads: Anthropologies of urgency in the time of COVID-19*. London: UCL Press, 222–242.

Bhakuni, H. and Abimbola, S., 2021. Epistemic injustice in academic global health. *The Lancet Global Health*, 9 (10), e1465–e1470. doi:10.1016/S2214-109X(21)00301-6.

Garcia-Iglesias, J., Nagington, M., and Aggleton, P., 2021. Viral times, viral memories, viral questions. *Culture, Health & Sexuality*, 23 (11), 1465–1469. doi:10.1080/13691058.2021.1976564

Gedela, K., et al., 2022. Antiretroviral drug switches to Zidovudine-based regimens and loss to follow-up during the first COVID-19 lockdown in Bali, Indonesia. *HIV Medicine*, 23 (9), 1025–1030. doi:10.1111/hiv.13298

Halperin, D.M., 1995. *Saint Foucault: Towards a gay hagiography*. New York: Oxford University Press.

Hegarty, B., 2021. The biosocial body: HIV visibility in an age of pharmaceutical treatment in Indonesia. *Ethos*, 49 (4), 460–474. doi:10.1111/etho.12325

Hegarty, B., Nanwani, S., and Praptoraharjo, I., 2020. Understanding the challenges faced in community-based outreach programs aimed at men who have sex with men in urban Indonesia. *Sexual Health*, 17 (4), 352–358. doi:10.1071/SH20065

Hegarty, B., et al., 2021. Chasing targets in a pandemic: The impact of COVID-19 on HIV outreach workers for MSM (men who have sex with men) in Jakarta, Indonesia. *Global Public Health*, 16 (11), 1681–1695. doi:10.1080/17441692.2021.1980599.

Kelly-Hanku, A., et al., 2021. From the researched to the researcher: Decolonising research praxis in Papua New Guinea. In S. Bell, P. Aggleton, and A. Gibson, eds. *Peer research in health and social development: International perspectives on participatory research.* London: Routledge, 20–32. doi:10.4324/9780429316920.

Kippax, S. and Stephenson, N., 2016. *Socialising the biomedical turn in HIV prevention.* London: Anthem Press.

Lazuardi, E., 2019. Navigating the social dynamics of HIV care: A qualitative study in urban Indonesia in the era of scaled-up testing and treatment (PhD dissertation). Sydney: Kirby Institute, UNSW Sydney.

Leclerc-Madlala, S., Broomhall, L., and Fieno, J., 2018. The "End of AIDS" project: Mobilising evidence, bureaucracy, and big data for a final biomedical triumph over AIDS. *Global Public Health*, 13 (8), 972–981. doi:10.1080/17441692.2017.1409246

Mallay, R., et al., 2021. One transgender community's experience of the COVID-19 pandemic: A report from Indonesia. *TSQ: Transgender Studies Quarterly*, 8 (3), 386–393. doi:10.1215/23289252-9009003

Manderson, L., Burke, N.J., and Wahlberg, A., eds. 2022. *Viral loads: Anthropologies of urgency in the time of COVID-19.* Embodying inequalities: Perspectives from medical anthropology. London: UCL Press.

Nguyen, V-K., et al., 2011. Remedicalizing an epidemic: From HIV treatment as prevention to HIV treatment is prevention. *AIDS*, 25 (3) 291–293. doi:10.1097/QAD.0b013e3283402c3e

Nugroho, A., et al., 2019. Client perspectives on an outreach approach for HIV prevention targeting Indonesian MSM and transwomen. *Health Promotion International*, 1 (19). doi:10.1093/heapro/daz075

Pinto, R.M. and Park, S., 2020. COVID-19 pandemic disrupts HIV continuum of care and prevention: Implications for research and practice concerning community-based organizations and frontline providers. *AIDS and Behavior*, 24 (9), 2486–2489. doi:10.1007/s10461-020-02893-3

Ponticiello, M., et al., 2020. 'Everything is a mess': How COVID-19 is impacting engagement with HIV testing services in rural Southwestern Uganda. *AIDS and Behavior*, 24 (11), 3006–3009. doi:10.1007/s10461-020-02935-w

Quilantang, M.I.N., Bermudez, A.N.C., and Operario, D., 2020. Reimagining the future of HIV service implementation in the Philippines based on lessons from COVID-19. *AIDS and Behavior*, 24 (11), 3003–3005. doi:10.1007/s10461-020-02934-x

Redman-MacLaren, M., Mills, J., and Tommbe, R., 2014. Interpretive focus groups: A participatory method for interpreting and extending secondary analysis of qualitative data. *Global Health Action*, 7 (1), 25214. doi:10.3402/gha.v7.25214

Samuels, A., 2020. Strategies of silence in an age of transparency: Navigating HIV and visibility in Aceh, Indonesia. *History and Anthropology*, 32 (4), 498–515. 10.1080/02757206.2020.1830384.

Scheper-Hughes, N., 1994. An essay: 'AIDS and the social body'. *Social Science & Medicine*, 39 (7), 991–1003. doi:10.1016/0277-9536(94)90210-0

Scheper-Hughes, N., 1995. The primacy of the ethical: Propositions for a militant anthropology. *Current Anthropology*, 36 (3), 409–440. 10.1086/204378

Syvertsen, J.L., 2020. Sharing research, building possibility: Reflecting on research with men who have sex with men in Kenya. *Human Organization*, 79 (2), 83–94. doi:10.17730/1938-3525.79.2.83

UNAIDS, 2022. Indonesia Country Slides 2022. *HIV AIDS Asia Pacific Research Statistical Data Information Resources AIDS Data Hub*. Available from: www.aidsdatahub.org. [Accessed 7 July 2023]

Wilkinson, L. and Grimsrud, A., 2020. The time is now: Expedited HIV differentiated service delivery during the COVID-19 pandemic. *Journal of the International AIDS Society*, 23 (5), e25503. doi:10.1002/jia2.25503

15 Equitable access and public attitudes to prevention of HIV and COVID-19 in Vietnam

Pauline Oosterhoff and Tu Anh Hoang

Vietnam's initial achievement in controlling COVID-19 in 2020 by tracking, tracing and quarantine was hailed as a global success story. While cases surged elsewhere and countries around the world mourned their dead, Vietnam was successful in keeping the virus at bay. The two of us, living in separate parts of the Netherlands at the time, watched videos from the country with envy: while the Netherlands' half-hearted measures ensured that lockdowns dragged on, we could see Vietnamese people going about their business freely. We reflected on how Vietnam's initial success in fighting COVID-19 echoed its track record dealing with other emergency health situations, such as avian flu, SARS-CoV and HIV (McKenna 2006).

We were filled not only with envy, but also with a sense of pride at having had the privilege of working in the past on infectious disease management with the Vietnamese government. The fight to get enhanced access to antiretroviral therapy (ART) and other important measures to manage, treat and curtail the spread of HIV, on which both of us worked, had been successful. We had faith that Vietnam would be successful again. Yes, we were hearing that freedom of movement was drastically restricted for those who were infected. But that meant that the rest of the Vietnamese population could have productive work and social lives. Meanwhile, we were saddled with the Dutch government, whose COVID-19 prevention policies included publicly encouraging single people to find sex buddies during lockdown, which may be laudable for acknowledging the importance of sexual health but offered a distraction from untransparent financial management by the government. The court of auditors reported later that no less than 5.1 billion Euros has been spent partly unlawfully on face masks, protective equipment or other materials.

However, by mid-2021 enthusiasm for Vietnam's approach was waning both inside and outside the country. The national response to the Delta variant was floundering, and COVID-19 cases surged in hospitals, residential communities and industrial zones. The Case Fatality Rate (CFR) was high, hospitals were overflowing and the whole public health system, including tracking and tracing, seemed on the verge of collapse. Vaccines, such as those developed by Pfizer–BioNTech and Moderna, had been authorised for approval in late December 2020, but production was slow, distribution

DOI: 10.4324/9781003322788-18

focused on rich countries and Vietnam's borders remained closed. After almost a year, one of us managed to return home to Vietnam to join family, colleagues and friends. But our infatuation with Vietnam's COVID-19 policy was over. And as with love affairs, a retrospective look revealed that we had ignored several questionable elements of the pandemic response.

Vietnam's successful HIV track record in the early 2000s, for example, was not due to strict tracking and tracing or quarantining of infected people or 'at-risk' populations. It was to a large extent based on establishing dialogue with hitherto heavily stigmatised groups such as injection drug users (IDUs), sex workers and their partners. Another key component, arguably the main one, was expanding access to free, good-quality ART after 2004. To access such medication, a person's HIV status needed to be recorded. Instead of isolating people, the overall direction (although with many detours) was towards what we would nowadays call an inclusive and comprehensive social approach combined with effective biomedical prevention, detection and treatment options.

The insights presented in this chapter are emerging and time-bound. Revisiting datasets can provide a richer and more nuanced account of history, yet interpretations of events are influenced by broader cultural and social factors that affect how we understand the 'data'.[1]

Almost two decades have now elapsed between the start of our involvement with HIV in the early 2000s and the COVID-19 outbreak. Over this time Vietnam's economy has grown rapidly and the country no longer qualifies for the levels of official development assistance (ODA) that a lower-income or poor country might have. Internal migration and urbanisation have turned both Hanoi and Ho Chi Minh City into megacities where motorbikes compete with cars, buses and subways.

Yet there are also continuities. Vietnam is still a one-party state with a strong central government and a strong and expansive state health system that co-exists with a vibrant private health sector. Since *Đổi mới* (renovation), and the opening up of the economy in 1986, Vietnam has witnessed rapid industrialisation, high levels of rural-to-urban migration and growing inequality. The growth of large cities has resulted in increased demands on public services, including access to health care. Vietnam has invested in universal health insurance, and as a socialist state, it promotes equality, including gender equality. But inequalities between citizens based on class, ethnicity, ability, education and gender have increased and become more visible. Against this background, this chapter offers some reflections on epidemic management and national response – both in the case of HIV and COVID-19. It does so with the goal of contributing to efficient and grounded policy within a global context in which zoonotic diseases and outbreaks are likely to (re)emerge.

Methods

Our analysis is based on our shared experiences as researchers and practitioners working together over a period of almost 20 years. Throughout this time, we have used participatory approaches and tools and combined these with qualitative and quantitative methods and techniques. This chapter offers an expert-led examination of large mixed-methods participatory research programmes and evaluations of both HIV and COVID-19. The work on HIV covers multiple programmes, some of which had multi-million-dollar budgets, and lasted over almost a decade. The work on COVID-19 took place over a much shorter timeframe, with more limited funding and data collection under very different conditions. The main programmes that our insights are based on are as follows.

Research on Equitable Access and Public Attitudes to Vaccination for Internal Migrants in Vietnam funded by the UK Foreign, Commonwealth and Development Office between 2021–2022. Our work adopted a mixed-methods approach and brought together both primary and secondary data. We reviewed Vietnamese vaccination policies and interviewed a stratified sample of 74 key stakeholders. These included professionals working in the public sector, policy makers and a wide range of internal migrant groups, many of them seeking work in the growing cities.

Research on access to Prevention of Mother to Child Transmission (PMTCT) including ART for mothers and children among ethnic minorities in Vietnam funded by the Dutch Directorate-General for International Cooperation (DGIS) and conducted between 2008 and 2011. A team of eight female researchers conducted in-depth interviews with 56 Hmong and 87 Thai women in rural and peri-urban areas in Ha Giang and Dien Bien provinces to understand birthing practices and access to PMTCT services. In addition, the team conducted focus group discussions and interviews with policy makers and health staff and undertook observation in communities and health-care facilities.

Research on PMTCT including ART for mothers and children in Vietnam funded by DGIS as part of a regional action programme conducted from April 2004 to the end of 2007. Building on an operational programme, we conducted in-depth interviews with health authorities, women and their families living with HIV, and undertook observations at service providers and support groups in Hanoi and in Thai Nguyen City. We interviewed 275 health workers located at many different sites in the two cities, as well as dozens of other service providers and policy makers. We interviewed a total of 153 persons living with HIV.

Research on access to PMTCT and ART for female drug-users and sex-workers funded by the Catholic Organization for Relief and Development Aid (CORDAID) and Aan't Roer and conducted between 2009 and 2012. In this operational research, a team comprised of two international researchers and a Vietnamese research assistant conducted in-depth interviews on access to PMTCT with 18 women with a history of opiate use who had been pregnant while using. The research complemented long-term interactions with several hundred female HIV-positive drug users as part of an international programme operating since 2005.

Our insights have also been shaped by other research jointly undertaken, including research on the rise of the lesbian, gay, bisexual, transgender, queer and intersex (LGBTQI) movement in Vietnam and on transgender livelihoods conducted between 2008 and 2011 in which we took a critical look at the role of HIV funding in shaping the work of the organisations that make up these movements.

HIV from prevention to treatment as prevention

A concentrated epidemic

The HIV epidemic in Vietnam was strongly concentrated in certain groups, with elevated rates among IDUs, sex workers and their partners in urban locations and along major traffic and transport routes. The first case of HIV was reported in Vietnam in 1990, four years after the introduction of *Đổi mới*. Since then, the HIV epidemic has grown in all population groups under surveillance.

In Vietnam, HIV has never been an emergency affecting the whole or large segments of the population. National prevalence of HIV remained low, at an estimated prevalence of 0.5% in 2006. Some provinces such as Hanoi, Thai Nguyen and Quang Ninh reported higher rates at more than 1%. Young adults between the ages of 20 and 29 accounted for over half of the HIV infections (Hein et al. 2001). Most reported HIV cases were among young male IDUs in urban areas, border regions and seaports (MOH 2006), and mainly related to needle-sharing among drug users.

Focus on condom use, clean needles and testing

Until the arrival of the United States' President's Emergency Plan for AIDS Relief (PEPFAR) in June 2004 and provision for ART in Global Fund, access to treatment in the early 2000s was limited to that provided by a pilot programme run through the Esther hospital partnership, an international initiative funded by the Government of France (Raguin and French ESTHER Network 2016).

Until the arrival of major international funding, public health campaigns endorsed condom use and clean needle use. The design and scary image of billboards confirmed discriminatory public attitudes towards drug use and sex work without offering practical alternatives. A World Health Organization (WHO) supported approach to PMTCT meant that women received low-cost opt-out HIV testing to access short-term ART to save the life of the child, but no further help to raise it. HIV testing for members of the general population was offered for a fee. The residents of some drug rehabilitation centres received opt-out HIV tests. Voluntary confidential testing (VCT) was seen as the basic standard of service for HIV prevention. When international funding became available, the state later allocated staff and facilities for VCT clinics.

Confinement of high-risk groups

Soviet-style re-education centres for IDUs and sex workers[2] have had a role in responding to the HIV and tuberculosis (TB) epidemics. A significant proportion of the IDU population in Vietnam spends mandatory time at one of these camps because of judicial/police action, family and community referral, and in a few cases voluntary enrolment. Health conditions are poor. Relapse rates are high. Thus, camp residents with recurring and chronic health conditions such as HIV and other infectious diseases such as TB move in and out of the wider community. They suffer from different forms of HIV-related stigma both within the family and in wider society (Khuat et al. 2004), with estimated prevalence rates well over 30% within and sometimes even higher outside the re-education centres (Hein et al. 2001).

HIV testing for IDUs in rehabilitation camps, as closed settings, was patchy and controversial, because members of the camp population could not freely give consent. Standard HIV testing in rehabilitation centres became especially questionable when treatment options outside them increased.

Protecting the family and the general population

In 2004, antenatal care (ANC) testing was introduced in some major hospitals shortly after prevention of mother-to-child HIV transmission was included in the National Strategy on HIV Prevention and Control.[3] Vietnam aimed to provide low-cost universal opt-out testing to pregnant women through a strong and decentralised maternal care system well before the US Centers for Disease Control and Prevention (CDC) and WHO/UNAIDS endorsed opt-out instead of opt-in testing in 2006 and 2007, respectively.[4] In Vietnam, opt-out testing as part of ANC made medical and social sense since it enabled staff and patients to save face by standardising the interaction (Oosterhoff, Hardon et al. 2008). The availability of HIV tests was concentrated in larger urban facilities. Pregnant women attending commune- or district-level facilities therefore needed a referral to access HIV tests, which reduced the uptake considerably (Nguyen et al. 2008).

Initially, HIV test results from state health facilities and from some rehabilitation centres were given to the household by commune-level health staff as a response to low post-test return rates, especially among IDUs. This meant that (positive) results were sometimes shared with household members without consent, leading to social stigma and the exclusion of infected individuals (Oosterhoff, Nguyen et al. 2008). With support from ODA, such as PEPFAR, the government created individual counselling rooms offering anonymous counselling and testing. But without treatment for mother and child, women avoided services for this highly stigmatising disease. Even when ART became available, they initially avoided those services and had less access to ART than men (WHO 2006). The relatives of IDUs, especially the mothers of young drug users, also complained that individual counselling removed the opportunity for families to support their children. Without family support and opiate substitutes, few male IDUs managed to access and adhere to treatment.

Gender

In comparison with IDUs and other risk groups such as men who have sex with men, many pregnant women knew their HIV status. Although the group of pregnant HIV-positive women was and still is small compared to IDUs, many pregnant women who took ANC tests accessed treatment. Women's reproductive duties and the social expectation to produce a child within a year after marriage facilitated the early detection of HIV in young women. In the early days of ART, a rapidly growing network of peer support groups provided support to HIV-positive people. In support groups for HIV-positive mothers, women could weaponise the social expectations of motherhood to organise collective action, even when government policy did not allow group meetings (Oosterhoff, Nguyen et al. 2008). Men who injected drugs did not have these gendered privileges.

By the end of 2014, an estimated 93,298 adults and children (60,435 male and 32,863 female) were receiving ART at 302 sites nationwide. Women made up less than one-third of the HIV-positive population over the age of 15, but one-half of this population was in receipt of treatment.[5] Data on women who have not been pregnant remain limited, but surveillance data and other research suggest that Vietnamese women, despite their disadvantaged socio-economic and cultural status, have gendered advantages in accessing ART (Oosterhoff 2008; Oosterhoff and Bach 2011).

Open borders and rural–urban migration

In Vietnam, the HIV epidemic followed major international and national transport routes for illegal heroin and other illicit drugs, which shaped the locations of interventions. The general lack of adequate policies and institutional programmes for migrants, and the residence-based nature of the health and social welfare provision, has generated inequalities between HIV-positive migrants and HIV-positive residents. These are structural systemic inequalities. Health system research has shown structural inequalities between migrant and non-migrant workers in health status and access to services (Pham et al. 2019). Rural–urban migrants who cannot register at their destination area face formal exclusion from many health services. Health staff do make exceptions to these rules to accommodate people: for example, children under age 5 are rarely turned away from vaccination programmes. Internationally funded programmes try to be flexible but operate within a system in which the state does not recognise the legal status of migrants in destination areas.

Growing civil-society dialogues and collaboration

Throughout the epidemic, civil society organisations (CSOs) have played a key role in changing ideas, norms and practices that shifted HIV from being a death sentence into a chronic disease. Discussions brokered by CSOs between government authorities, state services and HIV-positive persons and their families led to this change. Discussions concerned fighting against stigma and dismissive public attitudes and mobilising for comprehensive treatment access, as well as patient-centred approaches and meaningful participation.

National and international CSOs have collaborated extensively on advocacy, research and mobilisation of HIV-positive people and their families. Groups such as the Sunflower support group for HIV-positive mothers and their families grew from four members in 2004 to a national network with thousands of members in 2009. Dozens of groups have emerged focusing on treatment access and inclusion for IDUs, men who have sex with men, transgender people and sex workers, first in the largest cities and soon all over the country. The Vietnam Network of People Living with HIV (VNP+) was launched at the end of 2009. Over the years, some of these grassroots groups, initially funded in response to HIV, have maintained their relevance by changing their focus to related areas such as LGBTI rights, the rights of sex workers, and (as we will see) Vietnam's response to COVID-19.

Stigmatised, overburdened health staff

Health staff working with HIV in hospitals and rehabilitation centres have long faced stigma and discrimination from colleagues and family (Pham et al. 2012). Their work lacks prestige due to the low status of IDUs. Family members feared infection, the workload was high and the remuneration was low, resulting in high staff turnover (Oosterhoff 2008). Over time, however, treatment success, the renovation of health facilities, new equipment, stipends and international training have contributed to improving their status. Seeing patients recover with ART and rebuild their lives professionally and privately was highly satisfying for health staff in hospitals. But for staff in rehabilitation centres or prisons, which received less international support, HIV-related stigma remains (Ha et al. 2013).

Strong international collaboration

In 2000, the United Nations Security Council recognised HIV and AIDS as a security threat, changing the belief that HIV/AIDS was 'only' a health issue and spurring the international community into action. Given its low prevalence rates, and under the impact of *Đổi mới*, Vietnam received remarkable levels of international funding for treatment access and civil-society mobilisation. US PEPFAR support to Vietnam, as elsewhere, was a political choice made against the backdrop of ongoing economic negotiations, including Vietnam's bid for World Trade Organization (WTO) membership (Vieira 2007). Vietnam's double-digit annual economic growth rates and geographical location bordering China have made it an important country politically and economically for the USA.

In sum, in Vietnam, the HIV epidemic has affected a small, highly stigmatised section of the population. It has not ended, nor has HIV been eradicated. Rather, infection has been managed by internationally funded treatment and care in collaboration with the state and with civil society.

COVID-19

A global and general epidemic

In Vietnam, COVID-19 was quickly recognised as both a global and a national emergency. The causative virus (SARS-CoV-2) affected the whole population and caused high death rates among the elderly, a culturally respected group in Vietnam. The first case was confirmed on 23 January 2020, when a patient tested positive for a strain of the virus originating in Wuhan, in neighbouring China. Since then, the Ministry of Health has distinguished four waves, each with different variants (Minh et al. 2021). Until the arrival of the Delta variant in late April 2021, through the control measures implemented until then, Vietnam had successfully prevented a generalised epidemic across the country.

Prevention: Testing, tracking, tracing and the 5 Ks

Throughout the different phases of the epidemic, Vietnam has used a '5 K' approach: mask (*khẩu trang*), hygiene (*khử khuẩn*), distancing (*khoảng cách*), no gathering (*không tụ tập*) and health reporting (*khai báo y tế*). A positive test in a household could mean a lockdown for everyone living in that ward or commune. Testing, tracing and strict isolation echoed the country's track record in emergency health responses and in fighting outbreaks of SARS, A(H5N1), A(H7N9) and avian influenza (McKenna 2006; Herington 2010).

Vietnam closed its international borders in March 2020, shortly after confirming its first COVID-19 case. After that, it allowed only a few international flights per week for a select group of returning Vietnamese nationals, foreign experts and diplomats. A 14-day period of quarantine in designated hotels or government-run facilities was mandatory upon arrival. Vietnam's approach was seen as a lesson for other countries on how to fight COVID-19 (La et al. 2020; Van Tan 2021). By the end of 2020, approximately 730,000 individuals had been quarantined at one of the isolation centres across Vietnam, and 1.7 million people had been tested for SARS-CoV-2 (Van Tan 2021).[6] Given the cultural and political history of the country, few questions were asked about medical or public privacy. Maintaining the security and confidentiality of patient records has a lower priority than protecting the whole population.

But some members of that population are more equal than others. Migrants, many of whom work freelance, have suffered more from the pandemic than contracted workers in larger, formally registered commercial and state enterprises (Pham et al. 2022). Actions to prevent the transmission of SARS-CoV-2 such as social distancing, which prevented people from moving between provinces, or leaving or entering important cities such as the capital Hanoi, affected migrants more than registered citizens (Rather 2020; Tuoi Tre News 2021). COVID-19 tests were costly given the GDP per capita of 3,756.5 USD per year.[7] However, factories depend on migrant workers. Keeping them open was a priority. State, national and international businesses pressed labourers to work, sleep and eat where they worked, and factory-wide 'bubbles' made it possible to keep production lines moving. There was a determined push to get people vaccinated by the Vietnamese government, especially by US corporate executives and Japanese, South Korean and other Southeast Asian companies located in Vietnam (McNall and Dang 2022).

Across class, ethnicity and migration status the burdens of lockdown were disproportionately carried by women (McLaren et al. 2020). Schools had been closed early in 2020 before Lunar New Year, remained closed for months and were re-opened and closed for several years.

When the Delta variants in the fourth wave of the COVID-19 epidemic resulted in increases in cases at a pace that was beyond the tracking and tracing system's capacity, the 5 Ks were no longer relevant, effective or credible. The forced testing of all citizens in September 2021 did not help to contain the epidemic. Rather it resulted in social media images of unarmed citizens in pyjamas being chased and pushed to the ground by armed police which questioned the wisdom of the government's response. It became apparent that the remedy was worse than the disease.

Prevention: Vaccination

At a meeting on COVID-19 responses in February 2021, the government confirmed that vaccination was a key measure to control the pandemic while maintaining the 5 Ks. This prompt adoption was in line with Vietnam's public health history of speedily embracing immunisation through vaccination since the 1980s (Nguyen et al. 2019). The new strategy for the COVID-19 pandemic was '5 Ks +vaccine' (Suc Khoe va Doi Song 2021).

Vietnam initially struggled with shortages of COVID-19 vaccine. In February 2021, the government issued a policy that identified nine priority groups for free vaccination. In order of priority, these were:

- frontline workers (health workers, health volunteers, army forces, police) diplomatic (government diplomats, assigned for overseas missions during the pandemic) and customs officials (customs officers, working at the border and checking people in and out of the country)
- people working in supply chains of essential goods and services
- teachers and people working in public administrative offices
- people over 65 years old and people with chronic diseases
- people living in locations with outbreaks of COVID-19

- poor people and people receiving social welfare
- people assigned by the government to work or study abroad
- other people identified by the Ministry of Health

The list shows the priority of health and economic development targets in vaccine allocation. Later adjustments to the list continued to reflect those priorities, for example by including enterprises and workers from the private sector because of their key role in the economy (McNall and Dang 2022).

COVID-19 vaccinations commenced in March 2021 in Vietnam. People who were not on the priority lists had to pay to be vaccinated. One year later, more than 200 million doses had been given to 80 million people (covering 84% of the population). Of these, 76.7 million were fully vaccinated (79.5% of the population)[8] and 46.9 million had received a booster shot (48.7% of the population) (VnExpress 2022). This achievement echoed Vietnam's previous success in the use of vaccinations for other infectious diseases such as polio (Jit et al. 2015; Nguyen et al. 2019). Acceptance of and willingness to pay for COVID-19 vaccination are high in Vietnam (Nguyen et al. 2021; Huynh et al. 2021).

There was concern however about equitable access to vaccination for migrant workers due to the household registration system. But migrants, though not explicitly included on the priority list for COVID-19 vaccinations, were not explicitly excluded either. More importantly, they could access vaccination through membership of other categories such as workers in business enterprises and their family members, people providing essential services, or freelance workers and people working in industrial zones. Especially vulnerable people such as the poor, people living with HIV and people with disabilities were also listed. Migrants thus had a range of options (Hoang et al. 2023).

But intersectional individual and structural differences between migrants and their workplaces affected access for certain groups. Those working for larger or international companies in industrial zones belonged to a priority group, while those working in small or informal businesses did not. Vietnam's informal economy is estimated to account for 20.5% of the country's total GDP, but provides an estimated 80% of employment, mostly in small- and medium-sized family owned businesses (International Labour Organisation 2021).

Migrant workers employed by small and informal businesses were not a priority even when their employers tried to get vaccination for workers. Migrants who came to towns or cities for medical reasons, such as supporting an ill relative in a hospital, could not register for vaccination even when patients, including their relatives, would be vaccinated. Another group that encountered limited access were people living in the suburbs of Hanoi or in its neighbouring provinces. Before COVID-19, these people travelled to Hanoi every day to work and might not have identified themselves as migrants. During the COVID-19 pandemic, when Hanoi was in lockdown, they could not enter the city and thus could not be vaccinated even when they had been invited to do so (VietNamNet 2021). In contrast, some people lived in Hanoi but travelled to work in nearby provinces every day. Due to COVID-19 preventive measures, they had to stay at their workplaces in the provinces and could not return to Hanoi for their vaccination.

Limited dialogue with civil society

In contrast to HIV, strong central leadership prevented local CSO involvement during COVID-19. CSOs had very limited, if any, involvement in dialogues about the 5 Ks or the vaccination campaigns. The movements of staff working in CSOs and local non-governmental organisations (NGOs) were restricted during lockdowns, which meant meetings with colleagues or citizens did not take place for many months, weakening connections and relationships. In contrast, public belief in the state health system was strong because of the success in the first wave of the epidemic. Public beliefs changed in May 2021, however, when despite the harsh restrictions, the virus spread rapidly with a relatively high short-term case fatality in Ho Chi Minh City.

The government had made ensuring people's safety and health its number one principle in the country's efforts to contain the pandemic, followed by social and economic development objectives (Government of Vietnam 2021). The objective of the vaccination programme was to 'actively prevent COVID-19 pandemic by vaccinating people at risk and the community'. Equal access to vaccination was also identified as a key principle in vaccine distribution and rollout of the vaccination programme. People living on the margins, such as homeless people, were grateful to the state for the free vaccination (Hoang et al. 2023). There were scandals about government officials exempting themselves and sometimes their families from restrictions, but these did not result in reducing the overall positive view.

The vaccination programme was organised through the administrative system in Vietnam. In this system, villages in rural communes or resident groups (*tổ dân phố*) in urban wards are at the lowest administrative level. In each village or resident group, a village head or group head (*tổ trưởng tổ dân phố*) is responsible for people's safety and the normal functioning of the village or group. This person should also make sure that people can participate in local decision making (MOHA 2021). During the COVID-19 vaccination campaign, group heads were among the key people asked to implement the campaign. This gave them unprecedented power. But by the end of 2022 scandals about government corruption had become widespread, resulting in the arrest and resignation of many government staff, including the prime minister. Among the allegations made against government staff were procurement violations and corruption during the pandemic, often in combination with allegations of tax fraud.

Health staff: Underpaid, overworked heroes

Initially, health staff working on COVID-19 received unprecedented appreciation and recognition from policy makers and the public. Health workers were seen as essential frontline responders who faced a disproportionate increase in occupational responsibilities during the pandemic. Protecting staff was a state priority. The public clapped their hands for the health heroes. However, people also expected health staff to deliver other health services and restore citizens' health, an expectation which was not possible with the limited means. Few health staff working on the frontlines in hospitals agreed that 'their work was appreciated by society'. Staff shortages, high workloads and low remuneration were issues that affected the motivation and sense of appreciation felt by health staff (Pham et al. 2021). COVID-19 revealed and aggravated a crisis in the health system. Health centres faced high drop-out and turnover rates as staff found the support they needed was not forthcoming. Health staff emerged from the crisis exhausted and wondering about their safety given the constant mutations of the virus and the lack of treatment for conditions such as long COVID-19.

Discordancy in partnerships

Throughout the COVID-19 epidemic, international organisations and collaborations lost status and respect. The priority access to vaccinations enjoyed by staff working for multilateral organisations, the United Nations and international NGOs, which placed them ahead of the elderly, was not evidence-based and was widely perceived as hypocritical, especially by their Vietnamese partners. United Nations organisations helped with access to vaccination, but the damage to their public reputations had been done. In comparison, large international companies were not seen as hypocritical. They acted in line with their mission, vision and values even when the treatment of workers, who were confined in factories to work, live and eat, was exploitative.

Conclusion

HIV and COVID-19 are vastly different conditions, with different routes of transmission and affecting different populations, but both do not respect national boundaries, and both have triggered widespread fear, stress and anxiety. In addition, the allocation of scarce resources, whether it be for ART or vaccines, is always political. The creation of the PEPFAR emergency funding framework to tackle a concentrated HIV epidemic among a highly stigmatised population and the late arrival of vaccines in Vietnam were international political choices. The choices made by the Vietnamese government reflect to some extent two distinct international political and epidemiological contexts. But they were still choices with major consequences for citizens and for civil society.

The focus given to condom use, clean needles and testing in the case of HIV was largely ineffective in the absence of international funding for ART since it caused sick and infected people to hide. CSOs were recognised for their ability to re-establish and restore some of that trust in the state. The

HIV epidemic strengthened dialogue and cooperation between the state, citizens and civil society. In contrast, the centrally led 5 K approach to COVID-19 lacked civil society involvement and dialogue until the arrival of the Delta variant. Gendered inequalities and roles inadvertently created ART access advantages for women, contributing to gender equality. COVID-19 eroded gender equalities in all three spheres of women's triple burden – increasing productive, reproductive and community workloads for women.

In both epidemics, the involuntary confinement of citizens by the state to protect the family and the general population played a huge role in outbreak management. In both cases, citizens by and large complied with and accepted what were extreme restrictions to their freedom of movement and association to serve the whole population's needs. Tackling unequal access for migrants to public health goods and services has been on the health system reform agenda for decades. Structural reforms may not have materialised, but migrants were not totally excluded from access to COVID-19 vaccinations.

In Vietnam, the HIV epidemic has been largely managed with treatment. Civil society has played a key role in ironing out some of the conflicts between the state and populations living with HIV. Local NGOs, community-based organisations (CBOs), multilateral and bilateral agencies, and the United Nations together with HIV-positive persons have advocated for evidence-informed alternative approaches, ending the forced confinement of sex workers and legalising the provision of methadone. The COVID-19 epidemic has been managed by vaccination, but civil society was confined and weakened along the way. The privileges that Vietnamese policy makers and (I)NGO and United Nations staff took in terms of vaccine access and freedom of movement have weakened social cohesion and trust in the state.

Zoonosis is here to stay. Nobody knows what the next outbreak will be, or whether the zoonotic pathogens will be bacterial, viral or parasitic. The main lesson to be learned for future pandemics is the importance of building and maintaining trust to maintain a state that works for its citizens before, during and in the aftermath of an outbreak. Pandemics, extraordinary as they may be, are occasions when citizens' relationship to the state comes under scrutiny. The outcomes of such scrutiny can, as we have seen from these two examples, be very different.

In the case of HIV, at-risk groups and people living with HIV distrusted the state's moralistic, directive and inflexible approach. Confidential, accurate and personalised information, reliable access to ART, responsiveness and flexibility to accommodate different needs were instrumental in rebuilding this trust. NGOs piloted and pioneered programmes in collaboration with the state. Relationships and communication between marginalised citizens with HIV, NGOs and the state improved during and as a result of the HIV epidemic. Top-down inflexible restrictive COVID-19 management was initially accepted, but with the arrival of new and more infectious variants it became clear that the state had lost direction and had run out of ideas, but did not want to admit it. Rather than recognising complexity and entering into an open dialogue with citizens, communication broke down. The use of force, exceptionalism and lack of transparency about the allocation of vaccines exposed the state to allegations of corruption and diminished the trust of citizens. Many accomplishments, such as the impressive scale up of access to vaccinations, would probably have been more appreciated if this trust had been maintained. But instead, this time civil society was not invited to help restore relations between citizens and the state. Civil-society space in Vietnam is shrinking. And as this book goes to press, scandals and rumours about exceptionalism and the privileges given to a few during COVID-19 ravage and paralyse the Vietnamese state.

Notes

1 An example of how time changes insights is Jorge Semprún's retelling of his experiences on the road to and inside the Buchenwald concentration camp during the Second World War. He wrote *Le grand voyage* (1963) and *Quel beau dimanche!* (1980), both autobiographical but with fictionalised elements in which he reaches fundamentally different conclusions concerning the benefits and protective character of communism.
2 Compulsory rehabilitation in centres for sex workers was abolished in July 2013 https://namvietnews.wordpress.com/2012/10/11/vietnam-to-free-prostitutes-from-rehab/
3 Decision 36/2004/QĐ-TTg, issued 17 March 2004.
4 www.aidsmap.com/news/may-2007/whounaids-endorse-opt-out-hiv-testing
5 www.unaids.org/en/regionscountries/countries/vietnam
6 The Ministry of Health (2020) announced its ten achievements in health care and epidemic prevention and control in 2020 in Vietnam.
7 At that time, a PCR test cost VND750,000 (around 30 Euros) and a rapid antigen test around VND250,000 (around 10 Euros).
8 Fully vaccinated equals two doses of Moderna, Pfizer, AstraZeneca, Vero Cell; one dose of Johnson & Johnson; three doses of Abdala. In the context of this chapter, the word 'vaccinated'/'vaccination' often means having received the first shot of vaccine.

References

Government of Vietnam, 2021. *57/TB-VPCP: Conclusion of the Prime Minister Nguyen Xuan Phuc at the Government Regular Meeting on Prevention and Control of Covid-19 Pandemic*, 23 March.

Ha, P.N., et al., 2013. HIV-related stigma: Impact on healthcare workers in Vietnam. *Global Public Health*, 8 (Sup1), S61–S74. doi:10.1080/17441692.2013.799217

Hein, N.T., et al., 2001. Risk factors of HIV infection and needle sharing among injecting drug users in Ho Chi Minh City, Viet Nam. *Journal of Substance Abuse*, 13 (1–2), 45–58. doi:10.1016/S0899-3289(01)00059-1

Herington, J., 2010. Securitization of infectious diseases in Vietnam: The cases of HIV and Avian Influenza. *Health Policy and Planning*, 25 (6), 467–475. doi:10.1093/heapol/czq052

Hoang, T-A., et al., 2023. *Equitable access and public attitudes to vaccination for internal migrants in Vietnam*. IDS Working Paper 587, Brighton: Institute of Development Studies. doi:10.19088/IDS.2023.011

Huynh, G., et al., 2021. COVID-19 vaccination intention among healthcare workers in Vietnam. *Asian Pacific Journal of Tropical Medicine*, 14 (4), 159–164. doi:10.4103/1995-7645.312513

International Labour Organisation, 2021. *Informal employment in Vietnam: Trends and determinants*. Geneva: International Labour Organisation.

Jit, M. et al. 2015. Thirty years of vaccination in Vietnam: Impact and cost-effectiveness of the National Expanded Programme on Immunization. *Vaccine*, 33 (Suppl 1), A233–A239. doi:10.1016/j.vaccine.2014.12.017

Khuat, T.H., Nguyen, T.V.A., and Ogden, J., 2004. *Understanding HIV and AIDS-related stigma and discrimination*. Hanoi: ISDS.

La, V.P., et al., 2020. Policy response, social media and science journalism for the sustainability of the public health system amid the Covid-19 outbreak: The Vietnam lessons. *Sustainability*, 12 (7), 2931. doi:10.3390/su12072931

McKenna, M., 2006. *Special report: Vietnam's success against Avian Flu may offer blueprint for others*. Minneapolis: Center for Infectious Disease Research and Policy (CIDRAP).

McLaren, H.J., et al., 2020. Covid-19 and women's triple burden: Vignettes from Sri Lanka, Malaysia, Vietnam and Australia. *Social Sciences*, 9 (5), 87. doi:10.3390/socsci9050087

McNall, S.G. and Dang, L.Q., 2022. Neo-imperialism and the precarious existence of Vietnamese factory workers during the Covid-19 lockdowns in 2021. *Fast Capitalism*, 19 (1). doi:10.32855/fcapital.202201.006

Minh, L.H.N., et al., 2021. Covid-19 timeline of Vietnam: Important milestones through four waves of the pandemic and lesson learned. *Frontiers in Public Health*, 9, 709067. doi:10.3389/fpubh.2021.709067

MOH, 2006. *Decision 149/BC-BYT Five-year review workshop on HIV/AIDS prevention and control in 2001–2005 and action plan for 2006-2010*. Hanoi: Vietnam Hanoi Medical Publishing House.

Ministry of Health, 2020. Bộ Y tế công bố 10 sự kiện y tế và phòng chống dịch Việt Nam năm 2020. 30 December. Available from: https://moh.gov.vn/tin-lien-quan/-/asset_publisher/vjYyM7O9aWnX/content/bo-y-te-cong-bo-10-su-kien-y-te-va-phong-chong-dich-viet-nam-nam-2020 [Accessed 20 March 2023]

MOHA, 2021. *Circular 04/2021/TT-BNV on guidelines for organisation and operation of villages and neighbourhoods*. Hanoi: Ministry of Home Affairs

Nguyen, C.T.T. et al., 2019. Immunization in Vietnam. *Annali di Igiene: Medicina Preventiva e di Comunità*, 31 (3), 291–305. doi:10.7416/ai.2019.2291

Nguyen, L.H., et al., 2021. Acceptance and willingness to pay for COVID-19 vaccines among pregnant women in Vietnam. *Tropical Medicine & International Health*, 26 (10), 1303–1313. doi:10.1111/tmi.13666

Nguyen, T.A., et al., 2008. A hidden HIV epidemic among women in Vietnam. *BMC Public Health*, 8, 37. doi:10.1186/1471-2458-8-37

Oosterhoff, P., 2008. *'Pressure to Bear': Gender, fertility and prevention of mother to child transmission of HIV in Vietnam*, PhD thesis, Amsterdam Institute for Social Science Research (AISSR). https://hdl.handle.net/11245/1.302753

Oosterhoff, P. and Bach, T.X., 2011. Effects of collective action on the confidence of individual HIV-positive mothers in Vietnam. In P. Liamputtong, ed. *Women, motherhood and living with HIV/AIDS: A cross-cultural perspective*. New York, London: Springer, 215–229.

Oosterhoff, P., Hardon, A., et al., 2008. Dealing with a positive result: risks and responses in routine HIV testing among pregnant women in Vietnam. *AIDS Care*, 20 (6), 654–659. doi:10.1080/09540120701687026

Oosterhoff, P., Nguyen, T.A., et al., 2008. HIV-positive mothers in Viet Nam: Using their status to build support groups and access essential services. *Reproductive Health Matters*, 16 (32), 162–170. doi:10.1016/S0968-8080(08)32408-2

Pham, H.N., et al., 2012. Stigma, an important source of dissatisfaction of health workers in HIV response in Vietnam: A qualitative study. *BMC Health Services Research*, 12, 474. doi:10.1186/1472-6963-12-474

Pham, K.T.H., et al., 2019. Health inequality between migrant and non-migrant workers in an industrial zone of Vietnam. *International Journal of Environmental Research and Public Health*, 16 (9), 1502. doi:10.3390/ijerph16091502G

Pham, Q.T., et al., 2021. Impacts of COVID-19 on the life and work of healthcare workers during the nationwide partial lockdown in Vietnam. *Frontiers in Psychology*, 12, 563193. doi:10.3389/fpsyg.2021.563193

Phạm, V.Q., Phạm, V.H. and Đinh, Q.H., 2022. Sinh Kế Của Lao Động Di Cư Tự Do Tại Thành Phố Hà Nội Trong Đại Dịch Covid-19. *VNU Journal of Social Sciences and Humanities*, 8 (1). doi:10.1172/vjossh.v8i1.925

Raguin, G. and French ESTHER Network, 2016. The ESTHER hospital partnership initiative: A powerful levy for building capacities to combat the HIV pandemic in low-resource countries. *Globalization and Health*, 12 (12). doi:10.1186/s12992-016-0149-9

Rather, A., 2020. The impact of unplanned lockdown on migrant workers. *Countercurrents*, 22 May. Available from: https://countercurrents.org/2020/05/the-impact-of-unplanned-lockdown-on-migrant-workers/ [Accessed 20 March 2023]

Suc Khoe va Doi Song, 2021. Thủ Tướng: Thực Hiện Chiến Lược "Vắc Xin + 5k". *Không Vì Vắc Xin Mà Chúng Ta Chủ Quan*, 24 February [Accessed 9 February 2023].

Tuoi Tre News, 2021. Social distancing in Hanoi locks ethnic minority migrants in tight spots. *Tuoi Tre News*, 22 August. https://tuoitrenews.vn/news/society/20210822/social-distancing-in-hanoi-locks-ethnic-minority-migrants-in-tight-spots/62709.html

Van Tan, L., 2021. COVID-19 control in Vietnam. *Nature Immunology*, 22, 261. doi: 10.1038/s41590-021-00882-9

Vieira, M.A., 2007. The securitization of the HIV/AIDS epidemic as a norm: A contribution to constructivist scholarship on the emergence and diffusion of international norms. *Brazilian Political Science Review*, 2. doi:10.1590/S1981-38212007000200005

VietNamNet, 2021. Hà Nội 'Phủ' Vắc Xin, Người Đang Ở Tỉnh Ngoài Có Được Vào Thành Phố Tiêm? *VietNamNet*, 12 September.

VnExpress, 2022. Số liệu Covid-19 tại Việt Nam. *VnExpress*, 25 March [Accessed 9 February 2023].

World Health Organization (WHO), 2006. *Progress on global access to HIV antiretroviral therapy, a report on 3 X 5 and beyond*. Geneva: WHO.

16 COVID-19 stigma and discrimination in India

Parallels with the HIV pandemic

Shubhada Maitra, Shalini Bharat, and Marie A. Brault

Introduction

India's first known case of SARS-CoV-2 (COVID-19) was documented in late January 2020 (Gunthe and Patra 2020). Since then, the country has reported over 44 million cases, over half a million deaths, and administered over 2 billion vaccine doses (Government of India 2023). India attempted numerous mitigation measures, including the world's largest nationwide lockdown in terms of the number of people, from 25 March to 31 May 2020. The country experienced three spikes in cases and mortality, with the deadliest being the second wave caused by the Delta variant in April 2021, which triggered additional localised lockdowns. Similar to other countries, COVID-19 magnified health, economic and social inequities across India (Mukherjee 2020). New and long-standing forms of discrimination based on occupation, religion, ethnicity, age, gender, health status and economic status also emerged during the course of the COVID-19 pandemic in the country (Bhanot et al. 2020).

Over 30 years before COVID-19, India faced another emerging infectious disease – the human immunodeficiency virus (HIV). Researchers initially expressed concern that HIV would spread 'out of control' across India due to the size of the country and complexity of preventing infection among men who have sex with men (MSM), sex workers, injecting drug users, transgender individuals and other key populations (Ramasundaram 2002). Besides these sub-groups, married, monogamous women (Gangakhedkar et al. 1997) and male migrants (Saggurti et al. 2012) emerged as vulnerable groups following HIV surveillance and sexual behaviour research (Mane and Maitra 1992). Despite dire predictions, India has witnessed steady declines in HIV indicators since 2000 (Government of India 2022). Recent surveillance data suggest a national prevalence rate of 0.21%, with 2.4 million people living with HIV, and over 62,000 new infections in 2021 (Government of India 2022). However, notwithstanding declining trends, both internalised and perceived stigma remain barriers to testing and care for key populations across India (Bharat et al. 2014; Ekstrand et al. 2018; Chakrapani et al. 2022). Although decades separate the emergence of HIV and COVID-19, there are

DOI: 10.4324/9781003322788-19

parallels in the construction of health-related stigma and in the impact of stigma on prevention and mitigation.

The work of Goffman (1963) and Foucault (1995) is foundational for our analysis of the stigma associated with infectious diseases. Goffman (1963) views stigma as a trait that is 'deeply discrediting' and dependent on what is viewed as acceptable or 'normal' by others within a given social setting. He describes three types of stigma linked to: abominations of the body; individual characteristics inferred from a record of 'deviant behaviour'; and stigma related to race, nationality and religion that can be transmitted through lineage (Goffman 1963, p. 14). While Goffman focuses on interpersonal and social processes in the construction of identities and types, Foucault views difference and deviance within the context of culture, knowledge and power. Foucault's theorisation of the construction of knowledge and its relationship to power, particularly within the fields of psychiatry and biomedicine, has led to deeper understandings regarding the exercise of control by 'knowledge systems' over individual and social bodies. He highlights how the social production of difference (what Goffman defines as deviance) is linked to regimes of knowledge and power. When Goffman and Foucault's work is read together, it offers a compelling case for the significant role of culturally constituted stigmatisation in the establishment and maintenance of social orders (Parker and Aggleton 2003).

In this chapter, we build on these and other understandings to define stigma as processes of exclusion, disempowerment, othering and discrimination, whether enacted (actually experienced) or perceived, and whether externally directed (by other individuals, communities and the state) or internally manifested (in the form of self-stigma). While external stigma results from public perceptions of difference and leads to exclusion and isolation, self-stigma or internalised stigma occurs when individuals, groups or communities internalise societal beliefs and opinions about their differentness or deficit. Self-stigma can thus lead to feelings of self-blame or guilt about individual or group 'difference', be it linked to illness, disability, ethnicity, religion or sexual identity. Internalised stigma may also lead to feelings of powerlessness to change a situation and doubts about deservingness of care.

This chapter draws on three sources of information to describe parallels in the construction of stigma during two infectious disease crises in India. Data are derived from the literature, media reports and the first two authors' reflections on their work on HIV and experiences during COVID-19 in India. We examine this information through the lenses provided by Goffman and Foucault, plus the multidisciplinary work undertaken since then, to trace the emergence of culturally constructed stigmatised identities related to COVID-19 and HIV. We compare the drivers of stigma, the manifestations of stigma, and the experiences of those who were stigmatised in these two epidemics, and offer recommendations as to how India's COVID-19 response might learn lessons from the earlier HIV epidemic.

The drivers and emergence of stigmatised identities in HIV and COVID-19

The first known cases of HIV were diagnosed in India in 1986 by Suniti Soloman and Sellappan Nirmala, amongst female sex workers in Chennai, Tamil Nadu (Pandey 2016). Throughout the 1980s, HIV was portrayed globally and in India as a 'gay' disease and disease of sex workers affecting only those engaged in 'immoral and unnatural' sexual activities. Many in India asserted that, as a largely monogamous, conservative society, India would be unaffected by AIDS.

In India, as in other countries, HIV was initially and continues to be concentrated among communities that were considered to be 'high-risk' – MSM, transgender women, sex workers, male migrant workers and long-distance truck drivers, and injecting drug users. Due to cis-heteronormative attitudes, cultural prohibitions on extra- and pre-marital sexual activities and colonial-era laws prohibiting same-sex practices, these groups are highly stigmatised in the Indian context (Shankar et al. 2022). The pre-HIV othering of these groups combined with misinformation regarding the mechanisms of HIV transmission led to the perception that only those engaged in 'immoral' activities would become infected (Bharat et al. 2014). This perception served to obfuscate correct information about HIV, further stigmatise sex workers and members of the LGBTQ+ community and limit open communication concerning HIV testing, prevention and care, perpetuating misinformation and discrimination. This cycle of stigmatisation might have remained restricted to these key populations, were it not for the identification of married male migrants and the male clients of sex workers as 'bridge populations' for HIV infection in India (Saggurti et al. 2012).

As infections emerged among married women contributing to mother-to-child transmission of HIV (Gangakhedkar et al. 1997), narratives of blame and stigma shifted (Bharat and Aggleton 1999). National efforts to systematically scale-up HIV prevention and care were launched, followed by more intensive efforts for testing and treatment. In 1992, India's National AIDS Control Program (NACP) began developing plans to address HIV, to be implemented through the National AIDS Control Organization (NACO). These entities, with involvement of non-governmental organisations, launched campaigns to spread knowledge and awareness of HIV and approaches to prevention. Stigma due to AIDS was yet to be identified as a roadblock to prevention and care; it came about only after 2000–2001 following the publication of United Nations-funded research on the forms and determinants of HIV-related stigma in India (Bharat and Aggleton 1999). External stigma was found to be rampant and highly gendered, with women, female sex workers, MSM and transgender individuals blamed for moral failings that perpetuated HIV transmission (Bharat and Aggleton 1999; Van Hollen 2010; Sahay et al. 2021). While stigma towards cis-heterosexual men visiting female sex workers existed, it was less apparent due to patriarchal norms legitimising male sexual needs (Bharat and Aggleton 1999). Female sex workers were paradoxically expected to insist on condoms and blamed for transmission when they failed to achieve this goal. External stigma continues to be directed towards people living with HIV in India by family members, healthcare workers, employers/co-workers, community members and social institutions.

In addition to external stigma, perceived and internalised stigma continues to be pervasive among people living with HIV in India and hinders prevention and treatment in the era of enhanced prevention and treatment options (Sahay et al. 2021). Regardless of identity or social status, feelings of guilt, blame and anger are common among people living with HIV upon learning of their diagnosis and hinder engagement with the HIV care cascade (Chakrapani et al. 2022). Depression is also commonly associated with both self-stigma and external forms of stigma among people living with HIV (Charles et al. 2012).

As in the case of HIV, the novel coronavirus (COVID-19) that emerged globally in late 2019 also resulted in stigmatised identities and discrimination against groups perceived as vectors of transmission. The first case of COVID-19 in India was detected in an individual who had travelled to China and, because of this, international travellers became the first group stigmatised and accused of spreading the disease (Bhanot et al. 2020). This tendency to stigmatise members of populations who were initially infected with COVID-19 or perceived as transmission vectors has continued. Migrant workers moving between urban and rural areas in India, day labourers, frontline healthcare workers and police personnel have all been subject to suspicion that they may be spreading COVID-19 based on perceived higher exposure due to occupation and mobility patterns (Chandrashekhar 2020; Nath 2020). Discrimination towards ethnic minorities, especially individuals from Northeast Indian states, and religious minorities has also been heightened by COVID-19 (Bhanot et al. 2020).

Communal tensions and discrimination towards Muslims in India were reinforced in February and March 2020, as rumours and social media using the hashtag #CoronaJihad spread Islamophobic messages blaming the *Tablighi Jamaat* gathering in Delhi (attended by international visitors) for the spread of COVID-19 (Al-Zaman 2022). The timing of the events, when limited information concerning COVID-19 was available, perpetuated fear, building on the stigma and discrimination that existed long before COVID-19 (Bhanot et al. 2020).

Other structurally marginalised communities in India, such as the urban poor and day labourers, also faced 'othering' when the government announced a three-week national lockdown in March 2020, with less than a day's notice. Migrants attempting to access limited spaces on buses were harassed by police (Ellis-Petersen and Chaurasia 2020). As transportation closed, many migrants were forced to spend days walking home, only to be placed in quarantine or face discrimination when they reached their villages.

For individuals who tested positive for COVID-19, internalised stigma manifested itself in the form of psychological distress and resistance to testing, treatment and quarantine, as well as post-COVID-19 feelings of guilt and distress (Bhanot et al. 2020; Adhikari et al. 2022).

While the literature on HIV stigma in India has grown over time, data are still emerging concerning COVID-19-related stigma and discrimination. Until recently, research has tended to prioritise the biomedical aspects of the pandemic perceived as more immediate. In addition, the need for social distancing may have limited more nuanced social science data collection on stigma. However, based on the information available, we can highlight similarities and differences in the emergence and drivers of stigma in the context of these two health crises. The ways that stigmatised identities emerged in the two pandemics may have differed. For HIV, stigma was linked to cultural constructions of gender and sexuality, with those acting outside norms marked as morally deficient. Conversely, COVID-19 has not been associated with sexuality and gender, with discrimination more closely aligned to occupations, ethnicity, religion and economic status. In the case of both diseases, however, stigma arose from fear of an unknown disease and fatality in the absence of a medical cure, fear of testing positive, social understandings of what is preferred behaviour, personal risk assessment and inequitable power dynamics, supporting both Goffman's and Foucault's conceptualisations. Despite the similarities between the emergence of stigma in these two pandemics, stigma reduction lessons learned from HIV have not been adapted for COVID-19 in India, or elsewhere.

HIV stigma reduction efforts in India

In the late 1990s, as the international community's concerns regarding the HIV epidemic in India grew, multi-lateral organisations, bilateral agencies like the United States Agency for International Development (USAID) and the UK Department for International Development (DfID) and philanthropic foundations encouraged the Indian government to develop a coherent response to HIV. Organisations and donors began offering financial aid and technical assistance with policy and programme development. They also supported the attendance of Indian government officials and parliamentarians at the initial international HIV-related meetings in an effort to overcome their resistance and build their understanding (Mane and Aggleton 2018). These efforts prompted the launch of India's first National AIDS Control Programme (NACP 1992–1999), and the NACO to implement the programme. Subsequently, State AIDS Control Societies (SACS) were established in Indian states and union territories (Government of India 2018). By 2013, NACO matured into a robust organisation with an evidence-based and data-driven approach to HIV prevention, treatment and care in partnership with affected communities including large numbers of civil society organisations (Bennett et al. 2015).

The SACS promoted local awareness, sensitisation and training for the general population, government officials and healthcare providers. Early on, the emphasis was on public information campaigns to spread scientific information and awareness about routes of HIV transmission and ways to prevent infection, using a three-pronged strategy that came to be known globally as the ABC strategy: abstinence, being faithful and condom use. Advice to use safe blood products and disposable/sterilised syringes was also included as part of HIV prevention communication. Over time, the prevention of mother-to-child transmission of HIV also became an important focus. Civil society organisations and affected communities, supported by NACO, played a major role in reaching previously unreached populations to spread awareness about prevention and transmission of HIV. Efforts to track the epidemiology of the epidemic, which began under NACP, were also utilised by NACO to gain a better understanding of which communities to assist with resources and information (Kadri and Kumar 2012). Although sex workers gradually gained negotiating power to refuse unprotected sex through collective action, married women rarely had the same ability to negotiate the terms of marital sexual relationships. Furthermore, married women unaware of their husband's sexual activities could neither control their husband's extra-marital sexual relationships nor negotiate condom use.

Despite continued challenges, India's response to HIV resulted in several lessons learned. First, it forced 'conservative' Indian society to begin discussing sex and sexuality. Second, it highlighted the role of stigma and brought visibility to stigmatised populations and their vulnerabilities. Third, it facilitated Behaviour Change Communication (BCC) interventions, community organising and activism to support individual and structural changes in health behaviour and healthcare delivery. However, HIV interventions and the responses to HIV stigma in India differ from the responses to COVID-19 in important ways. Early in India's HIV trajectory, stigmatised groups became organised and were well-positioned to take advantage of government and international funding for HIV prevention. Programmes and interventions were developed for different groups, including sex workers, injecting drug users, MSM, transgender people and people living with HIV. In each case, resources were provided to develop networks of support and community groups, with an emphasis on empowering hitherto disempowered and marginalised populations (Blanchard et al. 2013). In many cases, this brought visibility to these same groups, helping dispel some of the myths about them that had fuelled earlier forms of stigmatisation and stigma.

Over time, key population networks and collectives have taken a leading role in HIV prevention and destigmatisation, through peer education promoting condom use, or by facilitating access to community-based pre-exposure prophylaxis (PrEP) for HIV. Needle exchange programmes were also developed and led by states with support from donor agencies, to promote harm reduction. Efforts to increase the visibility of people living with HIV and reduce stigma have also taken the form of recognising the rights of these groups to non-discrimination, collective action and organising to promote protection. People living with HIV also formally represented their communities in national and international forums and policy-making events. Advocacy organisations note that more is needed, but these actions were important steps towards reducing HIV stigma by shifting power dynamics and empowering hitherto disadvantaged communities.

Challenges adapting HIV stigma interventions to COVID-19

There is a sharp difference between the responses to HIV detailed above and those adopted for COVID-19. In the latter case, early interventions were focused on top-down approaches aimed at restricting the movement of individuals, without consideration of the practicalities of effecting behaviour change through mask wearing, social distancing and hand washing, and without concern for building social support among affected individuals. In the context of HIV, groups vulnerable to the infection gained visibility and support from government and civil society organisations and could thereby build community and access prevention and treatment services, while for individuals and communities perceived to be at risk for COVID-19 infection and transmission, a social distancing approach served to isolate them further.

Significant similarities can be found in the communication challenges and approaches used to initially address HIV and COVID-19 in India. Public health communications in the early stage of COVID-19 focused on promoting masking, social distancing and hand washing. However, many of these recommended practices were impractical in low-income urban slum communities, where living conditions are cramped and water and sanitation facilities are limited. These communities more often house stigmatised and marginalised groups, such as migrants. The initial campaigns around HIV prevention in India similarly stressed individual prevention practices, while ignoring the structural inequities in power and access to prevention practices. However, social support and collective action helped increase the demand for condoms and condom use in India (Piot et al. 2010; Ramanathan et al. 2014). During COVID-19, access to and uptake of masks and hand washing also increased as more resources were provided to support vulnerable communities. Thus, in both HIV and COVID-19 health crises, the public health messaging initially failed by emphasising personal safety measures that were inequitably accessible. The emphasis on personal safety also neglected structural factors and the role of stigma.

India began its COVID-19 vaccination programme roughly one year after detecting the first case of COVID-19. Here again, communication efforts failed to consider how stigmatised communities might receive the intervention. Hesitancy concerning the safety of the candidate vaccines emerged, as dissemination of factual information concerning the vaccine's safety and efficacy initially lagged (Ennab et al. 2022). Ethnic and religious groups initially mistrusted the government and the indigenously produced COVID-19 vaccine.

Some marginalised groups believed that the vaccine contained animal products prohibited by Islam, would modify human DNA or would cause infertility (Kanozia and Arya 2021). Receiving the COVID-19 vaccine also required the use of an electronic appointment system developed by the Indian government, which was difficult to access by older adults and those with lower literacy. The app also collected personal information which some people were wary of sharing. However, these experiences were not universal, and many hailed the app and the COVID-19 vaccine as significant innovations. Despite challenges and disruptions, 61% of the eligible population was vaccinated by the end of 2021 (Bhatnagar 2021).

Fear of testing positive and the subsequent isolation/quarantine resulted in people with COVID-19-like symptoms going underground. Misinformation, high fatality risk and limited complete knowledge in the initial stages of COVID-19 added to the fears. These fears in turn led to the stigmatisation and blaming of groups seen as 'spreaders' of the virus, similar to HIV. Cases of suicide and attempted suicide increased from 220 in 2019 to 369 during the lockdown period in India. According to news reports, COVID-19-related fear and isolation were mentioned in 128 cases of suicide and 29 attempted cases (Pathare et al. 2020).

However, there were differences in how blame was constructed in relation to HIV compared to COVID-19, which carried implications for stigma construction and reduction. Initially, HIV infection was attributed to personal behaviour and therefore viewed as a threat that 'others' faced rather than attributes related to external determinants such as travel or migration. Conversely, COVID-19 in India was initially portrayed as 'the enemy' and a war to be fought and won, which was brought by foreigners and foreign-returned nationals, leading to the sealing of international borders. With infections rising in cities, many states enacted restrictions to deny entry of people from states/districts with higher rates of infections. People could no longer move freely from one Indian state to another without a valid reason (such as a death in the family) and a COVID-19 negative test result. Restrictions were also placed on individuals transiting from cities to rural areas, creating a divide between supposedly uninfected insiders, and the 'outsiders' who would spread the infection with their entry into the state, city or village. This led to the stigmatisation of groups such as migrant workers, ethnic and religious minorities, and health workers, all of whom were seen as potential carriers of infection despite limited epidemiological data to support these perceptions (Ghosh and Chaudhury 2020).

Health system factors during the two pandemics

India's already fragile health system infrastructure came under severe pressure as a result of COVID-19, which some have suggested contributed to the perpetuation of discrimination and marginalisation (Adhikari et al. 2022). Although the health system response was largely centralised and co-ordinated during the first wave of the epidemic, state-level responses varied during the second wave, with some states facing widespread disruption in services including health and public transport (Hale et al. 2022). As a result, people were unable to or afraid to go to hospitals and clinics for fear of infection. Conditions in some poorly managed COVID-19 quarantine facilities led others to avoid those perceived to be infected (Dhar et al. 2021). In contrast, a few Indian states promptly responded to the pandemic, using previous knowledge and expertise in dealing with disasters. One example was the South Indian state of Kerala. Although the first case of COVID-19 was detected in Kerala in January 2020, the state reported the lowest mortality rate in the country in 2020–2021, at 0.4% (Hindustan Times Correspondent 2021). Kerala employed a multi-pronged approach, not dissimilar to that adopted with HIV. This included active surveillance through the establishment of district control rooms for monitoring; capacity-building for frontline health workers; risk communication and community engagement; and actions to address the psychosocial needs of vulnerable populations (Joseph et al. 2023). Strong political leadership, a robust health infrastructure, and positive health and demographic indicators were instrumental to Kerala and other states' successes in handling COVID-19 – similar to aspects of the Government of India's earlier response to HIV.

COVID-19 in India also saw the emergence of 'shadow pandemics' of domestic violence and mental health problems among already marginalised communities including LGBTQ+ individuals (Maitra 2021). As employment opportunities and non-COVID-19 healthcare declined during lockdown, the poor including marginalised LGBTQ+ individuals faced financial difficulties and challenges accessing healthcare for testing and existing medical conditions. For the latter, economic hardships together with their increased isolation from society, their continued fear of accidental disclosure of identity to family and their uprooting from conditions of shelter made them more susceptible to abuse and violence (Aljazeera 2020; Maitra 2021). The hijra community, in particular, whose members had previously made a living by participating in social events such as marriages, births and deaths, or by begging, were restricted from earning an income due to lockdown orders. Romantic relationships, particularly those in which the partners lived separately, were threatened. However, as the pandemic continued, tele-mental health, food distribution, cash transfers and other forms of social programming supported many vulnerable groups (Kumar et al. 2022; Joseph et al. 2023).

Conclusions and recommendations for the future

The HIV response in India was successful in ensuring the promotion of social, economic, political and legal rights for those affected by HIV. Much of the effort aimed at creating enabling environments for previously stigmatised and vulnerable groups to allow them to exercise agency to practise healthy behaviours and obtain social, financial and political support. These efforts ranged from decriminalising sex work, drug use and homosexuality, to reducing violence against women, girls and key populations, and challenging stigma and discrimination, which remain substantial barriers to the HIV response (Buse et al. 2020).

The social mobilisation of vulnerable and affected groups was less obvious during COVID-19 compared to HIV but may be attributed to the more generalised nature of COVID-19. Support and communication concerning prevention were scaled up as Indian and international communities gained greater insight into COVID-19 and rapidly disseminated information. Three years after COVID-19 arrived in India, people are still reeling from the devastating socio-economic impact of the pandemic. COVID-19 information has largely improved but there remains a strong need for additional research to understand and address COVID-19-related stigma in India. As COVID-19 variants evolve, new surges may produce additional disruptions, but India appears to be building capacity to meet these challenges.

Together, HIV and COVID-19 have shown that new infectious diseases provide the ideal environment for the reinforcement of pre-existing stigma and discrimination, as individuals and communities face existential threats to health and socio-economic status. Goffman's work on stigma and Foucault's work on knowledge and power provide us with insight into how these stigmatising responses to pandemics come about and the steps that might be taken to mitigate their effects. In moving forward, and in anticipation of future infectious disease pandemics, it is important to draw upon the lessons from HIV and COVID-19 to reduce, if not completely eliminate or prevent, the stigma and discrimination that arises out of limited information and uncertainty. Key to this approach is recognition of the structural inequalities – of gender, ethnicity, class, migration/mobility and sexuality among others – that are seized upon by the public and political leaders in 'making sense' of epidemic events, and the resulting forms of exclusion that emerge. As the international community attempts to recover from COVID-19 and face the next health emergency, stigma reduction and promoting inclusion, remain critical work for social scientists, public health professionals, community workers and policymakers alike.

References

Adhikari, T., et al., 2022. Factors associated with COVID-19 stigma during the onset of the global pandemic in India: A cross-sectional study. *Frontiers in Public Health*, 10, 992046. doi:10.3389/fpubh.2022.992046

Al-Zaman, M.S., 2022. A thematic analysis of misinformation in India during the COVID-19 pandemic. *International Information & Library Review*, 54 (2), 128–138. doi:10.1080/10572317.2021.1908063

Aljazeera, 2020. Coronavirus lockdown 'lonely' and 'dangerous' for LGBTQ Indians. *Aljazeera* [online], 22 June. Available from: www.aljazeera.com/news/2020/6/22/coronavirus-lockdown-lonely-and-dangerous-for-lgbtq-indians [Accessed 14 January 2023]

Bennett, S., et al., 2015. Monitoring and evaluating transition and sustainability of donor-funded programs: Reflections on the Avahan experience. *Evaluation and Program Planning*, 52, 148–158. doi:10.1016/j.evalprogplan.2015.05.003

Bhanot, D., et al., 2020. Stigma and discrimination during COVID-19 pandemic. *Frontiers in Public Health*, 8, 577018. doi:10.3389/fpubh.2020.577018

Bharat, S. and Aggleton, P., 1999. Facing the challenge: Household response to HIV/AIDS in Mumbai, India. *AIDS Care*, 11 (1), 31–44.

Bharat, S., et al., 2014. Gender-based attitudes, HIV misconceptions and feelings towards marginalized groups are associated with stigmatization in Mumbai, India. *Journal of Biosocial Science*, 46 (6), 717–732. doi:10.1017/S0021932014000054

Bhatnagar, A., 2021. Devastating 2nd wave, billion+ vaccinations: 12 charts show how India fought Covid in 2021. *Times of India* [online], 29 December. http://timesofindia.indiatimes.com/articleshow/88564472.cms?utm_source=contentofinterest&utm_medium=text&utm_campaign=cppst

Blanchard, A.K., et al., 2013. Community mobilization, empowerment and HIV prevention among female sex workers in south India. *BMC Public Health*, 13, 234. doi:10.1186/1471-2458-13-234

Buse, K., et al., 2020. COVID-19 combination prevention requires attention to structural drivers. *The Lancet*, 396 (10249), 466. doi:10.1016/S0140-6736(20)31723-2

Chakrapani, V., et al., 2022. Associations between sexual stigma, enacted HIV stigma, internalized HIV stigma and homonegativity, and depression: Testing an extended minority stress model among men who have sex with men living with HIV in India. *AIDS Care*, 34 (12), 1586–1594. doi:10.1080/09540121.2022.2119467

Chandrashekhar, V., 2020. The burden of stigma. *Science*, 369 (6510), 1419–1423. doi:10.1126/science.369.6510.1419

Charles, B., et al., 2012. Association between stigma, depression and quality of life of people living with HIV/AIDS (PLHA) in South India – A community based cross sectional study. *BMC Public Health*, 12, 463. doi:10.1186/1471-2458-12-463

Dhar, R., et al., 2021. Fault lines in India's COVID-19 management: Lessons learned and future recommendations. *Risk Management and Healthcare Policy*, 14, 4379–4392. doi:10.2147/RMHP.S320880

Ekstrand, M.L., Bharat, S., and Srinivasan, K., 2018. HIV stigma is a barrier to achieving 90-90-90 in India. *The Lancet HIV*, 5 (10), e543–e545. doi:10.1016/S2352-3018(18)30246-7

Ellis-Petersen, H. and Chaurasia, M., 2020. India racked by greatest exodus since partition due to coronavirus. *The Guardian*, 30 March. www.theguardian.com/world/2020/mar/30/india-wracked-by-greatest-exodus-since-partition-due-to-coronavirus

Ennab, F., et al., 2022. COVID-19 vaccine hesitancy: A narrative review of four South Asian countries. *Frontiers in Public Health*, 10, 997884. doi:10.3389/fpubh.2022.997884

Foucault, M., 1995. *Discipline and punish: The birth of the prison*. New York: Vintage Books.

Gangakhedkar, R.R., et al., 1997. Spread of HIV infection in married monogamous women in India. *JAMA*, 278 (23), 2090–2092.

Ghosh, A.K. and Chaudhury, A.B.R., 2020. Pandemic as a 'disaster': Assessing Indian state response. *ORF, Observer Research Foundation* [online], 5 September. www.orfonline.org/research/pandemic-as-a-disaster-assessing-indian-state-response

Goffman, E., 1963. *Stigma: Notes on the management of spoiled identity*. Englewood Cliffs, NJ: Prentice-Hall.

Government of India, Ministry of Health and Family Welfare, 2018. *National AIDS Control Organization: About us* [online]. http://naco.gov.in/about-us

Government of India, Ministry of Health and Family Welfare, 2022. *Technical Report: India HIV Estimates 2021* [online]. https://naco.gov.in/sites/default/files/India%20HIV%20Estimates.pdf [Accessed 15 May 2023]

Government of India, Ministry of Health and Family Welfare, 2023. *MoHFW Home* [online]. www.mohfw.gov.in/ [Accessed 15 May 2023].

Gunthe, S.S. and Patra, S.S., 2020. Impact of international travel dynamics on domestic spread of 2019-nCoV in India: Origin-based risk assessment in importation of infected travelers. *Globalization and Health*, 16, 45. doi:10.1186/s12992-020-00575-2

Hale, T., et al., 2022. *Indian state-level policy responses to COVID-19 during the second wave*. Blavatnik School Working Paper. Available from: www.bsg.ox.ac.uk/research/publications/indian-state-level-policy-responses-covid-19-during-second-wave [Accessed 15 June 2023].

Hindustan Times Correspondent, 2021. Kerala adds 28,514 new Covid-19 cases, hike in death rate cause for concern. *Hindustan Times* [online], 22 May. www.hindustantimes.com/india-news/kerala-adds-28-514-new-covid-19-cases-hike-in-death-rate-cause-for-concern-101621703818965.html

Joseph, J., et al., 2023. Who are the vulnerable, and how do we reach them? Perspectives of health system actors and community leaders in Kerala, India. *BMC Public Health*, 23 (1), 748.

Kadri, A. and Kumar, P., 2012. Institutionalization of the NACP and way ahead. *Indian Journal of Community Medicine*, 37 (2), 83–88. doi:10.4103/0970-0218.96088

Kanozia, R. and Arya, R., 2021. "Fake news", religion, and COVID-19 vaccine hesitancy in India, Pakistan, and Bangladesh. *Media Asia*, 48 (4), 313–321. doi:10.1080/01296612.2021.1921963

Kumar, A., et al., 2022. Government transfers, COVID-19 shock, and food insecurity: Evidence from rural households in India. *Agribusiness*, 38 (3), 636–659. doi:10.1002/agr.21746

Maitra, S., 2021. Mental health in the context of COVID-19 in India. *The Indian Journal of Social Work*, 82 (1), 5–16.

Mane, P. and Aggleton, P., 2018. Enabling positive change: Progress and setbacks in HIV and sexual and reproductive health and rights. *Global Public Health*, 13 (10), 1341–1356. doi:10.1080/17441692.2017.1401652

Mane, P.N. and Maitra, S.A., 1992. *AIDS prevention: The socio-cultural context in India*. Mumbai: Tata Institute of Social Sciences.

Mukherjee, S., 2020. Disparities, desperation, and divisiveness: Coping with COVID-19 in India. *Psychological Trauma: Theory, Research, Practice, and Policy*, 12 (6), 582–584. doi:10.1037/tra0000682

Nath, S., 2020. Communalising the migrants in the middle of Covid-19 crisis in India. *Cities*, 5, 16.

Pandey, G., 2016. The woman who discovered India's first HIV cases. *BBC News* [online], 30 August. www.bbc.co.uk/news/magazine-37183012

Parker, R. and Aggleton, P., 2003. HIV-and AIDS-related stigma and discrimination: A conceptual framework and implications for action. *Social Science & Medicine*, 57 (1), 13–24. doi:10.1016/S0277-9536(02)00304-0

Pathare, S., et al., 2020. Analysis of news media reports of suicides and attempted suicides during the COVID-19 lockdown in India. *International Journal of Mental Health Systems*, 14 (1), 88. doi:10.1186/s13033-020-00422-2

Piot, B., et al., 2010. Lot quality assurance sampling for monitoring coverage and quality of a targeted condom social marketing programme in traditional and non-traditional outlets in India. *Sexually Transmitted Infections*, 86 (Suppl 1), i56–i61. doi:10.1136/sti.2009.038356

Ramanathan, S., et al., 2014. Increase in condom use and decline in prevalence of sexually transmitted infections among high-risk men who have sex with men and transgender persons in Maharashtra, India: Avahan, the India AIDS Initiative. *BMC Public Health*, 14, 784. doi:10.1186/1471-2458-14-784

Ramasundaram, S., 2002. Can India avoid being devastated by HIV? *BMJ*, 324 (7331), 182–183. doi:10.1136/bmj.324.7331.182

Saggurti, N., et al., 2012. Male migration/mobility and HIV among married couples: Cross-sectional analysis of nationally representative data from India. *AIDS and Behavior*, 16 (6), 1649–1658. doi:10.1007/s10461-011-0022-z

Sahay, S., et al., 2021. Understanding issues around use of oral pre-exposure prophylaxis among female sex workers in India. *BMC Infectious Diseases*, 21 (1), 930. doi:10.1186/s12879-021-06612-8

Shankar, P., et al., 2022. Decolonising gender in India. *The Lancet Global Health*, 10 (2), e173–e174. doi:10.1016/S2214-109X(21)00523-4

Van Hollen, C., 2010. HIV/AIDS and the gendering of stigma in Tamil Nadu, South India. *Culture, Medicine, and Psychiatry*, 34 (4), 633–657. doi:10.1007/s11013-010-9192-9

Index

Pages in *italics* refer to figures, pages in **bold** refer to tables, and pages followed by n refer to notes.

www.ingramcontent.com/pod-product-compliance
Lightning Source LLC
Chambersburg PA
CBHW060251220326
41598CB00027B/4058

* 9 7 8 1 0 3 2 7 6 4 9 8 6 *